Twice Dead

CALIFORNIA SERIES IN PUBLIC ANTHROPOLOGY

The California Series in Public Anthropology emphasizes the anthropologist's role as an engaged intellectual. It continues anthropology's commitment to being an ethnographic witness, to describing, in human terms, how life is lived beyond the borders of many readers' experiences. But it also adds a commitment, through ethnography, to reframing the terms of public debate—transforming received, accepted understandings of social issues with new insights, new framings.

Series Editor: Robert Borofsky (Hawaii Pacific)

Contributing Editors: Nancy Scheper-Hughes (UC Berkeley), Philippe Bourgois (UC San Francisco), and Arturo Escobar (University of North Carolina)

University of California Press Editor: Naomi Schneider

Twice Dead

*Organ Transplants and the
Reinvention of Death*

Margaret Lock

UNIVERSITY OF CALIFORNIA PRESS
Berkeley · Los Angeles · London

University of California Press
Berkeley and Los Angeles, California

University of California Press, Ltd.
London, England

Grateful acknowledgment is made for permission to quote from
Richard Selzer's *Raising the Dead: A Doctor's Encounter with His
Own Mortality* (New York: Viking, 1993); letters by Thomas J.
Poulton and Gregory Liptak in *Journal of the American Medical
Association* 255 (April 18, 1986): 2028, copyrighted 1986,
American Medical Association; and Mark Kennedy's "Brain Dead
Donors 'Alive': MDs Debate Ethics of Transplant," *Ottawa Citizen*,
March 3, 1999.

Library of Congress Cataloging-in-Publication Data

Lock, Margaret M.
    Twice dead : organ transplants and the reinvention of death / by
Margaret Lock.
        p. cm. — (California series in public anthropology; 1)
    Includes bibliographical references and index.
    ISBN 0-520-22605-4 — ISBN 0-520-22814-6
    1. Transplantation of organs, tissues, etc.—Japan. 2.
Transplantation of organs, tissues, etc.—North America. 3. Brain
death—Japan. 4. Brain death—North America. I. Title. II. Series.
    QP89 .L63 2002
    617.9'5'0952—dc21
                                                    2001004110

Printed in the United States of America

10 09 08 07 06

10 9 8 7 6 5 4

To the memory of Nakagawa Yonezō

Contents

Illustrations

Acknowledgments

Ethnographic research thrives by making impositions on people, and I owe a debt of gratitude to the busy individuals who gave generously of their time. Intensivists, neurologists, transplant surgeons, and intensive care nurses working in Japan, Canada, and the United States, and transplant coordinators from Québec Transplant, put up with intrusions into their already overworked days. Observing them at work in intensive care units and in operating rooms was a special privilege.

Organ transplant recipients in Japan and Canada brought home the poignancy of this research when they permitted me to enter into their lives. I am especially grateful to those who had dealt with brain death in the family and who were willing to talk with me. Their courage is commendable, and I hope I have done justice to their accounts.

Special thanks go to Vinh Kim Nguyen, colleague, informant, and friend, and to Frank Carnevale, whose interest and support are boundless. This book would be the poorer without their help. To Aikawa Atsushi, Akabayashi Akira, Awaya Tsuyoshi, Ikegami Naoki, Kawai Tatsuo, Robert Nelson, Nudeshima Jiro, Ota Kazuo, Sakakihara Yoichi, Jean Tchervenkov, Abe Tomoko, and Stuart Youngner I am indebted for valuable experiences and insights. Christina Honde was my first collaborator and coauthor on the brain-death problem. Her enthusiasm inspired me to go forward. In recent years, the members of the International Forum for Transplant Ethics have created a lively format for argumentative reflection, and my colleagues in the department of Social

Studies of Medicine at McGill University have, as ever, been provocative and to the point in their criticisms.

Readers of the manuscript without exception gave invaluable comments and constructive criticism. Lawrence Cohen, Judith Farquhar, Helen Hardacre, Susan Long, Robert Nelson, and Stuart Youngner all labored through earlier versions of this book, and I cannot thank them enough for their contribution to the final product.

I have profited throughout this long endeavor from dedicated research assistants, who also provided thoughtful reflections. June Kitanaka extended herself tirelessly on my behalf and, thanks to her, Kitanaka Kenji, Toki Nobuko, Kawazoe Hiroko, and Doi Machi kindly undertook to do last-minute revisions on Japanese sources. In earlier years, Mukai Keiko, Nukaga Yoshio, and Kanaba Miuki put in generous amounts of time. Stella Zoccali helped me in maintaining some semblance of control over the final stages of preparation of this book. Heartfelt thanks also go to Naomi Schneider, Sue Heinemann, and Erika Büky, at the University of California Press, and to Rob Borofsky, the series editor.

While writing the manuscript I was privileged at various times to be resident at the Rockefeller Foundation Center at Bellagio, associated with the anthropology and ethnomedicine departments at the University of Vienna, and the Neilson professor at Smith College in Northampton, Massachusetts. Each of these locations provided a unique space for reflection.

The Social Science and Humanities Research Council of Canada provided six years of funding for this research. Their support is gratefully acknowledged.

Richard as usual kept things centered.

Preamble

Accidental Death

> Technology has extended and widened the notion of the
> accident. . . . Accidents are part of our daily life and their
> shadows people our dreams.
>
> *Octavio Paz,* Conjunctions and Disjunctions

This book does not make for comfortable reading. Some readers will
find the subject macabre, even repulsive, for the focus is on death and
the "harvesting" or, in the prevailing euphemism, "procurement" of
organs for transplant. Stories about organ transplants appear in myth-
ology and folktales, as well as in documents from medieval times (Barkan 1996), but only during the past twenty years have medical knowledge and technology advanced sufficiently for organ transplantation to
become routine, with surgeons performing thousands of operations each
year. In the majority of cases, the transplanted organs come from the
bodies of individuals diagnosed as "brain-dead."

A "living cadaver," as the brain-dead were first called, is created by
an accident and sustained by medical technology. Major injury to the
brain must occur, whether caused by an automobile or motorcycle crash,
a drowning, smoke inhalation, a major blow to the head, a "cerebral
accident" (stroke) in which the brain suddenly floods with blood, or
some act of violence, such as a gunshot wound. Most victims of severe
head trauma are kept alive by a relatively simple piece of technology—
the artificial ventilator. Solid organ transplants,[1] which depend on the
procurement of organs from brain-dead patients, could not have been
institutionalized without the existence of the ventilator and other life-

---

1. "Solid organ" refers to the internal organs, including the heart, liver, kidney, and
lungs, that have clearly defined anatomical boundaries.

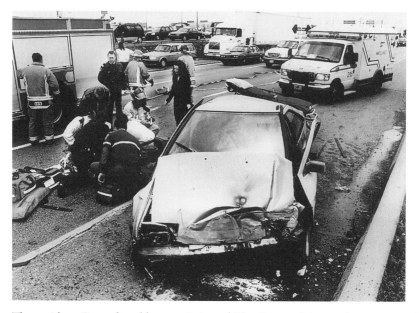

The accident. Reproduced by permission of *The Gazette,* Montreal.

support technologies. But this coincidence of new technologies and living bodies, some with irreversibly damaged brains, could not alone mean that organs could then be procured from these new entities: a new death had to be legally recognized before commodification of the brain-dead could come about.

Although clinical treatment for trauma is similar in virtually all countries where the necessary medical facilities are present, and the term *brain death* is used universally today, the consequences of this diagnosis vary considerably. Brain death is not necessarily equated with the death of individuals. This book explores the way in which developments in medical technology have forced a reconsideration of the recognized boundaries between life and death, and how these debates reflect deeply held social values and political interests. It is striking that in Japan, in contrast to North America and most of Europe, recognition of brain death as human death has proved to be an exceedingly contentious issue. By exploring in parallel the situation in North America and Japan, I hope to force some reflection about this problem in both locations: the one where the recognition of the new death was accomplished relatively smoothly and the other where it continues to prove deeply problematic. Quite simply, in the presence of advanced medical technologies, there remains disagreement as to what constitutes death, and little reason to believe that lasting resolution to the matter is in sight. While this situation exists, we cannot feel completely at ease about organ transplants that make use of brain-dead donors, although I am certainly not suggesting that we stop the practice.

I first became interested in brain death about ten years ago, while doing research in Japan on an entirely different topic. The subject was being discussed exhaustively in the Japanese media. Articles often included the results of polls inquiring whether the public was willing to accept brain death as the end of human life, and how people felt about organ donation from brain-dead patients. In the technologically sophisticated, literate economic superpower of Japan, the idea of this "new death" was clearly setting off alarm bells. Yet aside from an initial flurry after the first heart transplant in 1967, no similar concern has been apparent in North America or in most of Europe, where the media seem relatively untroubled by doubts as to whether brain death constitutes the end of life; instead, they focus on the saving of lives through organ transplants from brain-dead donors. The only worry is about a "shortage" of organs, the bittersweet outcome of success.

At first I limited my attention to the debate in Japan, where "the brain-death problem," as it is known there, has been the most contentious ethical debate of the last thirty years. Although the concept of brain death was medically recognized more than twenty years ago, and the diagnosis is used regularly in clinical practice, this condition was legally recognized as death in Japan only in 1997. Even now, brain death is equated with death only when patients have specified in writing that they wish to become organ donors and their families do not overrule these wishes. Brain-dead individuals who have not indicated that they want to become donors are not considered legally dead. As of the end of 2000, organs for transplant had been procured from only nine brain-dead donors in Japan; the organs from a tenth donor proved to be unusable.

In North America, by contrast, organs for transplant can be removed from bodies legally recognized as dead (including anyone diagnosed as brain-dead) if the individual's wish to become a donor can be reasonably assured. In theory, families may not overrule this intent. In several European countries, "presumed consent" allows transplant teams to procure organs from every brain-dead patient unless an individual has explicitly opted out of organ donation by signing a document to that effect.

After presenting my research findings from Japan to a variety of

North American audiences, it became evident that many people still assumed that the Japanese response to the new technologically created death is an anachronism, associated with religious beliefs and deeply rooted cultural traditions. Such assumptions persisted despite my energetic attempts to dispel this misconception. This prejudice highlighted two important and perplexing questions: in Japan, why did brain death become recognized as the end of life only very recently, and even then inconclusively? And why are organ transplants not perceived as an unequivocal good? Although shared values of long standing do indeed contribute to the debate, Japanese responses are exceedingly complex and defy any simple explanation.

Examination of the Japanese response raises another crucial question: why did we in the "West" accept the remaking of death by medical professionals with so little public discussion? The "gift of life" is a seductive metaphor, one that now seems natural to us, and it has proved effective in promoting the donation of human organs for transplant, but in adopting it we have glossed over questions about the source of these organs. Aside from discussion in a few academic and medical forums, we have chosen not to enter into debate about the new death.

Death would seem to admit of little ideological posturing, at least as an indisputable biological event. I suspect that the majority of us raised in the dominant traditions of Europe and North America understand death as an unambiguous, easily definable point of no return. Certainly the media lead us to think that this is the case. In contrast, discussion of brain death in Japan has caused considerable social angst, even though Japan, for the most part a secular society, is driven by the principles of rational order and scientific progress associated with modernization. What is more, many people in Japan apparently do not understand death as a straightforward event affecting only the physical body.

Clearly, these differences cannot be explained by a Japanese lack of education, technology, skills, or economic resources. Japan, in fact, utilizes and exports more complex medical technology than any other nation in the world. So "culture" must be at work, we assume, and we tend, as I did when I started this project, to look for features of Japanese, rather than North American, culture to account for this discrepancy. What concerns make Japanese resistant to the concept of a "new death" based on the condition of the brain? Is the difference to be found in attitudes towards nature—specifically, in a concern about tinkering with the bodies of the dying and the dead? Is Japan perhaps not as secular and rational, not as "modern," as its outward trappings lead us to believe? Are the majority of people in Japan unwilling to treat the body objectively, especially the body in death, as seems to be done in North America? An assumption implicit in this line of interrogation is that a secular society will strive to "save" lives if the technology is available. Hence we turn all too easily to searching for the relics of tradition, survivals from an archaic past lurking in Japanese modernity, that might account for this anomaly.

Several vocal Japanese commentators have invoked "tradition" when accounting for the reluctance to recognize brain death in their country, but they usually embrace an essentialized notion of culture as a positive force, one that protects the nation from unwanted change. These individuals draw on ideas and behaviors that they think of as uniquely Japanese, including characteristic ways in which human life and bodies after death are valued. They contrast this situation favorably with the perceived cultural vacuum of America, a nation overly preoccupied with individualism and insufficiently with history. This dearth of "culture," in their opinion, facilitates the implementation of medical technology without regard to ethical and moral implications. These commentators are insistent that Japan should not simply ape the "Other" of the West but should strive instead to ensure that contemporary moral order is infused with values associated with Japanese tradition.

The majority of Japanese with whom I have talked about brain death dismiss arguments that reify Japanese tradition. Nevertheless, many suggest that values common to a large number of Japanese, such as a concern about desecration of dead bodies, partially account for a resistance to a recognition of brain death as human death. But they make no claims about the uniqueness of their culture, nor do they assume that it is monolithic. On the contrary, they cite polls indicating that around half of the nation supports recognition of brain death in theory. Rather than focus on Japanese resistance, many of these individuals comment on the "culture" of the West. They suggest that the Christian tradition of charity has facilitated a willingness to donate organs to strangers, often adding that altruism is not well-developed in Japan.

Some academics and cultural commentators take yet another position. They argue that culture, by which they mean the "culture of tradition," is irrelevant to the impasse. Modern society is, by their definition, secular and rational and freed from culture, except of course for the "high" culture of the arts and the postmodern culture of fusion, into which aspects of tradition are selectively and self-consciously incorporated. Pockets of backwardness inevitably remain in any society, but these are, they assume, fast disappearing.

These commentators assert instead that patients rightly fear being subjected to abuses of medical power, especially when dying. People believe that their lives will be shortened by the medical profession's hunger for their organs. It is public mistrust of the medical profession that largely accounts for resistance to recognition of brain death as the end of human life. This group of critics, many of whom denounce "technological imperialism," also question the accuracy of the scientific discourse about brain death. Such concerns are not limited to Japan, but in Europe and North America only a minority has voiced them. Other Japanese, among them a good number of physicians and people waiting for transplants, lament that transplant technology is not freely available in Japan. They often describe their country as backward, irrational, and unreasonable in this respect. By no means does everyone in Japan fit neatly into this range of responses; some people change their opinions over time, and others maintain positions that are apparently contradictory.[2]

2. When polled, many Japanese claim, for example, that they are opposed to the recognition of brain death but that they are not in principle opposed to organ transplants. If, by organ transplants, respondents to these questionnaires have kidneys in mind, or possibly xenotransplants, then this position is tenable. It is possible that respondents do not recognize brain death as the end of human life and therefore do not want brain-dead patients used as organ donors, but that they are not in principle opposed to organ transplants. By far the majority of kidney transplants done in Japan, some liver transplants, and a very few lung transplants make use of "living related" donors. Otherwise, kidneys come from cadaver donors—that is, donors whose hearts have stopped beating, as opposed to brain-dead donors, whose hearts are still beating when the organ is procured. However, Japanese respondents who oppose organ procurement from brain-dead donors are taking the position, consciously or not, that no heart transplants and almost no liver or lung transplants can be permitted. It is also quite possible that respondents are thinking in personal rather than general terms: that they themselves would not want to donate organs, nor would they want family members to become donors, but they have no objection to organs being procured from other willing volunteers.

In the 1990s, between 400 and 500 kidney transplants took place each year in Japan using living donors (in the United States, with approximately twice the population of Japan, 4,493 living related donations took place in 1999). Another 150 to 250 transplants each year in Japan made use of kidneys procured from bodies in which the heart had stopped beating (these official figures almost certainly include the few cases in which kidneys were procured from brain-dead bodies).

As of August 2000, 46 Japanese patients were waiting for new hearts, 21 for lungs, 35 for livers, and 28 for pancreas transplants. Waiting lists for organs other than kidneys have existed for only three years, and this fact may account for these remarkably low numbers. The above figures make it clear that the United States is much more aggressive in the use of living donors than is Japan. This difference is largely explained by the lack of transplant surgery facilities in Japan, but it also suggests ambivalence toward the use of living donors.

In North America, discussion about brain death has been limited for the most part to a small group of doctors and an even smaller group of lawyers and intellectuals. The contribution of culture to this debate is virtually never raised, except perhaps to account for a perceived "lack of cooperation" among certain minority groups with the donation of organs. Periodically the debate has leaked into the media, usually when something newsworthy happens in connection with organ transplants. These reports are almost always positive and laudatory of medical heroics. Rarely has the assessment of brain death or the actual procurement of organs been given more than fleeting coverage.

Discussion of the institutionalization and legitimization of brain death as the end of human life, followed by its routinization across North America and much of Europe, has been dominated by two lines of thought. The first attempts to assign death to a scientifically deducible and verifiable moment, and thus to make it at once indisputable in medicine and recognizable in law. However, professional consensus has been lacking as to whether death is a moment or a process and how best to determine when it occurs. No consensus exists even as to whether a definition of death should be applicable to all living forms or whether there can be a death unique to humans.

Until the late 1960s this long-standing professional controversy had little effect on determining the death of individual patients, the precise timing of which is usually not important unless foul play is suspected. With the development of critical-care medicine, it became imperative to decide if and when it would be appropriate to discontinue life support for patients who were expected never to recover—who were in an irreversible condition that could end only in biological death. During the same period, organ transplants were becoming increasingly common. Particularly after the world's first heart transplant in 1967, many recognized that doomed patients on life support represented potential organ sources. However, these patients could not be diagnosed as dead in the usual way because their hearts were still beating, sustained by the ventilator. Doctors urgently needed to be able to formally declare death so that organs could be removed from brain-dead patients without legal repercussions. A new definition for death had to be established, one that located death in the brain; and its criteria needed to be uniform and objective.

The second line of argument about the new death, put forward most frequently by philosophers and bioethicists, is that if there is no possibility for cognitive function in an individual because of irreversible damage to the upper brain, then that person can be pronounced as no longer having any "individual interest." Such patients are neither clinically nor legally brain-dead because the lower brain remains intact. Nevertheless, supporters of "higher" brain death argue that because they will never recover consciousness, these patients are good-as-dead. This argument is not widely accepted by members of the medical profession and has not gained legal recognition anywhere, but it is increasingly being given serious consideration, for reasons that will be made clear.

In Japan, different sets of assumptions about death make it difficult to construct arguments reduced either to questions of scientific accuracy or to the demise of an individual. Efforts to assign death scientifically to a specific moment are frequently rejected outright by both medical and lay people. Dying is widely understood as a process, and cannot therefore be isolated as a moment. What is more, the cognitive status of the patient is of secondary importance for most people. If biological life clearly remains, even if an individual suffers from an irreversible loss of consciousness, many people do not recognize that individual as dead.

Most important, death in Japan represents more than the extinction of individual bodies: it is above all a familial and social occasion. Even when medically determined, death becomes final only when the family accepts it as such. It is not surprising, therefore, that in Japan it has proved very difficult to represent brain-dead patients as cadaverlike. In addition, many people repudiate the idea of tampering with newly dead bodies.

Of course, these values and behaviors can be conveniently glossed as cultural, and it is to such phenomena that Japanese refer when they argue that culture is implicated in the brain-death problem. But most people do not then go on, as does a minority conservative element in Japan, to incite nationalist sentiment by arguing that recognition of brain death goes against that which is "timeless" and "natural" to Japanese.

Setting aside the rejoinders of active nationalists, are the responses of most Japanese so remarkable? People anywhere, when actually confronted with a brain-dead body, may find it hard to think of the person as dead, because the body exhibits many signs of life. Only if the idea of the "person" is clearly confined to mind and brain can the destruction of the brain be equated with the death of an individual. On the other hand, if the concept of the "person" is diffused throughout the body, or even extends outside the body, then destruction of the brain is not easily reckoned as signifying death.

Influential individuals in Japan have drawn on what they believe are widely shared values to encourage doubt as to whether a brain-dead patient is indeed dead. These same doubts are widely disseminated in the media. The public debate, for many years biased against recognition of brain death, has ensured that a diagnosis of brain death has not displaced the view that death cannot be pinpointed in time, nor located in the brain. Cultural sentiments have been mobilized for political ends.

The Japanese legal profession has been opposed all along to recognition of brain death, making it unlikely that the concept would gain easy acceptance. And although the legal status of the corpse is not clearly defined, civil court decisions have nevertheless affirmed that those who conduct the burial rites and will directly succeed the deceased have rights over the body (Machino 1996:108). It is widely assumed that the family should make the final decision about donation, even overriding expressed wishes of the individual.

In clinical settings, in addition to the necessary technology, a cluster of concepts and associated values must coexist to facilitate organ transplants from brain-dead bodies. First, a dead body must be recognized as alienable:[3] specifically, this means it can be handed over or acquired for dismemberment for medical purposes. Commodification of the human body in the name of scientific progress has a long history in Europe and North America but a relatively short one in Japan.[4]

Concern about use of medical resources and money is also important. When ventilator support of a brain-dead patient is interpreted as a "waste," and continued care deemed futile, then it is a small step to visualizing how the body of such a patient, declared legally dead and therefore alienable, could be put to good medical use. Medical practitioners in Japan are less likely to subscribe to this utilitarian position than are clinicians and hospital administrators in North America. Health care expenditures in Japan have been rigorously controlled, and the single-tier socialized health care system accounts for a much smaller percentage of GNP than it does in the United States, Canada, or the United Kingdom (Campbell and Ikegami 1998). Pressure exists in Japan to eliminate "waste" in connection with medical activities, but the mat-

3. *Alienable* means legally available for transfer or sale. Current policies in North America and Europe treat the cadaver and body parts as "quasi-property," thus making them alienable, but their transfer may not involve payment.

4. I am using *commodity* here in its original sense, to mean something that has a use, advantage, or value and can therefore be exchanged. Monetary exchange is the norm but not the only medium of exchange.

ter is not considered urgent because the health care system has not been permitted to be improvident. In any case, a brain-dead patient surrounded by a distraught family is very unlikely to be regarded as wasting scarce resources.

In modern society, "accidents" have no satisfactory explanation and are particularly disturbing because they represent a loss of control. The argument that organ donation can make something worthwhile out of an apparently senseless death is therefore a persuasive one. Through the "gift of life"—the ultimate act of altruism—control is to some extent reasserted and the disruption created by the accident is partly corrected, making nameless strangers into heroes. In Japan, however, another ideology competes with this view. Gift-giving is deeply embedded in an economy of reciprocal exchange; thus the idea of giving objects of value to complete strangers with whom one has had no personal contact appears strange to many. This, too, is culture at work.

The coalescence of these values, weighted very differently in Japan and North America, informs clinical practice, in one case enabling organ procurement and in the other inhibiting it. Despite the existence of constraining values, a lack of legal support, and the negative forces at work in the public domain, the majority of Japanese with firsthand experience of brain death, notably medical professionals working in intensive care units, think of this condition as human death. So do a number of relatives of brain-dead patients who ask for the ventilator to be turned off, although it often takes them several days to reach this decision.[5] But even then, families may not be in favor of organ donation.

Because the transplant enterprise is heavily dependent on organs procured from brain-dead bodies, it has been unable to establish a strong foothold in Japan. The thirty-year hiatus following the first Japanese heart transplant, an event with long-lasting, bitter repercussions, was finally ended in March 1999, one and a half years after the Organ Transplant Law was passed. A second heart transplant was carried out, together with a liver and kidney transplant making use of organs procured from a single brain-dead donor. In North America and much of Europe, by contrast, the dispute is about a so-called shortage of human organs and the unfulfilled "needs" of waiting patients.[6]

5. It is impossible to estimate how many families request that the ventilator be turned off, but of the nineteen emergency medicine doctors I talked to in Japan, all but one of them had experienced this situation more than once.

6. Discussion of a shortage of organs is not entirely absent from Japan, but it takes second place to the discussion about the recognition of brain death.

Aside from the vast discrepancy in the numbers of transplants performed, the biggest difference between Japan and North America is public discussion of issues associated with the new death. Many people in Japan are acquainted with the minute details of brain death and have some inkling of the competing arguments; this dissemination of information has led, however, to an impasse. A good number of Japanese also possess media-filtered knowledge about organ transplantation and related issues in North America, Europe, and elsewhere. In North America, we may joke about being brain-dead, but many of us do not have much idea of what is implicated in the clinical situation and know little or nothing about the debate in Japan. The medical and legal professions and the media in North America have damped down almost all the public anxiety that was briefly evident in the early years of organ transplants. Recently, a few television programs have focused critically on the sale of organs, usually in India. In the late 1990s, the difficulties of determining brain death have been discussed occasionally in the media. But this coverage is a fraction of what Japanese citizens have been exposed to.

My research strongly suggests that the majority of Japanese live and work with ontologies of death that differ from those of North Americans. This difference invites examination of the way in which contemporary society produces and sustains a discourse and practices that permit us to tinker with the end of life. Even when the technologies and scientific knowledge that enable these innovations are virtually the same, they produce different effects in different settings. Clearly, death is not a self-evident phenomenon. The margins between life and death are socially and culturally constructed, mobile, multiple, and open to dispute and reformulation.

The culture of Japan does not fully account for the discrepancy between the two geographical locations on this issue, although this is commonly assumed to be so. This could be the case only if the North American situation were assumed to be "normal," culture-"free," and progressive, and that of Japan to be in effect culturally "conservative." Such a dichotomous argument renders the concept of culture unproblematic—a position to which I take exception. In trying to explain why the brain-death problem persists as a hotly disputed matter in Japan, I argue that the culture of tradition is self-consciously put to work to aid those opposed to the recognition of brain death. It is not surprising that nostalgia for the "good old days" should be mobilized in arguments that warn about the moral implications of institutionalizing biomedical technologies that tinker with the margins between life and death. But in Japan this strategy draws on what are assumed to be shared values from the past and mobilizes them as a brake on innovations believed to have potentially damaging consequences for the "uniqueness" of Japanese society.

Widely shared values are certainly implicated in the brain-death debate in Japan, although they are not always mobilized for political ends. These values are not passed down unchanged through the centuries, as "traditionalists" would have us believe; they are subject to reflection, dispute, and transformation. Knowledge about what takes place in the rest of the world, notably in North America and Europe, informs this debate. But culture and politics are also at work in the United States and in Canada. Death can never be entirely divorced from culture, and the brain-death discussion also has political dimensions in North America, even though most of the discussion has proceeded as though the redefining of death is simply a medical and legal matter.

In undertaking this comparison I have chosen not to set out the North American situation and then that of Japan, but instead I move back and forth between the two geographical settings. This strategy is designed to underscore the point that the technology and expertise are equal in both locations and derive from a common recent history of medical innovation. Moreover, the juxtaposition illuminates how the debate in Japan is influenced by knowledge about the Other of North America and Europe. The various Japanese responses to brain death have evolved in part from an awareness of being a powerful nation in a globalized modernity, but being modern does not mean the erasure of what many believe is a distinct Japanese culture, nor does it entail an unexamined aping of the West. Concerns about creeping economic determinism and technological innovation coming at the cost of human well-being exist in Japan as elsewhere.

My simultaneous inquiry into the Japanese and North American debates is also designed to create uncertainty. Why was brain death accepted with relative ease in North America and most of Europe? And what relationship does this easy recognition have to the increased commodification of body parts for many purposes beside organ transplants? Between chapters I have inserted vignettes or excerpts from newspapers and other publications involving brain death, organ transplantation, and other disquieting medical matters. I have added very few comments, in part because no straightforward answers exist to most of the disturbing questions these stories raise. The bad science, the errors, and the self-interest exposed in some of these cases in a sense are secondary matters. Doctors, like most other people, usually work and plan as carefully as possible, safeguarding what they think of as the best interests of those in their care; even so, no obvious, unequivocal answers emerge to the moral questions raised by this form of body commodification. It is inappropriate, even if it were possible, to suppress emotional responses to organ procurement in the interest of finding rational answers. We are scrutinizing extraordinary activities: death-defying technologies in which the creation of meaning out of sudden destruction produces new forms of human affiliation. These are profoundly emotional matters.

My task is not to determine the morally correct path; I do not believe any hard-and-fast answer exists, and I find it difficult to take unequivocal stands about the various aspects of this complex situation, in which saving the life of one individual cannot in practice be disassociated from the death of another (although in closing I make my position clear on several key issues). Nor is my purpose simply to contextualize and account for the Japanese story. Through technological innovations we grow increasingly competent at the manipulation of the human body, alive and dead. This expertise demands a scrupulous consideration of the social consequences of what we are doing. One way to enter into this debate is to examine how societies other than our own have approached the social and moral issues associated with emerging biotechnologies, among them the creation of a new death for accident victims.

Discharge Summary

Mr. Smith, 29-year-old male, was brought to the ER on 15 September at 00:33, having jumped in front of a metro train at McGill station. Ambulance notes state that witnesses reported that he was struck by the train. Patient was recovered from under the first carriage. At the scene, he was reported unresponsive but breathing spontaneously with a strong pulse; other events surrounding the accident remain unclear.

Trauma team present on patient's arrival. He had an oral airway and a cervical collar. On examination he had good bilateral air entry, with O_2 saturation at 97%; trachea was midline and there was no chest wall crepitus. Heart sounds were normal with no murmur. He had a #18 left brachial intravenous line. He was noted to have an open skull fracture. Right pupil was blown, left pupil sluggish. Glasgow coma scale was 3.

He was intubated at 00:42 with a #8 orotracheal tube, according to trauma protocol; paralyzed with 100 mg succinylcholine and administered 100 mg of lidocaine. Three more large-bore IVs were started.

For every patient who is admitted to an emergency medicine or trauma unit and does not survive, a discharge summary must be written, usually by the nurse in charge of the case. This summary is based on a real incident, but all identifying features have been removed, and some of the details have been changed. Discharge summaries use many abbreviations and incomplete sentences. I have had to change the language to make this summary even minimally comprehensible, but I have deliberately retained much of the technical language in the document.

Cefazolin 2 g and a 200 mg bolus of Propafol were also administered. Blood pressure remained stable, running at 140/80 in the ER. Neurosurgery present in the ER.

CAT scan of the head done in the ER showed multiple skull fractures with bilateral intraventricular bleeds, subarachnoid hemorrhage and hydrocephalus with a small left epidural hemorrhage. C-spine CAT scan showed a right lateral mass of C1 fracture, and a C4 pedical fracture. CAT scan of abdomen showed a left lung contusion. Pelvis was cleared by the radiology resident.

Patient was transferred to SICU [surgical intensive care unit] at 01: 50, where he was hyperventilated; a mannitol drip was started. Neurosurgeons installed an ICP monitor which showed a pressure of <15 mm mercury. C3 transverse process fracture on CT also noted. 20 G right radial arterial line installed. Triple lumen left femoral line installed. Patient assessed by orthopedics. At 02:20 blood pressure began to drop and inotropes were started. At 03:00 temperature was 91°F (33°C), and he was noted to have right pupil at 6mm and left at 3mm and nonresponsive, with no corneals and no gag reflex. At 03:00 decision was made to warm patient to 94.5°F (35°C) and bring pCO_2 up to 40 mm Hg. At 03:00 a decision was made to stop all sedation and do an apnea test, if toxicology screen negative. If no spontaneous respirations at pCO_2 60 mm Hg, and no brainstem reflexes present, then diagnosis of brain death would be confirmed, and so advisable to discontinue treatment.[1] At 06:00 exam showed right pupil 7 mm fixed and nonreactive, left pupil 4mm fixed and nonreactive. Tox screen negative for acetaminophen, salicylates, tricyclics; ethanol was 28. Ventilated assist-control 8 tidal volume 800. Nil acute on chest X ray. Still on Levophed drip to maintain BP. Hemoglobin 89. Diagnosis likely brain-dead; plan to do apnea test, maintain BP with Levophed, alert transplant team; social services to ID patient.

Social services saw patient, noted police report #47–99–134–98–093, contacted Constable Brown 330–9483.

At 18:00 no change in neuro exam, failed apnea test, no eye movements in caloric test, doll's eye test negative. Plan to repeat apnea test later. At 20:30 police came to claim patient's keys. At 23:00 patient identified by police as John Smith, born 14 April 1969, address, 1234

1. The absence of a breathing reflex in the presence of a high concentration of carbon dioxide in the blood, which would normally trigger breathing, can indicate lack of function in the brain stem. This condition is established by using the apnea test, one of a set of clinical tests used to establish brain death.

South St., phone 555–1234. Social services traced and contacted parents who came to ID patient at 04:30 on 16 Sept.

Seriousness of injuries explained to parents, but that patient not clinically dead at that time, but very close. Parents agreed that once apnea test was repeated and was positive they would consent to withdraw active treatment, including ventilator.[2] Parents informed that they would be approached about organ donation in the event that patient was confirmed brain-dead. Parents agreed to consider in that case. Québec Transplant notified of potential donor. Apnea test was repeated at 06:30 and was positive. PCO_2 before 40, after 10 min pCO_2 61. Parents present at declaration of brain death, met with transplant coordinator. Consented to donation. Transplant team notified.

---

2. In this case, the medical staff and parents agreed that the situation was so bad that there was no need to do a second apnea test. All recognized that there was no possibility of survival.

THE PROCUREMENT

The pager on the bedside table goes off at 12:30 A.M. Jarred from a deep sleep, I stumble into the next room and dial the number displayed on the tiny screen. The transplant surgeon answers immediately from his car phone: "I'm ten minutes from the hospital, we'll be starting a procurement in about half an hour."

I drag on some clothes, stuff tennis shoes and thick socks in a bag, and call a taxi. During the fifteen-minute journey to the hospital I feel apprehensive about being an intruder into the efficient, sterile space of the operating room, in particular because it will be to observe not a lifesaving procedure, but the "harvesting" of human organs.

The cavernous hospital, overflowing with patients by day, is strangely quiet, the long corridors empty save for one man dozing fitfully across two upright chairs, perhaps waiting for news. The elevator takes me up to the surgical unit on the fifth floor, where I pass through double doors into a deserted reception area. Fortunately, this is not my first time as an observer in the OR, and I know where to find a set of "greens" into which I change. I pull on the thick socks and tennis shoes, essential for standing in one spot for three or four hours. Thus prepared, I go through a second set of double doors into a transition area, the busy assembly point for successive teams of surgeons during the day. Here I put on plastic hair and shoe covers before proceeding to room 12, the only one lit up and in use at this time of the night. I tie on a face mask before entering.

The OR is a place of intense activity: three nurses prepare the instruments, swabs, drapes, and other accoutrements; a transplant coordinator is on the telephone; one orderly departs after delivering the "patient," while another prepares containers for the organs; a senior surgeon stands at the foot of the operating table. He chats with his two residents, both women, until the nurses are ready to clothe all three of them in sterile gowns. Two anesthesiologists confer among the monitors clustered at the head of the table. No one gives more than a brief glance at the body, connected to numerous tubes and lines extending to a battery of monitors, the diaphragm rising and falling to the rhythm of the artificial ventilator.

Preparations complete, the nurses turn to the patient and remove all the drapes, except for one covering the groin. They place the arms on supports at right angles to the body. The donor had recently painted her fingernails a bright red; now, in death, they appear incongruous. The nurses swab the entire torso with providone iodine to sterilize it before the surgeons make the long incision. The body is then draped again, leaving only the iodine-stained center of the torso exposed. The catheter, inserted to collect the urine that the donor's kidneys will produce until the moment they are removed from the body, is carefully checked. Meanwhile, a waist-high barrier of drapes has been erected to separate the body of the donor, recumbent in the sterile area, from her head and neck, in the nonsterile domain of the anesthesiologists.

Using a scalpel, the surgical team makes a single long cut from just below the sternum to just above the pubis. With a cautery, the team works its way through the layer of fat beneath the skin and the abdominal musculature; then they use their gloved hands to expose the liver, lying deep in the right upper quadrant of the abdomen, beneath the ribs. The disquieting smell of burning flesh fills my nostrils as the cautery cuts and seals off small blood vessels to minimize bleeding into the abdominal cavity. Nevertheless I feel relatively little discomfort as I peer, along with the surgeons and nurses, into the body. Fascination and curiosity overcome feelings of horror or repulsion.

Her phone calls finished, the transplant coordinator can now relax a little. She has made all the necessary arrangements for delivery of the kidneys to other hospitals to which prospective recipients, already alerted by their pagers that the "gift of life" is on its way at last, will be admitted as quickly as possible. Preliminary tests have revealed that the heart is not in good condition, and so it will not be used.[1] The liver will be transplanted immediately into another patient, already undergoing preliminary sedation in another room of this hospital.

The coordinator was formerly a nurse, and she tells me enthusiastically how much she likes her present work, despite the inconvenient hours. She says that the donor lying in front of us had gone that morning to her bank, where she had suddenly collapsed, never to regain consciousness. Rushed by ambulance to the nearest hospital while attendants pumped air manually into her lungs, she was then intubated: that is, tubes were inserted through her mouth into her trachea, to which a mechanical ventilator was then attached. The staff in the emergency room had struggled to stabilize the patient; warmed fluids were forced into her veins to maintain her blood pressure, but it was clear from the outset that something was terribly wrong. A CAT scan revealed that a massive hemorrhage had virtually destroyed her entire forebrain, indicating that nothing further could be done to save her life.

The possibility that this patient could be an organ donor was now uppermost in the hospital staff's minds. The various electrodes, tubes, catheters and lines monitoring and administering medication were kept in place in the body while two neurologists were summoned. As it was late morning, they were on hand in the hospital, and they came independently to an opinion that the patient met the criteria for brain death. A little later she was unhooked briefly from the ventilator, and the apnea test was applied to see whether spontaneous breathing would start, but after a few minutes, when there was no response, the ventilator was reconnected. The same neurological tests were repeated six hours later, as is commonly recommended when establishing brain death, and the diagnosis was confirmed. The death certificate was signed. By this time it was known that the patient had signed her donor card and that her next of kin supported donation.

With the patient legally dead, care of the organs, rather than of the person, became the dominant concern. The donor was transferred from the suburban hospital to the tertiary care hospital in the city center for

1. The heart is tested with an echocardiogram before the patient is taken out of the intensive care unit where brain death is declared. In many parts of North America, provided that the organ is in good condition, hearts are procured from donors up to sixty-five years of age. In some locations, fifty-five or sixty is regarded as the upper age limit. For the liver there is no upper age limit; for kidneys some centers have an age limit, but others prefer to judge by the condition of the kidney once it is removed from the donor.

the organs to be procured, but the body had to be kept stable and at an appropriate temperature during this journey.[2] Ventilation was continued manually, the tubes and lines kept in place so that medication could be administered, and the heart rate and blood pressure were monitored continuously. It was essential that the organs, precious commodities, remain in good condition.

Now, in the operating room, the liver is exposed, but on seeing it the surgeon lets out an expletive. He asks someone to call a pathologist to determine whether the spots on its surface are due to cirrhosis, in which case the liver will be of no use. "She only drank a little, did you say?" Turning to the transplant coordinator, the surgeon frowns behind his mask. "Looks like more than a little to me." The team continues with the meticulous, tedious work of removing the hepatic artery and portal veins attached to the liver, noting as they do so certain deviations from "normal" anatomy—which, they tell me, are not uncommon.

During this part of the procedure, I stand near the anesthesiologist, just behind the donor's head, and peer over the mind/body barrier formed by the drapes. In stark contrast to the half-hidden, pale, life-less face of the brain-dead person, the interior of the body is colorful and alive. The diaphragm, untouched by the surgeons, rises and falls as air is delivered to the lungs from the ventilator. Beneath the diaphragm, the continued activity of the heart is clear: blood courses through the vessels, and the liver has the burgundy hue of health, so that even the offending spots are no longer visible. From inside the massive incision, held apart by powerful retractors, a bright melee of colors spills forth: yellow, orange, red, cream, beige, white. The surgeons handle the omen-tum and the intestines with familiarity and move them deftly to expose the critical vessels and the bile duct, which are clamped and tied off one by one.

The pathologist arrives thirty minutes later and takes a small liver biopsy for microscopic examination. The surgeons continue working in rapt concentration, heartened by the good color of the liver. The pa-thologist returns about twenty minutes later to declare that there is no evidence of cirrhosis or any other pathology. After further careful dis-section and perfusion of the liver to preserve its condition, the blood

2. Transplant teams usually travel to the hospitals where brain-dead patients have been identified to procure the organs. Sometimes this involves dramatic, hastily arranged helicopter and small plane flights. On other occasions, especially within a city, donors are transferred from small centers to tertiary-care hospitals to ease the job of the transplant surgeon, particularly if he or she is already occupied with another case.

vessels all neatly tied off, the liver is snipped free from the still-breathing body with several centimeters of each blood vessel left intact.

The senior surgeon leaves the donor to the care of his residents and carries the liver to a bowl filled with ice and perfusion liquid at the side of the room. Here he conducts further, minute dissection of the blood vessels. This painstaking work is designed to ensure success several hours later, when he will be suturing the blood vessels to corresponding vessels in the recipient. The gall bladder, intimately associated with the liver, is delicately separated, black bile flowing out when it is deliberately punctured. The liver is then placed carefully into a large plastic bag with ice and liquid and placed in cold storage until it is transplanted into the recipient, a few hours later, by the same surgical team.

The residents meanwhile turn their attention to the kidneys. Here they systematically expose and isolate the blood vessels and the ureter, first on one side and then the other, while the senior surgeon rejoins them at intervals and praises their progress. The kidneys are removed as a pair, then separated and made ready for donation in the waiting bowls; this will be the end of their partnership, for they will go to two different recipients. Right and left kidneys, carefully distinguished, in turn will shortly be placed in plastic bags, put into containers, and handed over at the door of the OR to a driver who will transport them to other hospitals. One or two small pieces of spleen are taken as backup for cross-matching of blood and tissue, in case some accident should befall the blood samples already stored in tubes. At this point, the delicate and technical part of their work just about complete, people relax and start to talk—all except the senior surgeon, who remains apart, meticulously preparing the kidneys for donation. Watching the delicacy with which the surgeon handles the kidneys and the way an arriving surgeon goes straight over to admire these newly procured, mulberry-colored organs glistening with health, I am reminded that throughout this entire process it has been the organs, and not the donor, on which everyone has been concentrating. The donor is merely a container that must be handled with care.

The patient's family had reported that the donor smoked a pack of cigarettes a day. The procurement just about complete, it is decided to separate the sternum and take a look at the effects of this habit on the lungs and heart. The beating heart is enclosed in a layer of protective yellow fat. Its rhythmic throbbing seems mechanical as it continues to labor, exposed, amid the lungs, which are blackened from the years of tobacco use.

The ventilator is then turned off, followed by the monitors that have kept track of heart rate and blood pressure throughout. The anesthesiologists leave the room, the first part of their night's work complete. Breathing ceases, and the heart too gradually ceases to function, finally transforming the body into a cadaver. One of the residents sets to work returning the intestines neatly to the body cavity, which is carefully sewn together with large sutures, topped off by a long strip of surgical tape. The surgical drapes are removed and replaced by a single sheet covering the cadaver to its neck. Now that the head is clearly exposed again, and the body discreetly covered, my eyes are drawn to the strips of tape placed over the eyes some hours ago, before the donor left the ICU, to keep the corneas moist. An ophthalmic surgeon is expected at any moment to remove them for donation, and I find myself repelled by this last intrusion in a way that I had not expected. For me, it seems, removal of the eyes represents more of a violation than does procurement of internal organs. More likely it is simply that the tension in the room has entirely dissipated, and now that people are leaving, stripping off their surgical gear as they go, I am permitted to reflect on the enormity of what is, to them, a routine procedure. The procurement complete, the cadaver is wheeled out of the OR and thence to the hospital morgue, eighteen hours after the incident in the bank and eight hours after brain death was confirmed.

stripping off surgical gear, letting their guard down
Lock is now also letting her guard down

Symbolic way of stripping off the enforced, whether or not suppressed, that the operation nevertheless has on all parts of the team.
members

THE GIFT

It is 6:00 A.M. The patient is waiting, first heavily sedated and then rendered fully unconscious, while two surgeons meticulously wash their hands and go into OR 14 to join the nurses, one of whom assists them in donning sterile gowns.

The body is swabbed and draped, and then a large incision, an inverted V, is quickly made just below the rib cage. The disconcerting smell of burning flesh assails the nostrils for a while as the cauteries cut deep through the layers of skin and fat, stanching the blood flow with their heat as they cut. When I first see the jaundiced, angular face and thin body of the patient I think that he is a teenager, not yet fully grown, but this is the effect of the disease. At thirty-four, even though he has never smoked or drunk alcohol, he has advanced cirrhosis of the liver and ulcerative colitis caused by an unusual autoimmune disease known as sclerosing cholangitis. The patient has been sick for a long time, but recently things took a turn for the worse; internal bleeding suggested to the doctors that he would not live much longer without a liver transplant.

Large, metal retractors are applied, forcing the rib cage up and back. I wonder if patients' ribs are sometimes cracked by this procedure. The small frame of the man's chest is dwarfed by the apparatus, and I speculate whether, amid the plethora of uncomfortable sensations he will experience the next day, he will even notice a rib cage aching with five hours of being pulled out of position.

The patient had been on a waiting list for a liver for nearly three months; everyone in the operating room agrees that he could not have gone on much longer. The seriousness of his condition is quite obvious, even to an untrained observer, once the omentum and the intestines are set to one side and the liver exposed. The organ has none of the rosy hue of a healthy liver but is mud-colored and covered with raised black spots, tiny knots of blood vessels struggling to do their work.

Music is piped into the operating room, providing a background to the occasional words exchanged among the two surgeons and their senior fellow. They work efficiently, first isolating the hepatic artery. Only once is the nurse chastised for passing the wrong-sized instrument. A resident pops into the room, comes round to the patient's head, and briefly touches him. "How's he doing?" he asks. "He's such a nice guy, I can't wait for him to get this over with." During the five-hour liver transplant, in addition to the three doctors, the staff includes two nurses, one or two anesthesiologists (who take it in turns to pop out to nap, having been working all night), occasionally an orderly; and, for the first hour, two or three medical student observers.

With the hepatic artery clamped, the surgeons move on to dissect the bile duct; then they clamp first the superior hepatic vena cava, next the inferior hepatic vena cava, and finally the portal vein. Great care is taken to minimize bleeding while also leaving the blood vessels in good condition for suturing to the blood vessels attached to the new liver. After two and a half hours of meticulous work, with the gall bladder still affixed to it, the diseased liver is eased out of the body and tossed into a bowl, to be taken for a pathological examination. It is surprisingly large and ugly in its sickness.

In an adjoining room, another surgeon has spent over an hour preparing the new liver for transplant. The donor was a twenty-year-old man who suffered a brain aneurysm and was declared brain-dead shortly after arrival at a nearby hospital. The organ donor consent on his driver's license was signed, and his family agreed to the donation. The computerized tissue-matching system showed quickly that of the wait-listed recipients considered urgent cases, this was the best candidate to receive this particular liver. It would be ten hours in all between the procurement of the liver and its complete transplant into the recipient: over seven hours on ice once it was removed and more than two and a half hours being transplanted into its new owner.

The patient's blood pressure drops suddenly when the sick liver is removed, and it stays unstable, but never dangerously low, for the next hour. The new liver is set in place just below the rib cage; it is larger than its predecessor and has to be eased carefully into its new quarters. The surgeons set about suturing the blood vessels together in the reverse order from that used to remove the liver. In response to my query about the cause of the unstable blood pressure, the anesthesiologist informs me that this phenomenon is common and appears to be due in part to the patient's blood system working hard to dispose of the toxins accumulated in the new liver while it lay on ice. This accumulation occurs despite constant perfusion to keep the organ healthy—not surprisingly, given that one of the principal functions of the liver is to filter toxins from the body.

During the suturing of the blood vessels, the patient starts to lose blood. This is quietly and quickly dealt with. Most patients receive three or four units of blood during a liver transplant, and these days surgery usually takes about five hours (compared with fourteen hours in the early days), provided that at least two experienced surgeons are present. The final step before starting to "close" the patient is to make a new gall bladder; his own is vulnerable to the autoimmune disease. A small portion of his small intestine is cut, refashioned, and sutured in place as a substitute. This final stage of the surgery seems particularly rough and ready—a cut-and-patch job—and it occurs to me that transplant surgery, for all its public image as a high-powered, innovative technology, is nevertheless a massive intervention into the human body demanding manual precision and precise anatomical and physiological knowledge.

The patient goes home just eight days after surgery. He is doing exceptionally well and is discharged a day early, but he will have to take powerful immunosuppressants for the rest of his life to stop his own immune system from wreaking havoc on the new liver. These drugs will almost certainly cause side effects and put him at increased risk for other diseases. A few days later, I am surprised and delighted to hear how well he is doing. While watching the surgery, I wondered several times how his frail body could endure this massive onslaught. I also pondered whether I would opt for a transplant should I have a life-threatening disease, and concluded that at his age I almost certainly would have wanted one.

I still cannot answer what I would have wanted for my children should they have contracted an incurable liver disease at a young age. From this research I have concluded that it is very difficult to imagine what one might decide when confronted with making a choice about either organ procurement from or a transplant for a dying relative. It is an especially difficult choice in the case of a child, for whom a transplant may involve immense suffering with a long-term outcome that is far from clear.[1]

Wendy Doniger, a specialist in the history of religions, was, like me, a member of an interdisciplinary group, brought together by the psychiatrist Stuart Youngner, that met regularly from 1991 to 1993 to examine the human and cultural meaning of organ transplants. Doniger added a personal postscript to her essay in the book that resulted from these meetings. She notes that as her involvement in our project deepened, she began to have serious misgivings about the wisdom of organ transplants, and she had "more or less decided that [she] was against it all." During the course of our meetings, Doniger learned from her brother that her niece was suffering from advanced renal failure and had only a few days to live. Doniger began "instantly to pray" that a donor would be found. In the event, one was, and the operation went ahead. Several years later, her niece was doing well. Doniger concludes that the near-tragedy revealed unconscious feelings about organ transplants that were different from those of her consciously articulated opposition. She comes to understand her article as an attempt "to formalize the bridge between those two sets of feelings in me and, I would hope, in the reader" (Doniger 1996:218).

I have never been tested as Doniger has, but I firmly believe, as she does, that no amount of rational debate, no amount of abstract soul-searching, can provide conclusive answers to these intensely emotional questions. The "truth" of firsthand experience and of subjective, gut-level responses to the fearful dilemmas posed by organ procurement and transplant are as important as is measured discussion.

---

1. The four-year survival rate in North America for patients with liver transplants is over 73 percent. Figures for five years and longer are not available, nor are details about quality of life, but the longest-surviving liver transplant recipient has lived for more than twenty-eight years following the operation (United Network for Organ Sharing 1999).

He looked pale and underweight for a thirty-seven-year-old as we sat facing each other in the privacy of a small room in the transplant unit.

"For a long time I fooled myself that I wasn't sick, but actually I'd really been noticing things."

"Like what"?

"Lots of excess skin on my feet, putting on weight, big mood swings—just little things that you don't pay much attention to."

"Excess skin on your feet?"

"Yes, that's common, I discovered, with cirrhosis, but of course, at the time, it never occurred to me that it was a sign that something was wrong with the liver. I do a lot of rafting, and I thought I might have picked up something from the river. I kept meaning to go to a dermatologist."

"What made you go to the doctor in the end?"

"About six months ago I really started to put on a lot of weight. I looked as if I was pregnant! I still didn't go to the doctor right away, but finally I got a herniated belly button, so I went to a GP, who sent me right away to a surgeon, and he sent me on to a liver specialist. He made the diagnosis in no time at all, and things just kept going downhill from there. He said early on that I was going to have to have a liver transplant at some point in my life, and that his bet was that it would be sooner rather than later. They put me on a whole bunch of diuretics that didn't do anything for the weight problem really. The main thing they did was to drain the liver every so often, and that really helped.

"I was working and I didn't want to give that up. I was on the Hibernia project. Have you heard of that?"

"Off the Newfoundland coast?"

"Yeah. I was a drilling engineer, and it was a terrific job. I was about to move everything from Montreal to St. John's permanently, but they don't have a transplant center there. I persuaded my doctor to let me come and go between Newfoundland and Montreal more or less on a biweekly basis."[1]

"That sounds terribly tiring."

"Yes, the doctor didn't really agree, but I just did it anyway, until he said that he simply wasn't going to put me on the waiting list for a transplant unless I came and lived permanently in Montreal. So, a couple of months ago, I came back on a Sunday to the tiny apartment I keep here. On the Monday I went out and did some grocery shopping, stayed home for the rest of the day, and on Tuesday I woke up vomiting blood, but I was already too sick to really realize how serious it was. I just fell back to sleep, and when I woke up I thought it was the evening—too late to call my doctor at the clinic—although it was actually only 4 P.M. I couldn't even read the clock properly. I managed to call my girlfriend in Newfoundland, and she arranged everything from there. The downstairs neighbor here in Montreal is a good friend of ours. She called the ambulance, and they took me to the hospital. The last thing I remember was the doctor coming back into the room with a nurse carrying the long needle they use for biopsies. I must have fainted, or gone unconscious, and the next thing I knew, I woke up two days later, and the operation was all done!"

"So they were able to find a liver right away?"

"Yeah. It was blind luck. They told me afterwards they'd given me a day and a half or two at the most to live, so I went to the top of the list, and I hit the jackpot."

"Didn't anyone realize how serious things were long before the crisis?"

"The doctors knew for sure, and to be honest, I knew too. Every test I had, they told me that my liver was getting less and less operational. I hadn't really worked on the Hibernia project for three months; I had no energy left, and I was forced to take sick leave, but I didn't want to come

1. The distance is over 1,625 miles.

and sit in Montreal doing nothing, feeling miserable. I was in hospital once before when I came back to Montreal one time for tests, it turned out then I had an infection on top of the cirrhosis. When they let me out, I went right back to Newfoundland, but on long-term disability—and I think I knew then finally that I was dying, but it was funny, I hadn't really taken time to think about it until I hit that low spot.

"I'm divorced, and my ex-wife has custody of the three kids, and my daughter is causing a lot of trouble right now, so she came to stay with me. But she doesn't get on with my girlfriend, and she doesn't understand why I can't have her live with me permanently, so I've been really depressed about things for a year or two. I wasn't sure that I wanted to go through with this transplant operation at all, and so I suppose that was why I didn't really face up to things."

"How do you feel now?"

"Well, I'm thankful, of course. But even now—I'm fifty days past surgery—you still get times when you wonder what the future holds, especially because I'm in rejection right now.[2] It would have been really helpful to have a support group or something. As a matter of fact, they do have a group, but at the moment it's all in French. I'm from Alberta, so you can imagine how much French I know. I've been bugging them to start up an English group again. Of course, my girlfriend was here for a while, but she had to go back, and my Ma is here now, but she's going back to Calgary this weekend. She came to make sure that I ate."

"Do you have an appetite?"

"A bit. It's funny, because they must have cut some major nerves, and initially you can't tell if you're hungry and, what's worse, you can't tell when you have to go to the toilet. I mean, you've got to think about it, and say to yourself, 'Time to go to the toilet now.' The sensations are slowly coming back, but the doctor says it will be a year before everything is back to normal.

"With all the drugs, especially the cyclosporine, you're supposed to put on weight, feel hungrier than usual, and your hair is supposed to get thicker. None of that has happened to me. It's scary. It's awful. They don't know why.

"It's a huge scar, but it's more or less healed now, so I'm supposed to get into some exercise. I should do some swimming. But a bathing

2. Despite the use of powerful immunosuppressants, organ recipients often have episodes in which the patient's own immune system mounts a reaction against the new organ. With careful monitoring and adjustment of medication, patients usually survive these rejection events with the new organ intact.

beauty I'm not going to be from now on! When people ask me what happened, I've started saying that I'm a test driver for Mercedes!"

"How long did the actual surgery take, do you know?"

"They told me it was about seven hours, which is long, but time flies when you're having fun! Sometimes they can do it in five these days. Then I had three days in the ICU. I don't know what they were feeding me for painkillers, but it sure left pretty pictures on the wall. They had tubes in me all over the place, but they started to get them out after the first day."

"Then you were moved to the regular unit?"

"Yes, I was here as an in-patient for three weeks. Now I have to come back every week. More while I'm having this rejection. I'm supposed to stay in Montreal for six months, but I've got no work. I'm not doing too well right now, but they tell me I'll get over this rejection all right—it's not unusual to have ups and downs at first."

"Do you know anything about the donor?"

"They try not to let you know anything. I think it was a man, I don't know why. It was a car accident in this city, that's all I know."

"It's possible to write a letter of thanks. Did you do that?"

"Oh yes. The annoying thing is I don't know if they ever got it. Apparently some administrative department calls up the family and asks them if they'd like to receive a letter from the person who got their relative's organ. It's up to them. If they don't want the letter, then it's not sent on to them, and even if they want it, they're not allowed to reply to me. That's because the donor family sometimes wants to build up a lasting relationship with the recipient, and the authorities don't want that. Anyway, it was the longest note I've ever written in my life. It was really hard to write. I really wanted to say thanks, but also try to explain to them that something good had come out of the death of their relative. But I don't know if they got it, or if it went into the garbage. I'd really like to know more about the donor. I dream about it. I realize I'll probably never know anything more, but I've often wondered what it would be like to meet the family. I suppose it would just bring back a whole bunch of bad memories for them, knowing that the liver is mine now. Anyway, I feel really grateful. I feel an emotion for him that I can't even describe, and I don't think I want to lose that, ever."

"Are you religious?"

"No. I was hoping to find out what a near-death experience was like, though, but I went right into a coma. I was disappointed because, being an engineer, I wanted facts, so as I could explain what near-death is really like! But I must say I've wondered why I lucked out and got an organ just when I needed it. It makes you think about prayer and faith, but even so, I think I'm still waiting for a personally engraved invitation to come and have a chat with God before I really believe."

"By the way, do you have any thoughts about why you got cirrhosis in the first place?"

"Oh, yes. When I was a teenager, about thirteen or fourteen, I used drugs for a while. I contracted hepatitis B then. Now the doctors think I probably also got hepatitis C at the same time, and that it stayed dormant until now. I'll always be a carrier. It's incurable. So it may kill off this new liver too. My doctor said to me, "From now on you're married to the transplant unit."

"So now you live with uncertainty all the time?"

"Oh yeah. I still wonder whether I should have gone through with this operation. There's always going to be limits on me now. Maybe I won't have a transplant next time."[3]

---

3. From the surgeon's point of view, this patient has continued to do well in the five years since his transplant.

ONE

Boundary Transgressions and Moral Uncertainty

The exotic charm of another system of thought is the limitation
of our own, the stark impossibility of thinking *that*.

Michel Foucault, The Order of Things

In this book I show how brain death is associated with different sets of
assumptions about what constitutes the end of human life in Japan and
North America. I also highlight what conditions are thought by some
to be as "good-as-dead" and ask if and when it is appropriate to make
utilitarian use of body parts. Differing assumptions in the two regions
yield different answers to these questions. They touch on boundaries
between nature and culture, life and death, self and other, person and
body. Medical science is undoubtedly one of the principal arbiters of
these judgments, but it should not be thought of as inevitably determining decisions about human death.

Biological death is recognized in society and in law by the standards
of medical science, but what exactly constitutes death of a body, and
what does this death signify with respect to death of the person? Does
irreversible brain damage count as biological death, even if on occasion
signs of life remain in the brain and other parts of the body continue to
function, albeit aided by medical technology? And if irreversible brain
damage counts as biological death, does this mean that the person too
has died? Moreover, does the law recognize brain death as human
death? Only when consensus is reached on these points can a brain-dead
body be thought of as cadaverlike and made available for commodification.

The position of the North American public, largely ignorant of the
issues, remains obscure. Among North American physicians, brain death
has been broadly recognized as an indicator of both biological and per-

sonal death; in Japan, there is no consensus. In recent years, in several countries, a few clinicians (most of them neurologists), legal commentators, and philosophers have argued that irreversible brain damage should not be thought of as biological death, but that it nevertheless represents the end of meaningful life. I review here several of the key concepts that inform my critical reading of this entire debate.

Moral Economies of Science and Styles of Reasoning

A dominant approach in the "modern" world argues that nature, including the human body in life and death, functions according to scientific laws and is, therefore, autonomous and independent of social context and the moral order. When nature is understood this way, boundaries between nature and culture appear self-evident and pose few, if any, philosophical problems. Humans, however, are often characterized as tool makers, a pursuit that has permitted us over millennia to transform the natural environment and harvest its riches. The usual explanation given for such activities, this cultural modification of the natural, is that they are essential to meet "basic" human needs. In other words, nature *must* be reworked on the basis of intellectual and technological innovation, but nevertheless functions according to laws that ensure its continued autonomy from culture.

With the formation of the biological sciences in the nineteenth century, systematic examination, classification, and manipulation of the environment and of the "natural" objects that inhabit it, including human, animal, and plant materials, expanded enormously. By the second half of the century, the idea of improving on nature, and thus of providing for far more than basic needs, was firmly established. At the same time, the language of needs expanded into one of rights. Today, for people in the so-called developed world, lifelong good health is clearly included in these expectations (even though the vast majority of the world's population, including many residents of the United States and Canada, will not enjoy this assurance without major economic reforms).

The dominant ideology of an autonomous nature is increasingly challenged by philosophers, historians, social scientists, and natural scientists themselves. The making of stone tools and the laboratory replication of DNA alike require application of the human imagination. All knowledge about the natural world and its transformation must inevitably be mediated by our senses, making the conceptualization of nature, including the specification of its relationship to human society, contingent. Moreover, meanings attributed to both nature and society change through time and space (Cronon 1996; Daston 1992; Latour 1993; Lock et al. 2000). Cronon argues, for example, that nature is a human idea with a long and complicated cultural history that has led human beings to conceive of the natural world in very different ways (1996:20). Following this line of argument, the distinction between life (associated with culture) and death (associated with nature), although usually regarded as unproblematic, is necessarily blurred.

Sophisticated challenges to the epistemology of science, including that of biology, with its appeal to objectivity, do not dispute the reality of the material world. Nor is it asserted that morals, judgments, and assessments are present in every aspect of the scientific endeavor in exactly the same way as they are in other areas of human life. Scientific reasoning is not conceptualized by these critics, whose ideas I share, as a form of human conversation, as Richard Rorty has argued (1988), but neither is science understood as exempt from interrogation about its truth claims.

Lorraine Daston, a historian of science, posits what she calls a "moral economy" of science. She notes that the ideal of scientific objectivity insists on "the existence and impenetrability" of boundaries between facts and values, between emotions and rationality, but she insists that this ideal is based on an illusion (Daston 1995:3). Certain forms of empiricism, quantification, and notions about objectivity itself require a moral economy to sustain them. By moral economy, Daston means "a web of affect-saturated values that stand and function in well-defined relationship to one another" (1995:4). Objects or actions are valorized and form part of a balanced system of emotional forces, with equilibrium points and constraints. "Although it is a contingent, malleable thing of no necessity, a moral economy has a certain logic to its composition and operations. Not all conceivable combinations of affects and values are in fact possible" (1995:4). Daston is not arguing that ideologies or political self-interest inevitably penetrate the scientific endeavor (although, at times, clearly they do), nor is she suggesting that science is merely socially constructed. Even though moral economies in science "draw routinely and liberally upon the values and affects of ambient culture, the reworking that results usually becomes the peculiar property of scientists" (1995:7). This is, Daston argues, a special instance of hegemony, often solidified slowly but relentlessly over, sometimes, hundreds of years.

Moral economies are not limited to one particular discipline or subdiscipline of science. Belief in the powers of quantification, empiricism, and objectivity, agreement as to what counts as evidence, and so on, are common across almost all facets of the scientific endeavor. During the nineteenth century, once death was made into a medical rather than primarily a religious matter, the assessment of death was transformed into a rigorous scientific endeavor. In hospitals and other medical settings, individual death was stripped of much of its social significance and remade as a biological event. Doctors acquired the authority to pronounce death because lay people did not have the required expertise or objectivity. As chapter 2 shows, large segments of the European and North American public became deeply fearful of medical authority in this new domain. Anxieties abounded about premature pronouncement of death and burial alive. The medical world responded by attempting to apply science more rigorously. By contrast, in Japan, where medical authority over death has been relatively weak until recent years, the social significance of individual death has not been subordinated to a medicalized, objective death, even in medical settings and despite the fact that Japanese doctors participate in essentially the same moral economy of science as those in the West.

Whereas a moral economy is common across the sciences, the philosopher Ian Hacking focuses on a narrower perspective when he argues for a "disunity" of science. The sciences should be grouped together, Hacking suggests, "in terms of one of their disunities, their styles" (1996:74)—thus avoiding any absolute conception of reality. He asks what it is about certain styles of reasoning that make them endure while others falter, and how and why such styles of reasoning become authenticated as truthful and accurate. Because some arguments are clearly more effective than others, attention must be paid, Hacking insists, to the "self-stabilizing techniques peculiar to a given style of reasoning" (1996:73). Among the techniques characteristic of contemporary science Hacking includes modification of hypotheses, the rebuilding of instruments, reconsideration of data analysis, and so on. It is these self-stabilizing techniques, together with processes of vindication, that Hacking sees as distinguishing scientific reasoning from most humanistic and moral thought.

The philosopher Arnold Davidson, writing about the history of psychiatry, suggests that as styles of reasoning develop, they bring with them "new categories of possible true-or-false statements" (1996:79). He cites an example used originally by Ian Hacking to make this point:

Consider the following statement that you might find in a Renaissance medical textbook: "Mercury salve is good for syphilis because mercury is signed
by the planet Mercury which signs the marketplace, where syphilis is contracted." Hacking argues, correctly I think, that our best description of this
statement is not as false or as incommensurable with current medical reasoning, but rather as not even a possible candidate for truth-or-falsehood,
given our currently accepted styles of reasoning. But a style of reasoning
central to the Renaissance, based on the concepts of resemblance and simil-
itude, brings with it the candidacy of such a statement for the status of true-
or-false. Categories of statements get their status as true-or-false vis-à-vis
historically specifiable styles of reasoning.

(Davidson, 1996:79)

Davidson elaborates on how most psychiatrists working today ha-
bitually draw on familiar analogies and make predictable inferences significantly different from those used in earlier decades. However, when
it comes to the "soft" part of psychiatry, to the creation of taxonomies
of illness (attention deficit and hyperactivity disorder [ADHD], for example), and to psychotherapeutics, then different, competing styles of
reasoning and schools of thought within the discipline are apparent.

It is tempting to extend Davidson's argument cross-culturally. Styles
of reasoning then differ not only through time but also through space—
that is, the space of culture. But this is to oversimplify matters. Science,
including medical science, makes use in effect of a globalized moral
economy, and often styles of reasoning may be more or less commen-
surate around the world. My research in intensive care units (ICUs) in
Japan and North America suggests that the styles of reasoning used by
neurologists and intensivists[1] in these two locations to determine brain
death are remarkably similar. There is virtually universal agreement, for
instance, that the condition of brain death, accurately assessed, is irreversible (although continuing advances in trauma medicine may prevent
many patients from progressing to this state).

However, even this seemingly firm end point is sometimes seriously
disputed. In a recent report to a committee investigating the low rate of
organ donation in Canada, Ruth Oliver, a psychiatrist, claimed that she
was declared clinically dead twenty-two years previously. She insisted
that she is "living testimony that people survive clinical death and brain
death" even when labeled by some as " 'irreversibly and inevitably' dying." A perceptive newspaper reporter noted that Oliver would probably
not have been diagnosed as brain-dead today, thanks to improved in-

1. Intensivists are medical and nursing specialists who work in intensive care units.

vestigative procedures (McIlroy 1999). In this relatively short period the technology has not changed radically, but cumulative experience, and with it systematization of the methods and reasoning used to determine brain death, have. The reporter, not surprisingly, interprets this change as an "improvement," as progress, and these are changes in which neurologists in Japan, North America, and other parts of the world have all participated.

Beyond consensus about the irreversibility of brain death and how to determine it (guidelines in Europe, North America, and Japan show small methodological discrepancies), differences clearly exist about the *significance* of a brain-death diagnosis. However, they do not fall neatly along cultural or geographic divisions. It cannot be said categorically that Japanese neurologists and emergency medicine doctors see things one way and North American neurologists and intensivists another. Certainly the majority of North American neurologists agree that brain death represents both biological death and death of the person, whereas much less certainty exists among Japanese clinicians. But complete agreement does not exist in North America, and indeed recent empirical findings have introduced considerable disquiet into the discussion—so much that the fundamental reasoning may well have to be modified.

A recent editorial in *Neurology* argues, for example, that with technological developments permitting the survival of a few brain-dead patients for months and even years, "even the 'dead' are not terminally ill any more" (Cranford 1998:1530). A double meaning is at work here, because the definition of "terminally ill," at least in United States Medicare regulations, indicates that a patient will in all probability be dead in six months. Cranford may well be highlighting the ambiguity that these empirical findings raise both for being terminally ill and being dead.[2]

All along, the brain-death debate has hinged on several crucial questions: What is a person? What is the relationship of person to body? Does the person cease to exist when the physical body dies? And perhaps the most fundamental, most obdurate question of all: What exactly *is* death—physical, personal, and social? Obviously answers to these questions depend on values articulated in the broader social milieu. They do not involve conflicts in styles of clinical reasoning about the determination of brain death, but they do result in fundamental differences in clinical practice and patient care, and above all in conflicting ideas about the commodification of living cadavers.

2. I am indebted to Robert Nelson for this insight.

It is the ambiguity of the brain-dead body that permits such varied responses to it. The result has been a complex, messy relationship among clinical practice, the styles of medical reasoning common to neurologists, the moral economy of contemporary medicine, with its emphasis on objectivity, and the social milieus in which these clinical practices are embedded. Clearly, if ideas about the nature of persons, individuals, human essences, and souls are implicated, then we are concerned with beliefs and concepts of great historical depth, drawn from the humanities, religion, and metaphysics as well as from everyday commonsense and from medical science. These concepts are further complicated as they mingle over time and space. The idea of the person as an autonomous individual has its origin in Europe, for example, but it has made deep inroads into Japanese thought. Although such values and concepts are outside the style of reasoning fundamental to neurobiology, they nevertheless profoundly influence clinical responses to the brain-dead.

We must also be concerned with the way in which ideas about the worth of persons and bodies, alive or dead, are employed to legitimize arguments for and against the recognition of brain death as the end of human life. Once again, the ambiguity associated with a brain-dead body permits this type of rhetoric to flourish. Such rhetoric does not have the power of self-authentication that Hacking assigns to styles of reasoning used in science. For one thing it must be convincing to several audiences: politicians, lawyers, physicians, the media, and the public. Competing discourse and rhetoric in the public domain in turn influence the way in which brain death is debated, institutionalized, managed, and modified in clinical settings.

In North America it has proved possible to claim that brain death is, for all intents and purposes, the end of recognizable human life. In Japan, this view has been repeatedly challenged. Both medical objectivity and diagnostic precision have come under fire from the media, from the legal profession, and from medicine itself. Even though Japanese neurologists concur about the irreversibility of brain death, and the vast majority of them are convinced that they can diagnose this condition reliably, they nevertheless remain reluctant to cooperate with organ procurement. Even now, many hesitate to encourage relatives to think of brain-dead patients as dead. Thus, even though a reasonably stable and similar style of medical reasoning exists in the two locations (though always subject to challenge in light of new medical knowledge and technologies), this does not lead to a congruence of clinical outcomes.

Quite possibly the difficulty that I confront might not arise in physics, engineering, or chemistry.[3] But because medicine deals, by definition, with the human body, moral judgments cannot be set apart from scientific reasoning and clinical practice. Clinicians have a range of moral positions, irrespective of where they have been raised and trained; and they often defer to the judgment of patients or families about what is in the patient's best interests on such questions as radical mastectomies for women with a family history of breast cancer or the use of Prozac to tailor personality. More often than not in Japan, it is patients' families, not physicians, who decide when the ventilator should be turned off once brain death has been declared.

The Ambiguities of Blurred Boundaries

Making decisions about the clinical care of dying patients inevitably involves moral judgments. Such decisions very often determine the timing of the transition between life and death. It is difficult under these circumstances to maintain an argument that the natural world, to which biological death is usually assumed to belong, is entirely autonomous. Nevertheless, as I have noted, medicine has made numerous advances over the past two centuries by making just such an assumption.

For example, in England, to permit the legal dissection and autopsy of certain corpses, the Anatomy Act was passed in 1832. Corpses were valuable to Western medicine long before the nineteenth century, but their procurement for medical purposes had been for the most part clandestine. Alternatively, semilegal use was made of the bodies of executed criminals or of paupers (Richardson 1988). Hesitation about commodification of dead bodies and their use for medical purposes arose less from a concern about the moment of the departure of the soul than from reservations about desecrating the human body. Only when corpses could be conceptualized as neutral biological objects, as part of nature and therefore autonomous and without cultural baggage, was it possible (for medical men, at least) to divest them of social, moral, and religious worth; commodification for the benefit of scientific

3. It could perhaps be argued that physicists in Japan and America make use of differing conceptual spaces as a result of the way in which physics laboratories are structured, but Sharon Traweek's research (1998) suggests that this difference does not affect the theory or the practice of physics itself, but rather the community of physicists. In contrast, I am arguing for different interpretations and inferences drawn in Japan and North America from specific scientific measurements and printouts that then have a profound effect on clinical practice in connection with the brain-dead.

advancement then became not only legal but laudable (Mantel 1998). Richardson has shown, however, that for involved families the bodies of their relatives were not so easily divested of social meanings (1989: 52ff).

With recent innovations in biomedical technologies,[4] and the consequent proliferation of machine-human hybrids that has accompanied these advances, we cannot sustain the fiction of a radical dichotomy between the human and material worlds. It is important to ask why oppositional dualities continue to captivate the imagination of the majority. Do people find security, resolutions to ambiguous questions, and perhaps profit by ordering the world in this way?

The brain-dead patient-cadaver is a particularly complex hybrid, constituted from culture and nature while in transition from life to death; both person and nonperson, entirely dependent on a machine for existence. Technology—principally the artificial ventilator, but also other life-support equipment and procedures—is indispensable in the creation of living cadavers. Without them the machine-human hybrid could not exist. But it is the hybrid and not the machine itself that incites moral dispute, doubts, and angst. Although the ventilator influences discourse about the brain-dead and in this sense is an active agent—it permits a living cadaver to appear as though it is sleeping, for example, causing discomfort among inexperienced observers—it is not itself a decisive force in the formation of discourse and practices in connection with the brain-dead. The existence of the technology does not *determine* anything.

Bruno Latour refers to the conceptualization of hybrids as *either* human *or* nonhuman entities as a process of "purification" (1993:10). To expose this process, so characteristic of the scientific method, Latour calls for recognition of an "object-discourse-nature-society" assembly whose networks of entanglement we should follow (see also Haraway 1990). An awareness of concepts, reasoning, and practices that contribute to the determination of brain death, its management and significance, forces us to pay attention to the way in which this particular hybrid, a living cadaver, is assigned either to life or to death, and under what circumstances.

Technologies are usually understood as "enabling" scientific progress in addition to fulfilling human "needs." Legitimization of biomedical

---

4. For example, heart-lung and dialysis machines.

technologies is inevitably accompanied by rhetoric about their value. But of equal concern, as Marilyn Strathern (1992) has noted, is the opposition voiced against so many of the new biomedical technologies, such as the new reproductive technologies. Such opposition reveals how the resultant hybrids act as moral touchstones, especially in matters of life and death (Lock 1995).

The hybrid condition perpetrates anxiety by eliminating conclusive arguments for morally absolute categories. When claims about the epistemologically neutral status of nature and its rigorous separation from society are challenged by the existence of such ambiguous, technologically created entities—neither alive nor dead, both dead and alive—moralizing runs wild. Some physicians and philosophers insist that brain death represents no radical departure from death as we have always intuitively understood it. But this position is not tenable. It is irrelevant that from time immemorial some people have died of traumatized brains. It is the case that biological death has always been recognized on the basis of changes to the body that are judged irreversible; this is not new, but use of the ventilator means that the process of bodily dying can be extended for increasing periods, very occasionally for years. Before the ventilator existed, it was not possible to determine death on the basis of the extent of damage to the brain alone. Living cadavers, and the transformation of some of them into organ donors after legal declaration of death, are entirely new; the very existence of such hybrids is a potential threat to the moral order.

Defining death as that which occurs when the heart and lungs stop functioning may well have caused similar concerns when it was first routinely put into use at the beginning of the nineteenth century. Before that particular assessment of death could be widely accepted, it had to oust an older belief in putrefaction as the definitive sign of death. The point at which irreversibility can be confidently declared has been moved earlier and earlier over the years as a result of systematized application of medical knowledge and technologies. A worry that we were tinkering with dying—declaring people dead in order to appropriate their organs—was apparent for several years in the late 1960s and early 1970s, after the first heart transplant. Nevertheless, in North America and much of Europe, the medical world was given authority to institutionalize the new death on the grounds that it represented no radical departure from previous practice. In Japan, a significant number of people sensed that a radical change in practice was indeed imminent in that country, and at the very least they wanted public involvement before any changes were made in the diagnosis of death.

Moral disputes over the introduction and adoption of new medical concepts and technologies, similar to those associated with brain death, occur regularly both in what are taken to be rational, secular, scientific societies and in societies where other forms of cosmological order are dominant (Kaufman 2000; Lock and Kaufert 1998). These disputes are not uniquely associated with the "developed" or "developing" worlds. Disputes attract attention; but where silence resounds, and technologies are tacitly accepted, this should also be of concern. The task then is to name the hybrid, for it will usually be camouflaged, its ambiguous attributes will be suppressed, and it will appear to reside fully in either the domain of society, or that of nature. This, in effect, is what has happened to brain-dead organ donors in most of the countries routinely involved with organ donation: they are constituted as cadaverlike, their rights as members of society stripped from them.

Historical and multisited ethnographic research make plain the ambiguities and doubts that have surrounded living cadavers during nearly half a century of existence. This is a history that we in North America and much of Europe have suppressed in the interest of saving lives through organ transplants.

The Uses of Culture

Everyone knows what cultural anthropology is about:
it's about culture. The trouble is that no one is quite
sure what culture is. Not only is it an essentially
contested concept, like democracy, religion, simplicity,
or social justice; it is a multiply defined one, multiply
employed, ineradicably imprecise. It is fugitive, unsteady,
encyclopedic, and normatively charged, and there are
those, especially those for whom only the really real is
really real, who think it vacuous altogether, or even
dangerous, and would ban it from the serious discourse
of serious persons.

Clifford Geertz, Available Light

Sarcastic comments not withstanding, Clifford Geertz is a true believer in the concept of culture. The word may be ineradicably imprecise, but nevertheless it is of use when searching for clarity. Many people who appear in this book and whose views I report refer to "culture" to explain their feelings about brain death and other matters; their collective usage of it boils down to three ideas. Some people confine their use of culture to just one meaning; whereas others use it in more than one way: It is employed, first, as a dualistic contrast to that which is taken as "natural" and exists independently of human intervention; second, as conveying the idea of a group of people sharing behaviors and values (even when differences such as class, gender, and ethnicity clearly exist among them); and third, as a tradition representing the speaker's "authentic" heritage, one threatened by modernity. This third usage is often mobilized in political opposition to change. I too make use of culture as an explanatory device, but with hesitation, and with many provisos attached. I do not think of culture as real, as a "thing," in contrast to numerous people today who refer to it as an independent force.

Because brain death has not been recognized in Japan as the end of life until recently, a few Japanese who have needed transplants, rather than accept death, have gone abroad to obtain organs. The *Guardian Weekly* of August 4, 1996, reprinted an article from the *Washington Post* about twenty-three-year-old Kiuchi Hirofumi under the headline "Japanese are Dying for a Transplant."[5] Kiuchi had been flown to Los Angeles for a heart transplant, without which he would have died very soon. The $380,000 cost of the operation was raised through loans and by a fundraising campaign to which more than ten thousand Japanese people contributed. The article, which is unabashedly partisan, asserts that transplant advocates in Japan consider the situation there a national embarrassment: "Citing tradition, culture and religious concerns, Japan has rejected medical advances that have given thousands of critically ill people around the world a second chance at life" (Jordon 1996). It quotes Kiuchi as saying, "I feel that I was supposed to be killed by Japan, by the Japanese government, Japanese tradition, Japanese culture. If I had stayed there I would have died." Both journalist and patient seem to cast the problem as one of technology versus tradition. The issue becomes even more perplexing when, one year later, Kiuchi points out that his own mother has trouble accepting brain death as human death: "Even though a transplant saved my life, she's uncomfortable with the

5. There is some dispute about Kiuchi's age, which was reported as twenty-seven in 1997 (*Time* 1997).

idea of removing organs from someone whose heart is still beating" (Kunii 1997:20).

What exactly does this *Washington Post* journalist mean by Japanese "culture" and "tradition"? And can we generalize from the words of one citizen, however much his plight moves our sympathies? Should we perhaps give equal weight to the argument of the sociologist Nudeshima Jiro when he claims that opposition to acceptance of brain death as the end of life is attributable not to "culture" but to a lack of trust in doctors (1991a)? But then we must surely also ask why Japanese attitudes towards the medical profession should not be thought of as "culture," albeit tinged with politics? Clearly culture and tradition, concepts that are often used interchangeably, serve as rhetorical devices; their use frequently signals an opposition to the logic of modernity, that is, to that of science and technology and their associated institutions, which allegedly function without cultural constraint.

Secularization and modernization have followed different trajectories in Japan and North America. Japan, which has long been technologically innovative and adept, was clearly on a path to modernity by the mid-nineteenth century. The transfer of scientific and other forms of knowledge from Europe to Japan from the middle of the nineteenth century, and particularly after World War II, has been described by some Japanese commentators as a "kind of rape" (Morioka 1995:90). This cultural colonization has made many in Japan very sensitive about new concepts and technologies that appear radically foreign. The relationship between tradition and modernity is fraught, and the brain-death debate has brought this tension to the fore. But with the considerable variation in thinking and disputes within both Japan and North America, deterministic arguments about the force of culture are inappropriate.

In both locations, competing values and assumptions contribute to the meanings attributed to brain death. These disputed values are in turn intimately associated with past and present experiences of individuals; regional histories; political interest; and moral positions, which are often consciously or unconsciously infused with religious dogma and attitudes toward scientific knowledge and practices. Because the United States and Canada are so often held to be without a culture of tradition, except that fostered by ethnic minorities, it becomes a challenge to detect something that might be called "culture" at work in the acceptance of brain death. It is difficult to take issue with a cultural assertion of "no culture" when technological innovation is synonymous with progress and the greater good of all. On the other hand, it is all too easy to overdetermine the influence of culture in distant Japan, particularly when some Japanese and foreigners alike unabashedly cultivate nostalgia for the country's past.

In North America, legitimization of brain death as the end of human life has rarely been contested either by medical professionals or by the public. This suggests that hegemony is effectively at work. Brain death has been naturalized with little dispute; it is apparently logical to most of us that death can be located in the brain, and that consciousness is what makes an individual recognizably alive and fully a person. It also appears, from surveys about attitudes toward organ donation in North America, that a majority of people favor the utilitarian use of brain-dead bodies (although practice does not bear out this finding [Prottas 1994]).

In Japan, by contrast, naturalization of brain death has not been possible. Death is not readily located in the brain, nor is the essence or identity of the person; and commodification of bodies, dead or alive, creates angst. Medicine has not been able to claim hegemony over the new death; determination of boundary formation between life and death is hotly disputed, with the result that the clinical handling of brain-dead bodies is less uniform than in North America. Abortion, however, has long been routinized in Japan with relatively little public dispute. Ironically, Japanese feminists often oppose the form that institutionalized abortion takes, not because they are against it in principle but because it is legitimized under an outmoded eugenics law under which the rights of women are not sufficiently recognized (Norgren 1998; Hardacre 1997; Ueno 1997).

Anthropologists worry today that culture is too often understood as a totalizing, all-or-nothing concept amenable to appropriation by those with nationalistic interests. Culture can readily be turned into an "exclusionary teleology" (Daniel 1991:8), one that mobilizes the notion of an idealized shared past, a reinvented history. This is exactly what has happened in the Japanese brain-death debate. Dominguez argues that culture should be regarded as something invoked, not as something that simply "is" (1992:23). This applies equally to those who lay claim to participation in a culture and to those who make claims on behalf of others about their participation in or exclusion from a culture. Unequal relationships of power, of inclusion and exclusion, exist within virtually all sociocultural complexes, and assertions about culture are more often than not simultaneously moral and political claims.

In short, it is not appropriate to argue for essentialized cultural differences between groups of people, nor yet for essentialized similarities within any given culture. The culture concept can be understood as a *mise-en-abîme,* an endless series of self-reflecting regressions. (Pollack 1992:2); a fluid, contestable entity comprising sets of practices, ideas, imagination, and discourse, much of it barely available to consciousness. Culture in this fluid sense can be said to contribute to the brain-death debate in both Japan and North America. In Japan, culture is self-consciously called on by some as a rhetorical device to assert a moral position against recognition of brain death. But, as I have noted, it is rejected by others as having no significant influence; and still other people, perhaps the majority, argue that shared cultural values may well be activated to cause anxiety about the idea of brain death that the media then play up.

In North America, by contrast, arguments about death are usually assumed to lie fully in the medical domain and therefore to be objective. A moral economy and a style of scientific reasoning associated with brain death are safely ensconced. The law has supported this position, and so too have most philosophical commentators. The media have been essentially silent on the matter, and culture is rarely recognized as playing an active role as a limiting force. But if we readily believe that Japanese culture is at work in arguments for rejection of brain death there, then surely we should question the assumption that dominant values make no contribution to the acceptance of a new death in North America. Could there not be some premodern anachronisms lurking in our responses to the brain-dead?

Commodification of Human Body Parts

All forms of commodification involve a complex interaction of temporal, cultural, social, and political factors. The "commodity candidacy" of things is culturally determined, but at the same time the process is fluid and open to dispute both within and between localized systems of meanings (Appadurai 1986). With increasing globalization, the circulation of commodities, including human labor, cadavers, and body parts, transcends local meanings and regulations. Production and consumption often occur at a great remove; they are linked by a string of intermediaries, each with their own interests, leaving the original providers of goods and services subject to exploitation. This exploitation is evident in the sale of organs by the poor in the developing world (L.

Cohen, ms.). Today, the scale, form, and extent of commodification, particularly of body parts, are vast.

The use of human bodies in slave, wage, and sex labor has a long and tortuous history. It is only recently, however, that the body has gained commercial value as a source of spare parts and therapeutic tools (Hogle 1996). Until well into the twentieth century it was not technologically feasible to capitalize out of isolated organs and tissues.

From the 1940s on, following the refinement of knowledge about blood types and matching, human blood acquired value for use in transfusions. As Richard Titmuss has documented, almost overnight questions arose about demand and supply, accompanied by heated discussions as to whether the commercial exchange of blood would defile its sacred quality (1971). Since that time, in the United States, the sale and the donation of blood have both become customary; most European countries and Canada rely almost exclusively on donation.

The blood market has always been limited by the fear that blood offered for sale may be tainted, a perception fostered by the knowledge that paid blood clinics are usually located in inner cities. The possibility of transmission of AIDS and hepatitis C through blood transfusions has, of course, amplified these fears. The international market in blood and blood products and the brutal conditions under which some people are forced to "give" blood are less well known (Kimbrell 1993; Starr 1998). Blood is not the only human product that is sold: human sperm, eggs, embryos, cells, and fetal tissue are commodified, and so too are organs and tissue for transplant and experimentation, although the sale of organs is not legal in Europe, North America, India, Japan, and many other countries.

It has been argued that commodities should not be understood "as one kind of thing rather than another." In other words, an item is not necessarily always a commodity, and it may not originally have been created or produced for that purpose. Transformation into a commodity may be one phase in the life of some things (Appadurai 1986:17). Commodities, like humans, therefore, have a social life—a life history of sorts (Kopytoff 1986). Clearly, in their original function, body parts are not commodities, but they may become commodified. It is important, therefore, to consider how and under what conditions body parts accrue value, at times monetary value, and what local resistance there may be to the alienation of body parts.

Without transplant technologies, aside from possible use for experimentation, human organs could have no value other than to the individual in whom they reside, and then only if they remain healthy. Once transplants were routinized, vital organs rapidly became of immense value to other interested parties: physicians, transplant coordinating organizations, dying patients and their families. But for an organ to be of worth in this way, it must first be made into an object, a thing-in-itself, entirely differentiated from the individual from whom it was procured. Moreover, it must be healthy. Hogle has discussed how the procurement of organs has been standardized to ensure that the resultant "product" is of good quality (1995). The legal system, particularly that of the United States, supports this type of commodification in that the body, and by extension body parts, can be legally constituted as separate from persons (Hyde 1997:258).

In the English language use of the word *donation* with respect to property exchange is of long standing, but use of the term *donor* in connection with the anonymous release of body tissues and parts commenced only in the 1960s. Individuals who sign "donor" cards, some of whom eventually become organ donors, are in effect acquiescing in a form of depersonalization that is integral to the system of national and international organ-sharing networks. In my opinion this depersonalization constitutes a form of "euphemized violence" (Bourdieu 1990a: 85): a form of exploitation in which vital human organs are assessed as invaluable until the moment that culture intrudes, in the form of a skilled transplant surgeon. Organs are then transformed into precious commodities. I am not categorically opposed to the sale of organs, although I am opposed to human organs being placed on the open market, but I question why those who make "gifts" of their organs, and their families, should receive neither recompense nor recognition of any kind. Some donor families cannot even be sure their gift has not ended up in the slop bucket.

One cannot consider the commodification of body parts without returning to Marx, even though he was preoccupied above all with the way in which, under capitalism, commodities are transformed into money. Marx wrote about the "fetishism of commodities," whereby items come to be thought of as having inherent value, as they might have weight or color. The commodity—the object—is decontextualized in a capitalist system, and consumers know little or nothing about the social relations of production or of exchange. As Harvey puts it, "the grapes that sit upon the supermarket shelves are mute, we cannot see the fingerprints of exploitation upon them or tell immediately what part of the world they are from" (1996:232). What is produced by the labor of individuals appears before us simply as objects, or alternatively as just one object among others: this, for Marx, is fetishized commodification.

In commenting on often-cited theories in which technology is taken as autonomous, Bryan Pfaffenberger argues that fetishism of objects, so characteristic of contemporary society, renders invisible the social relations in which technologies as a whole arise and are applied (1988:242). By extension, human organs, crucial components of transplant technology, are transformed into decontextualized objects. Their previous social history is erased, and their value assessed solely in terms of their quality as organs for transplant: are they vital and healthy, and have they been well cared for during procurement? Furthermore, they have become *scarce* commodities, for they cannot be acquired fast enough to meet the ever-growing demand. To this end discussion has turned to new ways of procuring organs and to the possibility of procuring organs from classes of people other than the brain-dead. Chapter 14 deals with these developments.

The proclaimed shortage of organs is described as a public health crisis (Randall 1991). Transplant technology professionals are reminded repeatedly that many thousands of patients die each year waiting for an organ and that many organs "go to waste." In the United States, for example, more than 66,000 patients were waiting for transplants in 1999, and many of them were likely to die before having a transplant (United Network for Organ Sharing 1999). Those who need kidneys continue on dialysis (Arnold et al. 1995:1). In both the United States and Canada, the number of patients waiting expands each year, in part because an increasing number of very young and also elderly patients, as well as patients formerly considered too ill to undergo a transplant, are placed on waiting lists.

This shortage is exacerbated because, thanks to better technology and greater use of seat belts and other safety equipment, the number of fatal automobile accidents has been cut in half.[6] Nevertheless, organ donation (including live donors) has doubled in Canada since 1984 (Canadian

6. In the United States head trauma, including injuries from automobile accidents, is the primary cause of donor death at 46.2 percent, followed by cerebrovascular accidents and stroke at 42.1 percent. In Canada, by contrast, the most common cause of death is intracranial hemorrhage (cerebrovascular accident) at 44.1 percent, with motor vehicle accidents second at 26.2 percent. In consequence, Canada's donor population is on average older than that of the United States (Canadian Organ Replacement Register 1996).

Organ Replacement Register 1996) and increased by 57 percent in the United States between 1988 and 1997 (United Network for Organ Sharing 1999). In 1998 the number of organ donors in the United States was about 5,500 higher than in previous years. The repeated lament about the growing numbers of patients on waiting lists masks the fact that people in both countries are increasingly cooperating with organ donation appeals.[7]

Organ procurement agencies are particularly vigilant these days. Transplant coordinators give lectures and even provide small, nonmonetary incentives to medical personnel working in intensive care units to encourage procurement. By law, "required request" of potential donors' families is obligatory in many American states; in Canada this practice is less common. Procurement agencies monitor the success of intensive care units in obtaining organs. In the province of Québec, for example, admonitory letters are sent to units that fail to meet a quota based on the number of fatalities they have.

Although it is thus far not part of the monetary system in North America, an economy of organ procurement and disbursement is thoroughly entrenched, one that depends entirely on the benevolence of brain-dead patients and their families. Not only do we make organ donors anonymous, but we argue that their generosity should go unrewarded. Unlike other forms of philanthropy, organ donation is rarely memorialized (although living donors are often hailed as heroic). Nor is there social recognition of any kind; in Bourdieu's terms (1990b), there is no gain in symbolic capital. Recently this situation has changed a little in several parts of the United States, where local organ procurement organizations now have annual ceremonies at which memorial plaques are given to the families of donors.

Ethnographic Investigation of Biomedical Technologies

In studying new biotechnologies that transgress bodily, legal, philosophical, and spiritual boundaries, we must ask why in some locales such innovations raise little concern, whereas in others they create havoc.

Because the focus in most of Europe and North America has been almost exclusively on the heroics of organ transplants and the "gift

---

7. The donor rates per million population in the United States (17.7 percent) and Canada (12.2 percent), although on the increase, remain considerably lower than in Spain and Austria, where donation rates are over 20 percent. These European countries have a doctrine of presumed consent, which no doubt accounts for the difference (McIlroy 1999).

of life," little public reflection has taken place about the accompanying new death or on the ambivalence about donation so often manifested by relatives of brain-dead patients. These munificent citizens are rendered invisible. In Japan, by contrast, it is the suffering of people who wait for organ transplants, most of them in vain, that is often overlooked.

These differences suggest that disputes about the boundaries between nature and culture need empirical investigation in specific historical and geographical locations. Moreover, such boundaries, even when apparently established beyond dispute, may become fluid once again as a result of technological modifications, innovation in medical knowledge, or political contests. Given the rapid technological transformations and heterogeneous forms of contemporary society, it is doubtful whether demarcations between nature and culture can ever be settled. And social commentary can rarely keep abreast of the changes, let alone make predictions to inform official guidelines or policy.

Clearly, meanings attributed to brain death vary depending on whether one is near to death but still conscious; a close relative of a patient who is diagnosed as brain-dead; an intensivist trying to avert death; a transplant surgeon trying to procure organs; a cultural commentator writing for the media; someone who is devoutly religious or aggressively secular; an "average" Japanese or an "average" Canadian or American; a social scientist writing a critical commentary; or some combination of the above. In clinical settings these meanings are affixed, as Monica Casper suggests (with reference to fetuses), through "work practices" (1994). But they are also created through the subjective responses of those directly involved and by the social matrix that influences these responses—including the remarks of individuals not directly involved, among whom media commentators and academics are prominent.

From the subjective accounts of patients, relatives, and clinicians, the complexities and ambiguities of work practices, of making and maintaining boundaries in the clinic, are abundantly clear. Beyond the clinical setting, public debate reveals the politics and values invested in boundary making: in this particular case, whether living cadavers are assigned to the category of life or of death. My task as ethnographer is to go one step further: to consider why certain responses, decisions, and commentaries become dominant and "naturalized" and why other possibilities may be either openly disputed or completely beyond consideration.

Absent Subjects

It is impossible, for obvious reasons, to interview key informants about their experience with brain death. Moreover, I could not expect to interview families assembled around the beds of their dying relatives. Following accidents that culminate in brain death, events proceed very quickly. Decisions are made, some of them instantly, and relatives in a state of acute shock come and go from ICUs, leaving no possibility for any discussion that would not be callous. With a few notable exceptions, relatives, whether or not they cooperate with organ donation, are rigorously protected from the media and researchers, and rightly so. A further problem is that comparatively few people are ever confronted with making decisions about organ donation on behalf of a brain-dead relative. Without personal experience, it is impossible to imagine the situation in anything more than a superficial way. The anthropologist is therefore divested of some of her strongest research strategies.

Interviews with medical professionals working in ICUs, as well as with transplant surgeons and organ recipients in Japan, Canada, and America, make clear the differences in clinical practices for brain-dead patients. But the significance of these differences is impossible to evaluate without knowledge of the historical and political contexts of clinical practice. In fact, in the absence of such contextualization an observer may reach wrong and even dangerous conclusions. One American neurologist, told that Japanese families are not usually informed that the patient is dead the moment a brain-death diagnosis is confirmed, condemned the practice flatly as unethical.

In an effort to overcome these limitations, I draw not only on my own observations and on incidents that were recounted to me personally but also on second-hand accounts, the majority of which first appeared in professional journals, the media, books aimed at the general public, novels, and so on. More than one chapter of this book is devoted to the recognition and institutionalization of brain death and to media and medical responses in North America and Japan. I also include discussion—historical, anthropological, philosophical—about what constitutes the death of persons and bodies.

As a result of these excursions, I feel compelled to argue that if anything is peculiar or unusual, it is not the queasiness about recognition of brain death among many Japanese, and no doubt among many people everywhere. On the contrary, perhaps, it is the long and tortuous history of vivisection, cadaver dissection, and commodification of the human body in Europe—a history that surely facilitated the imagination necessary to conceptualize the retrieval of organs from one dying individual in order to "save" a second dying individual, that is peculiar. This tradition facilitates the argument that organs that are not retrieved go to waste, and that sick people have a right to organs for transplant.

Before going any further, I must make my own position on this difficult subject clear. Neither I nor my family has had any personal involvement with organ donation. My fascination with the subject was initially fired by my observations in Japan, and since that time it has been fueled not simply by intellectual curiosity but also by participation in symposia, workshops, and conferences on brain death. Several of these meetings were organized by Stuart Youngner, an American psychiatrist who has worked energetically to clarify the concept of brain death since it was first formulated, and who has influenced my thinking on the subject. Between 1994 and 2000 I have also been a member of the International Forum for Transplant Ethics. This group is composed of three transplant surgeons, an immunologist, a past president of the Royal College of Physicians of Great Britain (who is an endocrinologist), a lawyer, a philosopher, and myself. Its mandate is to incite some critical reflection about organ procurement of a kind that the international transplant community rarely undertakes. I have gained a wealth of knowledge from participation in this forum and have had my ideas profoundly modified by my coparticipants as, I hope, their views have in turn been modified by some of my own. We have also had major disagreements.

I am not opposed in principle to organ transplants. My donor card is signed. This research has made me acutely sensitive to the suffering of patients waiting to receive transplants and to the many more who live half their lives tied to dialysis machines. Nevertheless, I believe we should undertake some clarification, reflection, and reconsideration of what we are about, and the comparison with the Japanese experience is enlightening. There are no easy alternatives at present to the commodification of living organs, but I hope that transplants procured from brain-dead bodies will in the end prove to be a stopgap measure.

REANIMATION

Richard Selzer, the surgeon who retired early in order to write, died a few years ago but, fortunately for us all, rose again shortly thereafter. Rushed to an intensive care unit, Selzer, revived, narrates his own story. He wants neither his readers nor himself to be permitted the safety of distance from this experience:

> Let us look upon that cubicle of the emergency room: the stretcher upon which he lies is engulfed in nurses and doctors, each of whom is ministering to him at the same time. In a moment, his clothing is stripped from him. Because he is flailing about, his wrists and ankles have been restrained. From veins in his arms and groin endless ribbons of blood, dark from the cyanosis, are pulled into tubes. His head is steadied, his neck extended by mighty hands; the mouth of the man is pried open and an attempt is made to insert a tube into his trachea. But his agitation is extreme, like that of a man drowning. Or rather, that of a man playing the role of someone drowning in an old-fashioned melodrama. It has that jerky, staccato rhythm. Because of this, the intubation cannot be carried out. Medication is injected into a vein and the doctor at the head of the stretcher tries again.
>
> There. Now the tube is in his trachea, the cuff inflated to keep it from slipping out. Still not fully narcotized, the man shakes his frantic head from side to side, refusing what has been thrust in. He coughs, strains, his neck is a contraption of taut tendons and engorged veins. To the uninitiated it might seem a kind of molestation. At last the morphine reaches his brain; he subsides into flaccidity. His chest lifts, recedes, lifts again at the insistence of the rhythmic, squeezing fist of a perfect stranger. Ointment is squeezed from a tube into his eyes, and his lids are taped shut to protect the corneas. It is the

beginning of a long sleep. In the meantime, a catheter has been slid into his
bladder, another plastic tube into one of his nostrils to gain access to his
stomach. Already, long strings of blackish bile are staining the sheet on which
he lies. The cardiogram shows the rhythm of his heart to be precarious—
ventricular tachycardia. Drugs are administered, electrodes readied to apply
to the chest. An X-ray is taken; one of the doctors remarks that the chest is
not expanding symmetrically. The diagnosis is massive bilateral pneumonia
with toxic shock. . . . Is he going to die? No one knows. But there is more
than a hint of death here.

   Within minutes then, he is a preparation, something they have made and
whose every flicker and seepage can be measured precisely. . . .

   The martyrdom of the intensive care unit has begun . . . the man in the
bed is to be ventilated, dosed, defibrillated, probed, suctioned, and infused.
Most of his bodily functions will be taken over. No longer need he swallow,
chew, inhale, or exhale, cough, urinate, defecate, clear his throat, maintain
acid-base balance, cogitate, remember, sigh, weep, laugh, desire.

                                                    (Selzer 1993:30–32)

On day twenty-three Selzer informs the reader that it is now his "sad
duty to report to you his death." He has had a massive episode of ventricular tachycardia. Despite every effort at resuscitation, Selzer's electrocardiogram remains flat, with no heartbeat, for over four and a half
minutes. Eventually medical intervention is abandoned, and someone
declares that Selzer is dead. The attending nurse writes the time of death
on the chart and ten minutes later observes the characteristic "settling"
of the body, "the fixity that is incontrovertible." Then, unexpectedly,
the body shudders. "A moment later he draws his first breath. It is a
deep sigh that might be interpreted as one either of sorrow or of satis-
faction, as though one precious thing were being relinquished and another embraced." Soon, a tracing returns to the electrocardiogram, and
the breathing becomes regular. "The room, which had descended into
a subaqueous silence emanating from the corpse, is now fiercely active.
All the machinery is back in place, chugging, vibrating, clicking, ringing"
(44–45). Later, at the weekly conference, people question the judgment
of death, but the nurses persist with their claim that the EKG was flat
and that they could detect neither a pulse nor blood pressure.

   On the day of his discharge, Selzer fires a parting shot at his doctor:
"Next time hold a feather to my lips. It's more reliable" (99). Eight
months later, Selzer makes a final observation about his experience:

Only days ago, I noticed at some two-thirds of the distance between each
cuticle and the tip of the finger a fine, distinct transverse dent. Now, considering that fingernails grow at an average rate of one millimeter per week, and
considering that the length of the nail proximal to the crease measures two

centimeters, it cannot fail to occur to even the least suggestible that these lines were at the very nail bed itself some twenty weeks ago. That would be April, sometime during my comatose residency in the intensive care unit. What are these transverse creases if not the manifestation of some cataclysmic event that took place at that time?

Selzer takes these creases as evidence of his "death" and "resurrection." He asks for his doctor's opinion on the matter and is disappointed with the reply:

> "Oh those," said Gordon, yawning behind a fist. "Beau's lines. We see them after major medical disorders—a coronary, severe pneumonia." As if familiarity could diminish the miraculous.
>   "So you have seen them before?" I respond. "But can you explain why they occur?"
>   "No, I am afraid we cannot."
>
> (117–18)

Selzer's purpose is not to produce an objective account; he does not strive to tell us what "really" happened. We could, perhaps, dismiss this narrative as fanciful, but as Selzer unequivocally says himself, "The facts are not always where the truth lies" (115). Many people have struggled to make the assessment of brain death objective, factual and infallible. However, the "truth" about brain death does not reside in tests and measurements, but in what it signifies to its witnesses.

TWO

Technology in Extremis

What next, being alive when you're dead, whatever next?
Elias Canetti, Auto da Fé

Do you ever think of yourself as actually *dead,* lying in a box
with a lid on it? . . . It's silly to be depressed by it. I mean
one thinks of it like being *alive* in a box, one keeps forgetting
to take into account the fact that one is *dead* . . . which
should make a difference . . . shouldn't it? I mean, you'd
never *know* you were in a box, would you? It would be just
like being *asleep* in a box. Not that I'd like to sleep in a
box, mind you, not without any air – you'd wake up dead,
for a start, and then where would you be? . . . Eternity is
a terrible thought. I mean, where's it going to end?
Tom Stoppard, Rosencrantz and Guildenstern Are Dead

Breathing Machines

One vivid memory I retain from World War II is of an iron lung. This
massive, frightening contraption was standing at the entrance to the
hospital ward where I was taken by ambulance after the family house
was destroyed by what turned out to be almost the last German missile
of the war, fallen short of its London target. Tales about the iron
lung and who had died encased in it circulated amongst us children
as we traded our shrapnel collections, but I had never actually seen
the fearsome thing until that day. Together with the nightly air raids,
this machine made it clear that death lurked close by, and we told sick
jokes about the technologies of war and of medicine to hide our
terror.

The iron lung is a recent example of the principle of technologically
assisted ventilation, perhaps first described by Andreas Vesalius. Writing
in the sixteenth century, Vesalius reported: "But that life may in a manner of speaking be restored to the animal [a sow], an opening must be

attempted in the trunk of the trachea, into which a tube of reed or cane should be put; you will then blow into this, so that the lung may rise again and the animal take in air" (Vesalius, *de Humani Corporis Fabrica*, 1543).

It was not until much later that knowledge of this kind was systematically developed in Europe. In the eighteenth century "Humane Societies" were formed by concerned doctors and lay people to assist people who had met with accidents and appeared to be dead (Pernick 1988: 22). The original society was founded in Holland in 1767 to promote "newly discovered" life-restoring techniques, including mouth-to-mouth resuscitation, which other European countries then emulated. In 1786 Edmund Goodwyn of London received the Humane Society gold medal for his dissertation on the connection between life and respiration (Mörch 1985). He speculated in his writings that respiration enabled a beneficial chemical substance to be transmitted to the blood. In the same year, a humane society was established for the first time in Massachusetts. Physicians who joined these societies achieved respect for their widely disseminated publications on suspended animation (Thomson 1963), knowledge that formed the basis for the modern specialty of emergency medicine.

From the middle of the nineteenth century, numerous "breathing machines" were built that were designed to encase the entire body. These machines applied a negative pressure regularly to the chest surface, permitting the lungs, even when damaged, to continue their work of supplying oxygen to the bloodstream. Among the many forms of these machines, one group became known as "iron lungs." The version invented by the Danish physiologist August Krogh was used extensively from the 1930s for patients whose lungs had collapsed because of paralysis caused by poliomyelitis (Mörch 1985).

During the 1950s artificial ventilation was used for the first time in the treatment of patients with severe chest-crushing injuries. Since then close to four hundred different models of artificial ventilators have been developed, attesting not only to their widespread use but also to competitive marketing. Because artificial ventilation could maintain vital functions in patients who would certainly have died without it, the use of the ventilator eventually precipitated a reconsideration of the conventional medical understanding of death. An intractable debate as to what exactly constitutes death was rekindled. To this discussion was added an entirely new debate about whether death can be located in the

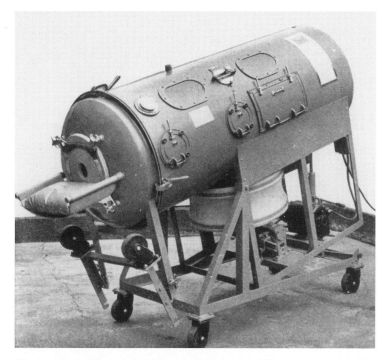

The iron lung. From Special Report Series 237, "'Breathing Machines' and Their Use in Treatment," Report of the Respirators (Poliomyelitis) Committee. Reproduced by permission of the Medical Research Council, United Kingdom.

brain instead of in the heart and lungs, and how best it can be determined.

Intensive Medicine

The formation of intensive care units from the early 1960s represents a coalescence of several medical specialties founded earlier in the century, the oldest of which were the postoperative recovery units of the 1920s. Specialized respiratory care units were established during the 1940s, largely as a result of polio epidemics, followed in the 1950s by "shock units" that focused on trauma and emergency medicine of various kinds—specialties that owed a great deal to the knowledge amassed from combat medicine earlier in the century. As early as the 1930s, it was recognized not only that the lungs could be kept functioning with

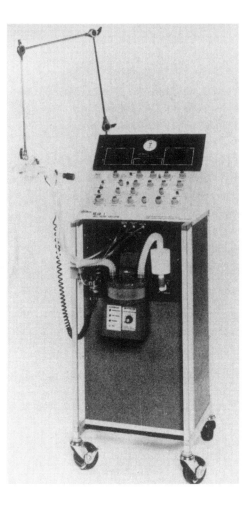

The artificial ventilator.
Courtesy of Thermo
Respiratory™ Group.

technological assistance but also that the heart could sometimes be re-started after it had stopped beating (Timmermans 1999). The development and application of electrocardiograms revealed that electrical activity continues in the heart for up to half an hour after "death" has been confirmed. The Berlin Medical Society commented: "There does exist a possibility of taking advantage of this persistence of the heartbeat after death to restore normality to the agitated movements upon which it has entered. . . . In this way it might be possible to recall a man to life—to raise him (in a manner of speaking) from the dead" (*Literary Digest* 1931). From these experimental beginnings intensive cardiac care was developed in the 1950s, including what is perhaps the most dramatic of interventionist technologies and the one given the most exposure in movies and television hospital dramas: that of defibrillation, applying electrically charged paddles to the chest to provide a massive jump-start to the heart.[1]

From these various specialties evolved the cross-disciplinary conglomerate of intensive care, which in large city hospitals is usually divided into medical, surgical, and neurological divisions. In the 1960s, only about one hundred intensive care units (ICUs) existed in the United States; today almost all hospitals with more than one hundred beds can provide intensive care (*Globe and Mail* 1999a). Acutely ill or injured patients who are first helped by the interventions of paramedics and emergency medicine specialists are stabilized and moved to intensive care units, where they receive round-the-clock care from staff trained in life support. Physicians who work in ICUs include specialists in neurology, cardiology, surgery, anesthesiology, and respirology. Nurses and respiratory technicians can also specialize in intensive care medicine. They are known collectively as intensivists.

Many intensivists think of themselves as individuals who work well under stress. As one nurse put it, "I enjoy the adrenaline rush of dealing with an emergency." Obviously, an aptitude for technology is also essential. Perhaps for these reasons, staff working in ICUs are often disproportionately young. When discussing his work with me, an experienced nurse pointed out that "care" of machines takes up a great deal of working time—about fifteen minutes in every hour. Reading printouts and checking machines is routine and monotonous work; nevertheless, most of the machines are considered "user-friendly." The ventilator is among the more temperamental and difficult ICU machines to operate, and for this reason is handled almost exclusively by respirology technicians. Writing in a standard text on mechanical ventilation, F. Trémolières insists that technological advances have improved the "efficacy" of ventilators but notes that "a ventilator cannot be operated as easily as, say, a washing machine" (1991:1).[2]

Technology is indispensable not only for supporting the respiration of critically ill patients but also for feeding them, administering medication, and monitoring body functions. It ensures that patients in ex-

1. The 1990 movie *The Flatliners,* directed by Joel Schumacher, is perhaps the best-known example.

2. Over the years ventilators have become highly precise in terms of the pressure they generate and the velocity with which they deliver oxygen. Damage to the lungs caused by ventilators is much less than was formerly the case (Franco Carnevale, personal communication, 1999).

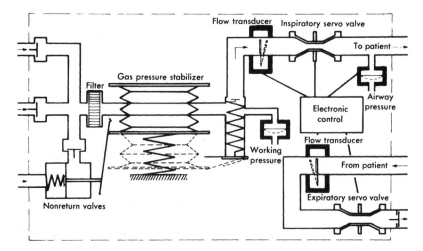

Functional flow diagram for Servo ventilator 900B. Courtesy of Siemens Canada Limited.

cruciating pain do not have to be touched or moved very much or endure frequent needle pricks. In short, technology takes a good deal of the unpleasant and disturbing work out of the care of badly damaged patients while also providing the ability to monitor body chemistry and physiology. "Normalcy" is "produced and regulated by detailed and ongoing surveillance" (Kaufman 2000:70), and, with improvements in technology, many more patients survive severe physical trauma than formerly.

The turnover in ICUs is rapid; a patient's stay is usually a few days or weeks. Many patients are kept unconscious or heavily sedated. Among those who are partially or fully conscious, a condition known as ICU psychosis is quite common. Patients suffer a complete loss of control; their bodies are penetrated in almost every available orifice and pierced in numerous places. They are subjected to a ceaseless overload of noxious stimulants, among which sound and light appear to be the most troubling; poor pain control is another key source of distress.

To an outside observer the ICU, with its central monitoring station and beds ranged around the walls, all surrounded by machines quietly doing their work, appears calm. Except for moments of temporary upheaval when new patients are wheeled in, or when a machine indicates that a patient's condition is spinning out of control, the medical staff move quietly and efficiently about the unit. However, for semicomatose, severely damaged patients, the continual movement and hum of human

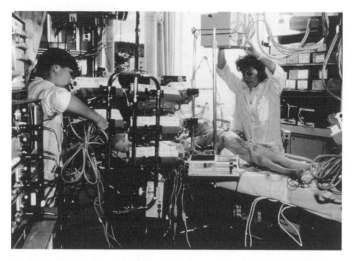

Technology dominates in the ICU. Courtesy of Frank Carnevale, Montreal Children's Hospital.

conversation, phones ringing, and the high-pitched ticks, beeps, and pings of the various machines, create a cacophony of sound. The units are windowless, and the lights remain on all the time, although, barring emergencies, they are dimmed at night. Soothing and comforting stimuli are in short supply.

Obviously great potential exists for dehumanization of patients in ICUs. More than a dozen tubes, lines, or leads may be inserted in or attached to patient's bodies—a concatenation of technology that demands constant attention. These tubes and leads link the patient to an array of monitors and machines, among them the indispensable ventilator. However, the effects of technology are buffered, especially in pediatric intensive care units, by the constant nursing that patients receive and by the frequent presence of family members.

Most intensivists, doctors and nurses alike, report that they are as concerned almost as much for families as they are for patients, and spend a great deal of time talking to and comforting relatives and close friends. Despite this human buffering of the technological assault, one intensivist describes the numerous printouts, traces, films, and X rays that result from the close monitoring of patients as a kind of "displacement." The subjective experience of the patients—their "personhood"—is unavoidably discounted and replaced by a medical narrative composed of graphs and traces.

Of course, in the ICU, where so many patients are unconscious or nearly so, the displacement of vocalized subjectivity is unavoidable. But nurses and families at the bedside often deduce things about patients that machines do not register, among them subtle changes in skin texture as death approaches. Not surprisingly, given the tenets of contemporary medicine, this interpretation of subjectivity, although not dismissed entirely, is usually not given much credence in diagnoses and decisions about treatment.

Although many patients, even after sustaining quite severe head trauma, are "weaned" off the ventilator to make a full recovery, for others the stabilization process is ineffective. The blood pressure drops, leading rapidly to cardiac arrest and death. There is a third class of patients for whom resuscitative measures are only a "partial success" (Ad Hoc Committee 1968). With the aid of the ventilator, the heart and lungs of such patients continue to function, but the brain is irreversibly damaged. These patients remain betwixt and between, both alive and dead; breathing, but suffering from a permanent loss of consciousness. Without the artificial ventilator this category of patients could not exist. The machine permits the technological creation of a space for the living dead, a space that can be medically monitored and managed. Even with life support and intensive care, however, such patients survive for only a few days or weeks, or very occasionally for months, because their hearts give up or their blood pressure cannot be sustained. Over the years survival rates have lengthened (Shrader 1986), and several exceptional cases have been reported of over a year's duration (Shewmon 1998). However, there are no professionally documented cases of anyone recovering from this state.

The Birth of Organ Transplant Technology

Patients with a diagnosis of "irreversible coma," as this condition was originally termed, would probably not have received much medical attention were it not for the simultaneous development of biotechnologies permitting solid organ transplants in humans. The work of Alexis Carrel, the 1913 Nobel Prize winner for medicine, along with several other scientists, provided the foundations for transplant technology. Carrel and his colleagues showed that cells and tissues could not only be kept in suspended animation, as was well known by the turn of the century, but could be made to function and reproduce independently of the donor body. Two fragments of chicken heart suspended in an appropriate medium pulsated and grew rapidly. After a few hours, these fragments approached each other and coalesced (Hendrick 1913:309). One specimen grown this way increased in size and pulsated on a microscope slide for 103 days. It was claimed that Carrel's experiments had demonstrated that cells need not necessarily die and that under certain circumstances they are "immortal" (Hendrick 1913:306). It was a short step to experimentation with vital organ transplants in animals (the usual testing ground prior to human use).

During the 1950s, developments in immunology facilitated kidney transplants in humans from both cadaver and living donors, but it was still disputed whether these procedures were experimental or therapeutic (Fox and Swazey 1978). The failure rate of such operations, aside from transplants done between identical twins, was very high. Transplant technology was not destined to a routine therapeutic regimen until the late 1970s, when powerful immunosuppressants were developed that significantly reduce the rejection of donated organs.

Despite the equivocal success of kidney transplants, several surgeons carried out experimental liver and heart transplants on animals during the 1950s and 1960s. In 1967 the flamboyant South African surgeon Christiaan Barnard took the world by storm when he performed what was touted as the world's first human heart transplant. It was at once clear to the involved surgeons that if transplants were to become part of regular clinical care, then organs for transplant would have to be made available on a regular basis, and they could not come from ordinary cadavers. Almost overnight, the organs of the irreversibly comatose had become targets for procurement.

Only between 2 and 5 percent of patients in ICUs are eventually declared brain-dead (in all, approximately 10,000 to 12,000 cases each year in the United States, a number that is actually declining).[3] The organs of brain-dead donors were, from the outset, a scarce resource, and it was evident that the urgent need for organs might threaten the presumption that every effort should be made to preserve human life.

Hard on the heels of the South African transplant, an editorial in the *Journal of the American Medical Association (JAMA)* voiced the major

3. This figures varies with location. In neurological ICUs or major hospitals with large trauma centers, it is higher (on average 6.4 percent in nine major centers in Cleveland and Pittsburgh between 1994 and 1998 [Meckler 1999]). In some pediatric ICUs in the United States, which treat both abused infants and adolescent patients who have been victims of violence, the figure may be between 15 and 24 percent. In a Montreal pediatric unit, the figure for 1998 was 7 percent (Franco Carnevale, personal communication, 1999).

dilemma posed by vital organ transplants: "It is obvious that if organs [such as the liver and heart] are taken long after death, their chance of survival in another person is minimized. On the other hand, if they are removed before death can be said to have occurred by the strictest criteria that one can employ, murder has been done." The editorial went on to argue that it is "mandatory that the *moment* of death be defined as precisely as possible" (emphasis added) and concluded: "When all is said and done, it seems ironic that the end point of existence, which ought to be as clear and sharp as in a chemical titration, should so defy the power of words to describe it and the power of men to say with certainty, 'It is here'" (*Journal of the American Medical Association* 1968a:220).

Since the 1960s one of the tasks of medical experts has been to determine this "moment" of death. They must also clarify whether the patient has indicated in writing or verbally an intent to become an organ donor and, further, if the family is prepared to support this intent.[4]

Artificial Resuscitation and Premature Burial

Martin Pernick, in an article titled "Back from the Grave," shows that medical concern about establishing the time of death has emerged repeatedly throughout history, most often in the wake of medical discoveries in connection with experimental physiology, resuscitation, and suspended animation (1988:17). When, in the eighteenth century, the humane societies were founded to teach resuscitation techniques and artificial respiration, one consequence was increased fear about premature burial among both the medical profession and the public. Although it was recommended that a physician be present at the time of death (before the eighteenth century, physicians were expected to leave the room when last rites were administered by priests), many doctors remained uncertain whether they could accurately pronounce death. Until the beginning of the twentieth century, eminent practitioners continued to have doubts about their ability to objectively assess death and insisted that "nothing short of putrefaction could distinguish death from life" (Tebb and Vollum 1905; Pernick 1988:22).

Other eighteenth-century physicians were opposed to this extreme position. The French surgeon Antoine Louis argued that a physician

---

4. Family agreement to donation is not legally required in most of Europe and North America; even so, without this agreement a transplant would rarely go ahead.

who could not detect the unequivocal signs of death could not be trusted to understand the signs of a complicated disease: "The uncertainty of Medicine necessarily follows from the uncertainty of the signs of Death" (Louis 1752:22).

In Europe, a fear of being buried alive was evident from at least the fourteenth century, exacerbated by outbreaks of plague and other infectious disease. This fear was widely acknowledged in the eighteenth century, and physicians, patients, and governments resorted to new and sometimes bizarre measures to prevent premature burial. The Code Napoléon required a waiting period of twenty-four hours before anyone could be buried, and in Frankfurt and Saxony this was extended to three days (Pernick 1988:31). For the wealthy in Europe, "waiting mortuaries" were built, where bodies could be laid to rest and carefully observed. An early twentieth-century book on premature burial describes the London waiting mortuaries as gloomy, especially in comparison with those in Germany, which were elegantly decked out with floral tributes (Tebb and Vollum 1905). Some individuals were buried with devices such as lights, flags, and noisemakers designed to alert their families if burial had indeed been premature. Others left instructions that before burial the blood should be let from their bodies or that their bodies be mutilated, embalmed, or even decapitated to prevent any mistake.

In Japan, by contrast, for many centuries cremation and burial have both been practiced.[5] With the growth of densely populated urban areas and an increasing shortage of land, cremation followed by interment gradually became customary. Crematoriums were at first built in temple precincts, but in the mid-eighteenth century cholera epidemics placed a great strain on these facilities, and complaints about pollution resulted in their removal to the margins of cities. Toward the end of the nineteenth century, during one of the periodic movements to revive "pure" Japanese tradition, several key intellectuals argued that cremation was against Japanese custom, and in 1873 it was outlawed. Two years later, after a lack of space proved the law impossible to implement, it was

5. One or two accounts dating from the tenth century, or perhaps earlier, depict priests who had themselves buried with bamboo tubes inserted into the lids of their coffins that permitted air to enter; bells were often included as well. This practice was not, it is argued, a precaution against premature burial, but part of a formalized ritual ensuring entry into the Buddhist heaven. Someone close to death was appropriately laid to rest, and when the bell could no longer be heard and nothing emanated from the tube, it was assumed that death was complete (Matsumoto 1993). Premature burial does not appear to have been of great concern in Japan, although a proverb states, "Don't put up the gravestone too soon." (I am indebted to Helen Hardacre for drawing my attention to this proverb.)

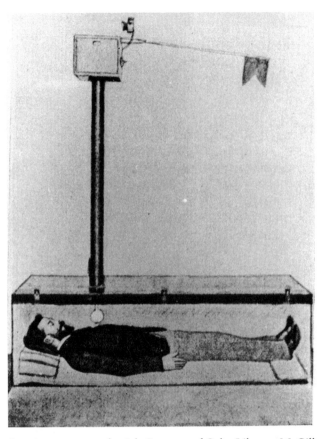

Averting premature burial. Courtesy of Osler Library, McGill University, Montreal.

repealed. In 1897 a second law was passed making it obligatory to cremate those who died from infectious diseases, among which tuberculosis was the most common. Local governments were required to build crematoriums, and the rise in infectious disease among the crowded urban population, together with increasing land pressures, made cremation a common practice. Despite nineteenth-century edicts about cremation, as of 1925 only 43 percent of the population had their relatives cremated (Kōseisho seikatsu eisei kikakuka 1988). Today the figure is just under 99 percent (Kōsei tōkei kyōkai 1998), largely because of the shortage of space in densely populated urban Japan.

The practice of cremation in urban areas may have forestalled the kind of anxiety about premature burial that was so widespread in nineteenth-century Europe. Panic in Europe was heightened by newspaper accounts of successful resuscitation attempts by the humane societies (Richardson and Hurwitz 1997:6). Cases of premature burial also received considerable public attention. The physician Alexander Wilder notes several that had come to his attention, including the following: "A six year old boy who was exhumed after 25 years and found to have the arms bent over the skull, one leg drawn up and the other bent over it. Another case is of a man, 35, who was buried 48 hours after the diagnosis of death from scarlet fever. He was exhumed two months later. The coffin was found to have the glass front shattered, the bottom kicked out and the sides sprung. The body lay face downwards, the arms were bent and in the clenched fists were handfuls of hair" (Tebb and Vollum 1905:81–82).

The Wilder cases and numerous others were compiled in a book by two physicians, one of whom, Perry Vollum, had himself experienced what he describes as "a very narrow escape from a live sepulture,[6] having been pronounced dead from drowning, and prepared for internment, when consciousness happily returned spontaneously" (Tebb and Vollum 1905:18). They also report that a Dr. Franz Hartman received sixty-three letters from May to June 1896 from people who claimed to have escaped premature burial at the last minute.

Folklore, macabre literature like the writings of Edgar Allan Poe, and urban myth are replete with similar accounts. Today we continue to titillate ourselves with stories of deaths that are out of the ordinary. Television and the newspapers regale us with accounts of people coming back to life after being determined dead. The Japanese media are filled with similar accounts, but in Japan the overriding concern is that such deaths, including hospital deaths, are at a remove from the family and therefore out of place.

The Science of Death

Scientific interest in trance, ecstasy, and other similar states encouraged new lines of thought in the mid-nineteenth century about the relationship between mind and body. It was argued that the body could remain alive, in a zombielike state of suspended animation, without consciousness or will. Researchers identified various conditions in which verification of death was clearly problematic, including extreme cold, drown-

6. *Sepulture* is the archaic form for *sepulcher*.

ing, opiate use, stroke, and severe head injury (Pernick 1988:23). An
article on death in a comprehensive nineteenth-century French medical
encyclopedia reveals how much effort was put into systematizing diagnoses of death: twenty-seven major signs of death and many more minor
signs are discussed at length.

The physician G. Tourdes wrote in 1875 about the complexity of
diagnosing death and the need for specialist expertise: "The public desires a single and infallible sign that everyone can observe, as the best
guarantee against premature burial. But this guarantee is illusory if the
observation of the sign is left to a non-physician. The best sign can be
poorly established. The risk of error is greater when observation concentrates on only one point" (cited in Alexander 1980:30). Alphonse
Devergie, the founder of the Paris morgue, cautioned similarly against
"vulgarizing" the signs of death: "Suppose for a moment that a sign of
death obvious to the whole world were discovered. What would happen? *Persons wouldn't call a physician to verify death.* . . . Let us
therefore abandon the unfortunate idea that the signs of death must be
vulgarized" (cited in Alexander 1980:30).

In mid-nineteenth-century physiology laboratories, death was increasingly systematized and determined by means of new instruments
for calibrating bodily motion. Respiration, blood flow, and the electrical
activity of the heart were recognized as critical signs of life. Ken Arnold
notes that many of these new technologies used pens hooked up to ro-
tating drums wound with paper to record vital signs. Scientifically speaking, death was now to be represented as a flat line on a graph (1997:
19), although physicians at the deathbed continued to establish death
on the basis of clinical examination rather than technology.

One test frequently described is the response of a dead body to being
burned. Several books from around the end of the nineteenth century
document that in a dead body a burn produces an areola—a burn
mark—but not a blister, as it would in a living body (Brouardel 1897;
Tebb and Vollum 1905). This test has long since fallen into disrepute in
Northern Europe and America, but I was told by a doctor who had
worked in the 1970s in Argentina, in crowded and chaotic emergency
rooms, that he had been taught this technique.

Nineteenth-century physicians acknowledged that "increasingly complex combinations of highly technical and invasive death tests won medical acceptance in large part because they were too complicated for lay
people to perform" (Pernick 1988:43). Their authority was backed up
indirectly by the intervention of the state in the seventeenth century,

when mortality statistics were first compiled. These figures were essential to the state's effort to take control and improve the well-being of the entire population. By the mid-nineteenth century, official medicolegal procedures included death certificates, records of postmortems, and regulations about the storage of dead bodies. Corpses were of interest not solely to grieving families but also to medicine, as specimens for autopsy (practiced since the eighteenth century) and to the state, in its new undertaking of the surveillance of society (Foucault 1980; Hacking 1990).[7]

By the end of the nineteenth century, physicians had reached a consensus that the irreversible loss of heartbeat and respiration could be assessed with certainty. The 1915 edition of *The International Classification of Disease* was the last to use "worn out" as a cause of death in old age. Death had been successfully transformed into a condition caused by specific diseases rather than simply a "natural" event (Fagot-Largeault 1989).

As in Europe prior to the twentieth century, death in Japan was usually managed within the family, sometimes with support from religious institutions; dying did not fall into the medical domain until recently (Sakai 1982). In *kanpō*, the medical system practiced in Japan for over a thousand years, three to ten types of death pulse (*shi myaku*) were described in the medical classics. However, it is doubtful that these subtly differentiated states were put to much use in clinical practice (Yasui Hiromichi, personal communication, 1999).[8] Herbal doctors schooled in these classics were never in sufficient number to be routinely called to attend dying patients.

Routine medical involvement with death diagnoses commenced in Japan only after European-style medicine became dominant in the late nineteenth century. Japanese medical texts did not discuss death until the 1970s, and it was not until the brain-death debate sparked a public outcry that people realized that death had become a medical matter (Sakai Shizu, personal communication, 1998).

This situation may well have contributed to the worry often voiced in Japan today that new technologies have made death "invisible" and therefore turned it into an event that the family can neither fully partic-

7. Tebb and Vollum, in their book on premature burial (1905), insist that until the early part of the twentieth century medical certificates were signed by anyone on hand, often without a medical examination, thus throwing the accuracy of mortality surveillance into some question.

8. In *kanpō*, various pulses associated with several of the major body organs are recognized, and pulse taking is a subtle, highly developed form of diagnosis.

ipate in nor verify. Even though hospital death was becoming increasingly common when the brain-death debate first erupted, it remained less frequent than in North America. The sentiment that death is a family matter, that one should go home "to die on *tatami*," persists in Japan.

Locating Biological Death

By the beginning of the twentieth century in Europe, fears about premature burial apparently declined, and a rosier view of death emerged. Death was even lauded by popular biologists as being of "benefit to the race." Life, it was claimed, is "enriched" through sex, reproduction, and biological adaptation, and "Death . . . in the divine economy of nature is introduced as a means of life, of ever-increasing and happier life" (Newman Smith, cited in Dallas 1927:355).The concern did not disappear entirely, however, and as late as 1940 an article in *Scientific American* stated that "frequent" errors in diagnosing death remained the cause of premature burial (Newman 1940).

Despite this continued worry, dying was often unremarkable, and pronouncement of death, whether in a hospital or at home, does not appear to have posed a problem to the medical profession. Ken Arnold and his colleagues found that among fifty texts dealing with physical diagnoses published in the first half of the twentieth century, only one has an entry discussing the methods and techniques for diagnosing death. An informal survey carried out by the same authors in the 1960s revealed that, among a large groups of interns and residents from fifteen medical schools in the United States, not one could remember being instructed in how to determine death (Arnold et al. 1968:1951).

This apparent security was destroyed with the introduction of the artificial ventilator. The existence of living cadavers revived unsettling questions of very long standing. Observers of death from antiquity on had been perplexed by the survival of vital signs in the bodies of decapitated animals and people. Anatomy and vivisection investigations in sixteenth- and seventeenth-century Europe provided clear evidence that the heart, lungs, and brain could function independently for a short time. This revelation posed the conundrum of when an organism as a whole ceases to exist, as opposed to its parts. Also at issue was the question of when "personal existence" ceases (Pernick 1988:27).

For several centuries, the heart was usually (though not exclusively—see Le Goff 1989) understood as the organ that governed human life and all vital principles. During the eighteenth and nineteenth centuries a powerful counterphilosophy of decentralism held that the vital principles were distributed throughout the body. As Pernick notes, the idea of a mind/body dichotomy was increasingly challenged by developments in experimental physiology. For example, Robert Whytt, an Edinburgh physician, concluded, on the basis of experiments with decapitated animals, that the soul and its "vital principles of sensibility and irritability" are physically dispersed throughout the nervous system rather than associated with a single organ, the pineal gland, as René Descartes had suggested (Pernick 1988:28). Georges Buffon, the early eighteenth-century French naturalist, proposed that all creatures are composed of living "molecules" and that the life of the organism is therefore a summation of the organization of these separate entities.

The late eighteenth-century physiologist Marie François Xavier Bichat, by contrast, made efforts to demonstrate that the body consists of discrete vital tissues. He distinguished between what he called the "organic life" of the heart, lungs, kidneys, and other organs, and the "animal life" associated with the brain, which produces sensation and volition. Bichat observed that following a stroke, a patient "may live internally for several days after he has ceased to exist beyond himself" (cited in Pernick 1988:29). These arguments about the location of the essence of the person, and when and under what conditions person and body cease to exist, persist today in discussions in both North America and Japan about whether brain death represents the end of human life.

A second debate—as to whether death is an event or a process—is also of long standing. Those who hold a one-organ "centralist" position as the key to life usually argue for death as an event, although centralists today, as did Bichat, almost unanimously locate the principle of life in the brain rather than in the heart. Decentralists usually argue that because different parts of the body stop functioning and die at different times, death must be a process. Karen Gervais, a philosopher who writes about brain death and seeks to reconcile the discrepancy between centralists and decentralists, observes that to speak in terms of a moment of death "presupposes that one moment in the biological process of the dissolution of the organism has greater significance (for metaphysical and moral reasons) than the others" (1986:4).

In law, it has been expedient to regard death as an event. From the 1930s, several court decisions in connection with traffic accidents and gunshot deaths, both of which were becoming more frequent, make it clear that the legal death of a person is considered to be the "exact moment" of physical death. This was sometimes timed, for the benefit of the court, to the precise second, as in cases in which the order of decease of a married couple in an accident was important to the settlement of a will. Medical consultants, usually pathologists, have frequently been called on to testify as to the precise moment of death.

The legal debate often revolves around the question of whether death occurs when the heart stops beating or when the brain is destroyed, which occurs earlier. Prior to the late 1960s, decisions were made in favor of the heart (*Vaegemast v. Hess; Gray v. Sawyer; C. Smith v. A. L. Smith; Schmitt v. Pierce),* but once the concept of brain death was recognized, brain-dead victims were counted as legally dead, even when their hearts continued beating. Without this construction of the law, organ transplants from brain-dead bodies could never have been routinized. Medicine and law were jointly involved in the recognition of the new death, and the position taken by each profession no doubt reinforced that of the other.

Although human organs and body parts can be kept alive even when fragmented, dispersed, and prosthetically transformed, a good number of contemporary physicians consider that the arguments about biological death, its physical location in the body, and the moment of its occurrence have been settled once and for all: "The brain will be accepted as the critical system of the human organism, and brain-death as irreversible destruction of that system" (Korein 1978:28). Yet when the ventilator becomes a simulacrum for the defunct brain stem and its activities, unsettling ambiguities arise about "which signs of life are sufficiently important that their loss constitutes the death of the patient, while other signs of life persist" (Youngner 1996:45).

In a recent article in the *Lancet,* Powner and colleagues sum up the complexities of unresolvable questions about the determination of death:

- Does the "vital principle" of life reside in, or is it produced by, a single organ or part of a single organ . . . or is the "soul" represented throughout all organs, tissues, or cells? That is, does death occur and unique "personhood" end when a small number of organs, or perhaps only one, permanently cease(s) to function, or must the entire organism go through such a process before death is defined?

- How can a falsely positive diagnosis of death, however defined, be excluded with maximum certainty? "Apparent death" historically, "confounding factors" currently, and the modern potential for organ resuscitation/transplantation have provoked fear that the physician's life-sustaining duty may not be met.

(Powner et al. 1996:1219)

These authors conclude that these fundamental issues remain unresolved because key concepts that we recognize as life, such as personhood, cannot be measured by medical devices. The work of doctors in the early twentieth century to medicalize death and make foolproof its assessment have not withstood the test of time or the invention of the artificial ventilator. A new style of reasoning has had to be standardized and institutionalized so that medical death can now sometimes be located in the brain.

The new death, with its ambiguous figure of the living cadaver, has rekindled doubts about error and premature declarations of death. But because of the interests of the transplant enterprise, entirely new questions and concerns are also raised in connection with the procurement of organs from entities that are alive, but who will never again be conscious. Although there is a broad consensus that the new death is in practice uniformly and objectively determined, disputes continue as to what brain death represents in terms other than those of basic biology.

Concern about "bad" deaths—those that are unnatural, accidental, or untimely, or repugnant—is a universal, age-old preoccupation. Technologically orchestrated deaths appear intuitively to many people to be unnatural. We worry that individuals who die bad deaths suffer unduly, and, even though most of us consider such thoughts irrational, even some health-care practitioners may be harrowed by the idea that this suffering will come back to haunt the living.

In contemporary medicine the concept of futility (permitting the discontinuation of treatment when nothing more can be done therapeutically), combined with an economically driven vigilance about use of scarce medical resources, creates space for doubts about medically managed deaths. With the expanding commodification of human body parts, including those wanted as "living substitutes"[9] for "defective" or diseased organs, these doubts are exacerbated.

In Japan, anxiety about the new "unnatural" death has given rise to the publicly disputed "brain-death problem." The ambiguous nature of a living cadaver is evident in the discrepancies between Japanese clinical discourse and practice. In North America, we have apparently repressed worries about the source of organs for transplant and have instead focused on the heroics of this technology.

---

9. I am indebted to Judith Farquhar for this turn of phrase.

NARROW ESCAPES

According to a 1989 newspaper article distributed by the Canadian Press Associates, doctors in an Ottawa hospital had declared seventy-nine-year-old Mr. Cybulski to be brain-dead ten weeks after an emergency operation on his heart. The patient was about to be taken off life support and receive the last rites from a priest when, in response to his two-year-old grandson yelling at him from the door of his room, Mr. Cybulski sat up and stretched out his arms to the child. Mr. Cybulski was described as not only alive but exceedingly well one month after this incident. According to the newspaper story, his doctors cannot account for this case; they confirm that the patient's brain scans showed "almost" no activity, and they assumed that he had suffered "irreparable" brain damage. One doctor is quoted as saying, "With all our modern technology, it is still difficult to determine when or if a patient will come out of a deep coma" (*Montreal Gazette* 1989). Since "deep coma" and "brain death" are not the same diagnosis, we are left to wonder whether it was the newspaper or the doctors, or both, who were confused.

· · ·

In 1996, a British newspaper, under the headline "Thwarting the Grim Reaper," reported the case of a sixty-one-year-old woman who collapsed on New Year's Day and was pronounced dead by a doctor called to the scene. Once in the mortuary, the woman started to breathe again and eventually recovered (*Guardian Weekly* 1996b).

The following week a letter appeared in the same newspaper: "A woman is pronounced dead by her doctor. . . . When transferred to the mortuary, she is found to be living, and medical services hasten to find out what's wrong with her. Shouldn't they be finding out what's wrong with the doctor?" (*Guardian Weekly* 1996c).

• • •

Cases such as these are unusual—very unusual—but they are newsworthy, and their faithful recounting by the media fuels public misgivings about the new death. But these misgivings have not been sufficient to provoke systematic scrutiny of organ procurements by the media or any official investigative body.

THREE

Locating the
Moment of Death

For some time thoughtful men have been increasingly troubled
by the present attitude in the medical profession: "You're
dead when your doctor says you are."

Desmond Smith, The Nation

At the end of the 1960s, when transplant surgeons first contemplated
the systematic use of patients believed to be irreversibly unconscious as
a source of human organs, a new legal definition of death was urgently
needed to prevent physicians from being charged with murder. It was
essential that the new death be a diagnosable event and that it be timed
to allow the removal of organs while they remained "fresh" and reasonably well oxygenated. No longer based on the commonsense notion
of the end of life—a failure of the heart and lungs—the new death is
determined by the condition of the brain alone, even though the body
clearly remains biologically alive, albeit with mechanical assistance.

Identification of the moment of brain death was designed primarily
to avert legal complications, but it was also necessary to reassure the
public. The very existence of ventilator-dependent patients raised two
concerns: first, the fear of being counted dead before one's time and
overhastily designated an organ donor; second, the fear of being kept
alive too long, as a "vegetable," with severe, irreversible brain damage,
but not technically brain-dead (Pernick 1999:4).

Although this development has depended on technological innovation, it is rarely attributed to technology alone. The ventilator is simply
a tool at our service. It is the moral status of "living cadavers" as alive
or dead that has been troubling. Yet discussion among health care professionals over the past thirty years has nevertheless been reduced repeatedly to disputes about what constitutes *biological* death. Efforts to

come to terms with the ambiguous status of the living dead have usually been cast as though this matter can be settled if only we can get the facts of death straight. In part this view stems from the assumption that life and death are unequivocal, dualistic categories. But it derives also from the belief that extensive debate of this kind will increase anxiety and compromise public trust in medical judgment about death. The transplant enterprise, with its dependence on the goodwill of donor families, will then be in jeopardy.

Transplanting Hearts: Medical Hubris on Display

Medical, legal, and media debates on organ procurement and transplants that took place in the English-speaking world throughout the 1960s and 1970s reveal the disquiet that reigned at that time about organ recipients who would be walking around with someone else's spare parts in their bodies and, even more, about the condition of potential donors as dead or alive. When the remaking of death was first discussed in the 1960s, many transplant surgeons feared repercussions from an anxious public who would refuse to cooperate with organ donation (Shapiro 1969a:50; Schmeck 1969; Paton 1971:163). The public had to understand that potential donors would be protected from any attempts to snatch their organs (Reeves 1969:406).[1]

Four years before the first heart transplant was carried out, an editorial in the *Annals of Internal Medicine* explicitly raised the specter of a spare-parts technology, which continues to plague the transplant enterprise:

> Cannibalizing was the term applied to a practice that unhappy circumstances spawned in some of the more remote areas of action in World War II. This process consisted of combining parts of a number of damaged vehicles to make one whole vehicle that would function. Such a practice in medicine has not quite arrived but we are moving in that direction. Every day the press, lay and professional, brings us news of the borrowed use of some organ, natural or artificial, to shore up some damaged human "vehicle" and put him on the road again. The analogy may be a bit stretched, but the possibility of such human cannibalizing is implicit in the development of artificial internal organs and in the experimental transplantation of natural organs from one human being to another.
>
> (*Annals of Internal Medicine* 1964:309)

---

1. The analysis presented in this chapter is largely restricted to North America. The responses of Denmark, Sweden, Israel, and Germany, among other countries, are distinctly different (see, for example, Hogle 1999; Machado 1996).

The editorial inquires whether patients are in danger of being denied the right to die with dignity and with the least possible suffering. It further dramatizes the case against transplant technology by listing the outcomes of kidney transplants carried out during the 1950s. Of 28 transplants between identical twins, 21 recipients survived at the time of the survey; but among 91 patients who had received a kidney from a living blood relative, only 5 remained alive one year after the operation. And among the 120 patients who had received kidneys from living, unrelated donors or from cadavers, only one had survived more than a year (311).

Heart transplants did not begin with Christiaan Barnard. In 1964, physicians at a Mississippi hospital removed the heart of a chimpanzee and transplanted it into a sixty-eight-year-old man with severe myocardial disease. The patient had been expected to die in the next day or two. The publication that followed this experiment gives a graphic account of the removal and handling of the ape's heart, its treatment once placed inside the recipient, and the condition of the diseased heart removed from the recipient. Readers are not informed that the patient died but simply told that the transplanted heart "ceased to function two hours after stabilization in the recipient." The experiment was described as having "far reaching significance" because it showed that a heart could be kept functioning by perfusion alone for at least an hour. The physicians lamented that the human donor they had hoped to use had not died soon enough, and in consequence they were forced to use a chimpanzee heart that was too small. It was also asserted that the recipient was so sick that he was "perhaps the major factor in eventual failure of the transplant" (Hardy and Chavez 1968:777).

The more celebrated occasion of the first human-to-human heart transplant involved a certain amount of public relations choreography. Physicians on both sides of the Atlantic recognized that South Africa might be a suitable location because it was known to be less sensitive about ethical issues than either the United States or Great Britain. Even so, it was evident that the first donor must not be "colored." When, in December 1967, Christiaan Barnard carried out "the ultimate operation, " he is reported to have said that the recipient, Louis Washkansky, could go home in a few weeks (*Saturday Review:* 1968). The recipient experienced acute rejection and lived for only eighteen days.

Despite the failure, other heart transplants rapidly followed (*Time* 1967). On the same day as Barnard's surgery in South Africa, a heart transplant described as an "unequivocal failure" took place at Maimonides Medical Center in Brooklyn. This operation involved an anencephalic infant donor and a nineteen-month-old recipient.[2] Fifteen months later, 118 heart transplants had been performed in eighteen different countries, with a surgical mortality rate of just over 50 percent (that is, over half the patients died less than thirty days after surgery), and a cumulative six-month mortality rate of 88 percent (Cooper and Mitchell 1969). In the United States the cost of surgery ranged between $30,000 and $50,000. A number of people remarked not only on the expense but also on the strain that this type of surgery would place on the supply of blood for transfusion. Richard Titmuss reports that on one occasion over three hundred pints of blood were needed for an American heart transplant (1971).

On the day following Barnard's first transplant, the *New York Times* carried a long feature article on the operation (1967a). One week later, Barnard was featured on the front cover of *Time*, and a five-page article in the same issue effused unqualified praise for heart transplants. The road accident of the Cape Town donor, Denise Darvall, the declaration of her death by Barnard himself,[3] and the procurement of her organs were recounted in detail. Details about the surgical procedures used in the South African transplant were minutely reported. The article concluded with assurance that the worldwide acclaim given to Barnard in the weeks following the surgery would ensure that more people will be willing to "sanction the gift of a heart to help an ailing fellow man" (*Time* 1967:72). It also noted that in the Brooklyn case, the New York parents of the anencephalic baby had no regrets about their decision to donate, despite the complete failure of the transplant.

The *New York Times* of December 5 meticulously reported that at least one of Denise Darvall's kidneys had been donated to a ten-year-old "colored" boy who was doing well (1967b). A separate article in the same issue pointed out that the recent operations dramatized a situation that was already a cause for concern among many doctors: "the shortage of organs for transplant." The article concluded that "many specialists . . . are convinced that the day is fast approaching when the vital human organs will simply be too valuable to be used for just one life alone" (1967c).

Immediately following Barnard's transplant, the *South African Med-*

2. An anencephalic infant is born without cerebral hemispheres: that is, the upper part of the brain is entirely absent. Such infants, with very few exceptions, die shortly after birth.
3. Declaration of death by the transplant surgeon was shortly thereafter recognized as a conflict of interest and no longer permitted.

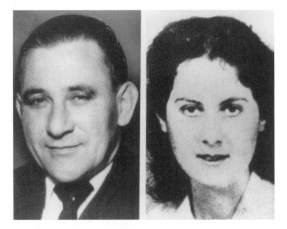

Louis Washkansky and Denise Ann Darvall, recipient and donor of the world's first heart transplant. Their photographs were published side by side after the operation. Reproduced by permission of AP/Wide World Photos.

ical Journal published an article by a professor of forensic medicine reviewing the significance of the "moment of death." This article supported the idea that resuscitation should be abandoned in hopeless cases in which the brain was irreversibly damaged and "life slips through the fingers." Whether death is certified as "the first, second or third arrest of vital functions is immaterial so long as that is the *finally accepted end of all hope and effort*" (Simpson 1967:1191, emphasis in original).

The following issue of the journal carried a brief notice of regret about the death of the recipient, Mr. Washkansky. The courage of Mr. Darvall, the father of the donor, was noted, as was that of Mr. Washkansky. Despite his death, the operation was repeatedly deemed a success (Louw 1967:1257).

By mid-December, however, the tone of media coverage was beginning to shift. Two *New York Times* editorials described the Barnard surgery as a historic experiment—"one of the peaks of modern scientific achievement"—but voiced concerns, which grew during the following months, about the way in which this technology inextricably linked the death of one person with the survival of another.. Although this was not the first time that a corpse had been "cannibalized" to aid the living, the editorial commented, the symbolic significance of the heart required a major shift in "habitual thought-patterns." People now had to recognize that Miss Darvall's heart was continuing to "live and work though she is dead" (1967d).

A second *New York Times* editorial appeared immediately after the death of Mr. Washkansky in late December. In defense of transplants, it noted that the patient had died of pneumonia and not because of the rejection of the transplanted heart. It argued for changes in the law and an educational campaign to encourage people to give "advance permission" to use their organs for donation. The editorial was concerned, however, to assure the public that a donor's death would not in any way be hastened, nor a life "sacrificed prematurely for the benefit of another," and it raised disturbing questions:

> One need not be a science-fiction writer to envision the possibility of future murder rings supplying healthy organs for black-market surgeons whose patients are unwilling to wait until natural sources have supplied the heart or liver or pancreas they need. More prosaically, shall people near death be allowed to sell their heart or liver to the highest bidder or shall the future use of such vital "spare parts" be decided by some agency set up by society?
> (*New York Times* 1967e)

The editorial expressed concern as to how society would make choices about allocation of this new, scarce resource, fearing that decisions might simply be left to market resources unless action was quickly taken.

By January 5 the tone of articles in both *Newsweek* (1968a) and *Time* (1968a) was clearly less supportive of transplants. Barnard had by then appeared on the popular television show *Face the Nation* explicitly to win public support; after the show he was "feted like a second Pasteur" (Smith 1968). *Newsweek,* under the headline "Surgery and Showbiz," stated that during the second heart transplant performed by Barnard in early January, "the medical significance of the feat was nearly obscured by a circus atmosphere with Marx Brothers overtones" (1968a). A freelance photographer had gained access to the gallery of the operating room. NBC-TV obtained a court order to stop him from selling his pictures; the TV company had a $50,000 agreement for exclusive interviews with the transplant recipient and his wife, as well as for coverage of the actual surgery.

In the event, NBC was kept out of the operating room but went ahead with exclusive interviews before and after surgery. Its rival company, CBS, paid Barnard's way to the United States to appear on *Face the Nation* and contributed handsomely to the surgeon's research fund (*Newsweek* 1968a).

The *Saturday Review* was scathing about these new surgical procedures, and even more so about Barnard himself. It noted that in heart transplants carried out by Barnard on dogs, under the tutelage of an

American surgeon, all the dogs had died (1968). However, *Ebony* described the first operation as a success, as did Barnard himself, and for the same reasons, namely that the transplanted heart continued to beat strongly throughout the eighteen days it resided in the recipient's chest. The fact that the patient died of pneumonia was, *Ebony* noted, "of little consequence" (1968).

Ebony exhibited even more interest in Barnard's second heart transplant, carried out in the first days of 1968. The editorial noted that "in blatantly racist South Africa," Barnard had transplanted the heart of twenty-four-year-old "Colored" Clive Haupt into the body of a white Jewish retired dentist, aged fifty-eight. The dentist, Philip Blaiberg, had been asked just before going into surgery if he had any objection to receiving a "colored" heart. He had none, and the operation went ahead. *Ebony* speculated in its editorial:

> If Dr. Blaiberg completely recovers and again walks the streets of Cape Town, a most ironic situation will ensue. Clive Haupt's heart will ride in the uncrowded train coaches marked "For Whites Only" instead of in the crowded ones reserved for blacks. It will pump extra hard to circulate the blood needed for a game of tennis where the only blacks are those who might pull heavy rollers to smooth the courts. It will enter fine restaurants, attend theaters and concerts and live in a decent home instead of in the tough slums where Haupt grew up. Haupt's heart will go literally to hundreds of places where Haupt, himself, could not go because his skin was a little darker than that of Blaiberg. (*Ebony* 1968:118)

The surgery might work medical miracles but not lasting political ones: the editorial cautioned, "It is doubtful . . . that the transplant of a Colored heart into a white man will have any positive effect upon the rigidly segregated life of South Africa" (1968:118).

By spring 1968, media ambivalence was rampant. In April, *Life* described Barnard as an "international folk hero—and a center of medical controversy." It noted that of 218 cardiologists interviewed, half of them said they would not undergo a heart transplant (Rosenfeld 1968). In May 1968 *Newsweek* expressed considerable surprise that four more heart transplants had recently taken place in three different countries, even though five out of the six recipients who had gone through this new invasive treatment were dead. This magazine suggested that a moratorium was appropriate but pointed out that Philip Blaiberg was "doing well" three months after his surgery and that this second operation had assumed enormous significance. The article cited Barnard as saying: "The patient himself seems to have answered the critics more ably than

I could" (*Newsweek* 1968b). When describing his first two cases in the *American Journal of Cardiology,* Barnard stated: "The first patient died 18 days after the operation, and the second patient is still alive after six months. Thus the technique evolved has so far carried a direct mortality of zero" (1968).

Raymond Hoffenberg, the physician for Clive Haupt, the donor for Barnard's second heart transplant, remains troubled by the media's role in the event. When I interviewed him in 1998, he recalled that transplant surgeons were "hanging around" the ICU where he was looking after Haupt and that he had to send them away, insisting that the patient was not dead. He decided to wait overnight before making a decision as to whether there was any possibility that Haupt could survive. Hoffenberg pointed out that, because at that time no concept of brain-death existed, it was exceedingly difficult to know when exactly to declare the deaths of patients on ventilators. When Hoffenberg returned to the unit in the morning, in his estimation, Haupt was no longer alive, but he cannot recall exactly when the death certificate was signed.

Hoffenberg is still shocked about a photograph showing Philip Blaiberg, the recipient of Haupt's heart, "swimming" at a Cape Town beach several months after surgery. He recalls that Blaiberg was never able to walk independently after the surgery. For the photograph he had to be taken down to the water's edge in a wheelchair, carried into the ocean, photographed, and then hauled out again.

By December 1968, one year after the first heart transplants, the initial euphoria had all but evaporated. The *Nation* published an article that month headlined "The Heart Market" in which they asked if someone was playing God; they asserted that a "shocking international heart transplant race" was under way. This article also reminded readers about the ambiguity of the donor's condition and stressed that, "contrary to the general impression, few doctors can predict the so-called 'moment of death' with certainty" (Smith 1968:720). It presented findings about a group of 120 head-injury patients who were unconscious for more than a month at Cambridge University Hospital in England. Sixty-three of them survived, leading the writer to the conclusion: "As the need for donors grows larger, the definition of death must be carefully redefined. When are you dead *enough* to be deprived of your heart?" (Smith 1968:721).

Media publications of the time yield a striking contrast with contemporary practices: photographs of organ donors (taken before their accidents) appear alongside photographs of recipients. The donor is usu-

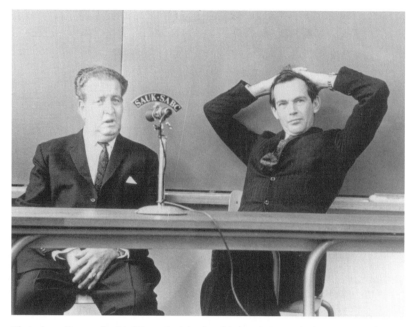

Christiaan Barnard with Pieter Smith, the third recipient of a heart transplant, carried out on September 7, 1968. Photo courtesy of Cloete Breytenbach for *Life* magazine.

ally young and exuberant, and the recipient looks middle-aged and exhausted. In one photograph, the wife of the first heart recipient is looking sympathetically at the grieving father of the donor, who had lost not only his daughter but also his wife when they were hit by a speeding car (*Life* 1967). However, by 1969 photographs of donors no longer appeared in the media; donors became cloaked with anonymity as the ambiguity of their condition drew attention.[4]

After one hundred heart transplants, media opinion was consistently against transplantation. Three eminent U.S. cardiologists had called for a moratorium on transplants in 1968, but Albert Rosenfeld, writing in *Life*, was convinced that Barnard would not abide by one. *Life* echoed *Newsweek*'s earlier surprise that no moratorium had been placed on this type of surgery (Rosenfeld 1968). There was at least one call, from

---

4. The media continue to report sporadically on individual, named patients who are waiting for organs, but graphic reports about the sudden, often violent death of those who donate organs was deemed early on as not appropriately newsworthy and perhaps overly macabre, even for the tabloids. In short, donor deaths go unnoted except when they are compiled into statistics about traffic accidents and the increased suicide rates of youth.

a professor of biology, for Barnard to be disbarred permanently from medical practice (Schmeck 1969).

The Ultimate Operation: Consolidation and Dissent

In July 1969 Barnard arranged for an international meeting in Cape Town of surgeons who had carried out heart transplants. Most of the conference was devoted to surgical and postoperative techniques, diagnosis of organ rejection, and findings from recipients who had died. The first part of the meeting, however, was given over to the "selection and preparation" of donors and recipients. Barnard asked "our neurosurgeon, Dr. de Villiers," to describe when a patient could be thought of as a potential donor. De Villiers responded that in light of recent developments in transplant technology, it had become necessary to redefine what is taken to be a cadaver, and he insisted that the termination of treatment should be exclusively a medical decision: "I don't believe we can share this responsibility even with relatives. We may not ask consent of the relatives; it is entirely a technical medical decision, nor should we be circumscribed in this decision by legal authority" (Shapiro 1969a:40).

The ensuing discussion emphasized that if the "conventional point of death," namely cessation of the heartbeat, was the earliest possible moment to declare death, "proper preparation" of a heart for transplant was impossible. At the same time it was argued that "for social and legal reasons," the introduction of "radically new concepts" of death should be avoided.

Adrian Kantrowitz, the American surgeon who had attempted to transplant the heart of an anencephalic infant into a nineteen-month-old baby, reminded the group that, as shown in canine experiments, transplants that make use of a still-beating heart have a much greater success rate than those using a heart that has stopped beating. If the heart has to be resuscitated, it does not "perform as well." Kantrowitz stressed that treatment of the donor should be terminated at the point when "irreversible brain-death" has been established (one of the first occasions when the term *brain death* was used). Denton Cooley, a transplant surgeon also from the United States, commented:

> Neuro-surgical colleagues at times have used terms which should be avoided. In the first place—I think that we should avoid the words "alive" and "dead" as synonymous with brain function or cardiac function. "Alive" and "dead" are such nebulous and vague terms, so ill-defined that they will never be defined, since no one understands either the meaning of "life" or "death". One should say the heart is contracting, or beating, but not "alive." . . . In

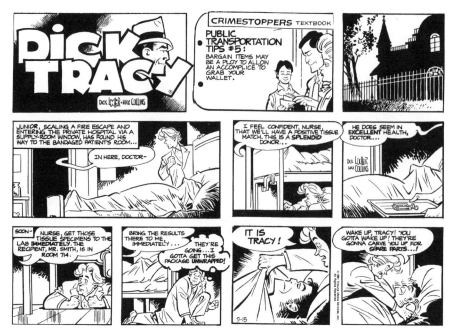

A healthy donor. Comic strip © Tribune Media Services, Inc. All rights reserved.
Reprinted with permission.

> my opinion the clinician can become too pre-occupied with the rights of the
> dead, namely the donor, at the expense of the recipient. We should not jeop-
> ardize the possible survival of the recipient while we are waiting around to
> make a decision whether the cadaver, as you call it, is dead or not.
>
> (Shapiro 1969a:45)

It was pointed out that France and Great Britain already had guidelines for diagnosis of "irreversible coma" and that the decision to discontinue treatment had been taken out of the hands of transplant surgeons and placed in the domain of neurosurgeons. Barnard and
Kantrowitz both took exception to these guidelines, stating that the well-
established reliability of physicians obviated the need for formal criteria.
Barnard went on to declare: "I think we can say we now have a donor,
i.e., a potential donor. On the whole, people will agree that there is no
need to wait for conventional death . . . if you have a patient who can
fulfill the criteria for becoming a potential donor once you stop the
respirator, you can also be certain that the patient will die, so why wait
until the heart stops beating?" (Shapiro 1969a:50).

Defining Irreversible Coma: The Harvard Committee

One month after Barnard's first heart transplant, with the recipient dead for just over a week, Henry Beecher, an anesthesiologist, approached the dean at Harvard medical school with a request. Beecher, well known for his ethical concerns about medical experimentation, wanted a group formed to discuss what he regarded as urgent issues associated with the "hopelessly unconscious" patient. The dean responded enthusiastically to Beecher's request and appointed him chair of the "Ad Hoc Committee of the Harvard Medical School to Examine the Definition of Brain Death." This committee was composed of ten physicians (whose specialties included transplant surgery, anesthesiology, neurology, and psychiatry), one lawyer, one theologian, and one historian. Mita Giacomini, who has worked extensively with unpublished documents produced by this committee, notes that most of its members were already well acquainted (1997). After six months of meetings, the group produced a report that was published in the *Journal of the American Medical Association* under the title "A Definition of Irreversible Coma" (1968).

The report opens with a statement that was to be frequently cited in future discussion:

> Our primary purpose is to define irreversible coma as a new criterion for death. There are two reasons why there is a need for a definition: (1) Improvements in resuscitative and supportive measures have led to increased efforts to save those who are desperately injured. Sometimes these efforts have only partial success, so that the result is an individual whose heart continues to beat but whose brain is irreversibly damaged. The burden is great on patients who suffer permanent loss of intellect, on their families, on the hospitals, and on those in need of hospital beds already occupied by these comatose patients. (2) Obsolete criteria for the definition of death can lead to controversy in obtaining organs for transplantation.
> (Ad Hoc Committee of the Harvard Medical School
> 1968:85)

Given that in 1968 no patient survived in a brain-dead condition for more than a few hours or days, it can be assumed that point 2 is of greater interest to the committee. The report describes the characteristics of "irreversible coma," including complete unreceptivity and unresponsiveness, an absence of movements, of spontaneous breathing, and of reflexes. The diagnostic procedures to be used in establishing the condition of a permanently nonfunctioning brain are described; an electroencephalogram (EEG) is said to be of "great confirmatory value." The report concludes that all relevant tests must be repeated after a twenty-four-hour interval, at which time, if the patient's condition has not changed, death can be declared and the ventilator turned off. It is made clear that only a physician can make the diagnosis.

A legal commentary is included in the report, confirming that judgment of the criteria for irreversible coma is a medical and not a legal issue. It also states that, if the medical community as a whole is supportive, the recommendations could become the basis for much-needed change in the legal concept of death. It cautions that patients should be declared dead before any effort is made to unplug the respirator: "The reason for this recommendation is that in our judgment it will provide a greater degree of legal protection to those involved" (1968:87).

Following the legal commentary, the report refers to an address by Pope Pius XII in 1958 titled "The Prolongation of Life." The Pope declared that it is not within the competence of the Church to determine the moment of death, and that while it is essential for a physician to take all reasonable means to restore vital functions and consciousness of patients, it is not obligatory to continue the use of extraordinary means in hopeless cases (*The Pope Speaks* 1958:398). From the outset, then, the Harvard group was reasonably assured that the debate over death would not open up vicious disputes, as the abortion question had done.

Martin Pernick suggests Beecher considered it a blatant waste of resources to keep patients on ventilators when their condition is deemed irreversible. Such patients could perhaps be made into experimental subjects, avoiding the ethical problems associated with experiments on fully alive patients (1999:10). But it was clear that organ transplants were uppermost in the minds of the committee. The report states: "The question before the committee could not simply be to define brain-death. This would not advance the cause of organ transplantation since it would not cope with the essential issue of when the surgical team is authorized—legally, morally, and medically—in removing a vital organ" (cited in Giacomini 1997:1474).

Pressure was on the committee to work quickly, and meetings proceeded behind closed doors. An early draft of the report proposed that before life support could be terminated, signs of death must be reaffirmed at twenty-four-hour intervals over three days. Giacomini notes dismay on the part of at least one of the involved transplant surgeons at the prospect of having to wait so long before organ procurement would be possible. The waiting period was eventually reduced to twenty-four hours, and a much shorter interval has since become usual. As to whether transplant surgeons should be banned from making diagnoses of death, it was decided in the end not to keep them from the bedsides of comatose patients who are potential organ donors.

Indeed, the committee struggled over whether its mandate was to try to redefine the concept of death or simply to define irreversible coma. At issue was whether "a patient [should] be declared dead, or merely hopeless, in order to qualify as a vital organ source" (Giacomini 1997: 1476). The committee was sharply divided, with one transplant surgeon arguing that the word *death* should be used, with no qualification. A neurologist, by contrast, cited two cases of patients in his experience who had made good recoveries after many months of "complete unresponsiveness," and as a result he argued for a much more cautious approach. The final report uses both *irreversible coma* and *brain-death*.

Noting that the committee report cites very few publications or conventional forms of scientific evidence to substantiate its statements, Giacomini argues that the committee set out to construct brain death as a verifiable fact by establishing first and foremost the technical features of brain death as medical phenomena and deliberately setting aside all philosophical "speculation." Although diagnoses more or less synonymous with brain death were already being applied in medical practice at several hospitals—as committee members must have been aware—they deliberately ignored current practice. Instead, they crafted their document as though the committee meetings constituted a historic event, the result of progressive medical insight that crystallized for the first time while they sat around the committee table.

Giacomini concludes that the committee marked out a new space between the living and the dead in which "the irreversible comatose body became a territory over which sometimes competing, sometimes cooperating technological interests negotiated their claims" (1997: 1478). The committee shifted arguments away from earlier concerns about the *meaning* of death to defining it in instrumentally measurable terms. "Redefining death was not simply a technical exercise, but an aesthetic act to fit the hopelessly comatose, the dead, and the organ donor into the same clinical picture" (1997:1480).

In 1969, Henry Beecher published a commentary in the *New England Journal of Medicine* defending the committee report. He lamented lawyers' reluctance to recognize irreversible coma, which had made hospital administrators hesitant about acting on the new view of death. Although the legal profession was apparently content to leave the actual determination of death in the hands of doctors, some lawyers nevertheless retained doubts. Beecher, well-known for his dislike of lawyers, insisted, "Once the decision is made to terminate the situation, to turn off the respirator, what difference does it make whether the heart is stopped by inexorable asphyxia or by removal?" He concluded that it is doubtful whether "we as a medical society have yet achieved enough emotional and sociologic maturity to handle this question boldly," but failure to do so "verges on the unethical" (1969:1071).

Quickening the New Death

The Harvard committee in fact accomplished little that was entirely new. A Boston medical examiner, William Brickley, in a talk to the Massachusetts Medical Society in 1941, stated that he had spent many years trying to establish the precise time of legal death. He concluded that this task is extraordinarily difficult because not all the parts of the body die at the same time. Brickley noted that while "science" has various definitions of death, in his opinion, "Life is over when brain waves cease" (*Time* 1941:62).

The first serious attempt to redefine death on the basis of the condition of the brain was made in 1959 by French neurophysiologists, who coined the term *coma dépassé* (beyond coma) to describe this condition (Mollaret and Goulon 1959; Jouvet 1959). The Harvard committee ignored the French publications. *Coma dépassé* was recognized as a new type of coma, a stage of life beyond the cessation of all vital functions: the foundling of life-support technology. Mollaret and Goulon argued that this condition creates an overwhelming temptation for the physician to pull the plug and stop the ventilator (1959:41). They clearly recognized that the presence of this "dark zone" made the redefinition of death essential.

The debate had also been opened earlier in the United States. According to a 1966 article in *Time*, "Many physicians now believe that the question 'Is the patient dead?' should be answered largely on the basis of his electroencephalograph (EEG or 'brain wave' tracings)." The words of a Boston neurosurgeon were cited: "The human spirit is the product of man's brain, not his heart" (*Time* 1966). Criteria for establishing brain death were set out in this article by Robert Schwab, a neurologist who later participated on the Harvard committee.

The article also reported on a Swedish cardiac surgeon who had recently caused a furor by suggesting that a person should be declared dead when a flat EEG shows that "his brain has definitely and irrevocably ceased to function." France, the article noted, was also in uproar because its National Academy of Medicine had supported the idea that a patient was dead if no brain activity was exhibited on the EEG for forty-eight hours. *Time* concluded that modern medical technology had rendered the current laws and the traditional precepts and practices of physicians "out of date" (1966).

From the early 1960s transplant physicians, who believed that their work was being impeded because brain death was not widely accepted, pushed to place their new enterprise on a firmer footing (Moore 1964). A 1966 Ciba Foundation symposium titled "Ethics in Medical Progress: With Special Reference to Transplantation," involving twenty-eight participants from Europe and North America (the majority of whom were physicians and surgeons), dealt extensively with increasing impatience toward conventional ideas of death. Among the questions addressed were the following:

> For how long should "life" be maintained in a person with irrevocable damage of the brain? [D]oes a parent always have the right to accept or refuse treatment of his child? [W]hat special protection might be given to minors, people of low intelligence, or prisoners, in regard to clinical trials or donation of tissues? [W]hen does death occur in an unconscious patient dependent on artificial aids to circulation and respiration? [A]re there ever circumstances where death may be mercifully advanced? . . . [D]oes the law permit operations which "mutilate" the donor for the advantage of another person?
> (Wolstenholme and O'Connor 1966:vii–viii)

Thomas Starzl, soon to become well-known as the most experimental and aggressive of liver transplant surgeons, revealed his confusion at this early symposium. He commented: "I assume that when kidneys are removed from 'living cadavers,' only one organ is removed, so that the patient is not thereby killed" (1966:155).

The conference revealed that no consensus existed as to whether death should be redefined. Several participants were concerned about protecting the reputations of transplant surgeons. At one point the discussion focused on Starzl's controversial use of prisoners as "volunteer" live kidney donors. Several participants stated that "dead" donors are more acceptable than living ones. Opponents of organ procurement from living donors invoked the Hippocratic imperative "First, do no harm," arguing that such practices constitute an "assault" (Kilbrandon,

1966:2). This concern was countered by a recurrent worry that tinkering with the process of dying could easily be interpreted as an expedient move to make organs available for transplant.

It is evident from the language used that participants were sensitive to the ambiguous status of the patient-cadaver. Scare quotes were placed around words such as *dead* and *irreversible* to qualify their meaning. During the conference and in the years to follow, several physicians invented cumbersome, sometimes graphic terms for patients suspended between life and death: "dead but in a state of artificial survival" (Hamburger and Crosnier 1968:42); "living cadaver" (Starzl 1966:70); "heart-lung preparation" (Alexandre 1966:156); "potential cadaver" (Revillard 1966:70); "reanimation patient" (Bessert et al. 1970), "respirator brain" (Korein 1978:9; Moseley et al. 1976), and "neomort" (Gaylin 1974:23). The struggle to define a clear transition between life and death, to create discrete boundaries, is apparent. It is equally obvious that the "need" to find organs for transplants gave an edge to the discussion, causing certain participants, usually transplant surgeons, to appear impatient and fractious. Others, most often neurologists, are much more tentative, concerned with describing accurately the "scientific" condition of "neomorts" as either living or dead.

Toward the end of the symposium, a urological surgeon argued that "as our thinking about transplantation of human organs develops, people must become enlightened enough not to think of this as a horrible experiment, or indeed as an experiment at all, but learn to accept it as a normal event" (Goodwin 1966:211).

Popular ambivalence was evident in comments by intellectuals. In an article originally published in *Daedalus* in spring 1969, the philosopher Hans Jonas was among the first of a string of intellectuals, neither physicians nor lawyers, to criticize the new definition of death. Jonas emphasizes that his quarrel is not with those who must decide when the "artificial prolongation of life" is futile. If a diagnosis of "brain-death" were used simply for that purpose, then it would present no problems. At issue for Jonas is the need to *"advance"* the moment of the declaration of death while keeping the respirator turned on, "thereby maintain[ing] the body in a state of what would have been 'life' by the older definition (but is only a 'simulacrum' of life by the new)—so as to get at his organs and tissues under the ideal conditions of what would have been 'vivisection' "(1974:129, emphasis in original). Jonas is above all concerned about protracting the process of dying and doing violence to a body conveniently redefined as dead. He insists that we do not know the "exact borderline between life and death" and that only the most stringent criterion of death will do: "The patient must be absolutely sure that his doctor does not become his executioner" (1974:131).

Jonas detects the classical "soul-body dualism" of Enlightenment philosophy at work in efforts to reformulate death:

> [In] its new apparition . . . the dualism of the brain and body . . . holds that the true human person rests in (or is represented by) the brain, of which the rest of the body is a mere subservient tool. Thus when the brain dies, it is as when the soul departed: what is left are "mortal remains." Now nobody will deny that the cerebral aspect is decisive for the human quality of life of the organism. . . . The position I advance acknowledges just this . . . [but] the extracerebral body [has] its share of the identity of the person. The body is uniquely the body of this brain and no other, as the brain is uniquely the brain of this body and no other. What is under the brain's central control, the bodily total, is as individual, as much "myself," as singular to my identity (fingerprints!), as noninterchangeable, as the controlling (and reciprocally controlled) brain itself. My identity is the identity of the whole organism, even if the higher functions of personhood are seated in the brain.
>
> (Jonas 1974:139)

Although it was intellectuals, rather than medical commentators, who first raised the question of the demise of the person, it has been increasingly taken up within the medical world. Today, despite advances in scientific knowledge about the brain, neurologists continue to write and openly worry about the death of the person. The ambiguous condition of the living cadaver leaves even these medical experts confused.

The Medical World Divided

Early in 1968, a patient was brought to a hospital in Richmond, Virginia, with a severe head injury. Despite intensive treatment, over the next twelve hours it became clear that the patient would not recover. The possibility of donating organs was discussed with the patient's family and with the medical examiner. Both parties agreed to donation, the respirator was turned off, and the heart and kidneys were removed. The heart was used in the first heart transplant to be performed in Virginia. Shortly thereafter the transplant surgeon, David Hume, stood trial on a charge of wrongful death, because it was asserted that the individual's death was caused by the removal of her heart (Pollock 1978:4). The jury eventually declared Hume and his associates not guilty. In reporting this case in the *American Journal of Surgery* ten years after the event, the author, a surgeon, was clearly shocked that a "law book" definition of death might take precedence over a medical definition.

In 1972, also in Virginia, four years after removal of Bruce Tucker's beating heart and its transplantation into a waiting patient, the four surgeons involved were acquitted of wrongful death charges. Tucker's brother, who had brought the case, alleged that the donor had not been dead when his heart and kidneys were removed, and that it was the removal of the organs that caused his death. Tucker had been diagnosed as irreversibly unconscious, but in 1968 no systematic criteria existed for this diagnosis.

On the basis of preliminary comments by the judge, the prosecution was considered likely to win the case, but apparently the judge's mind was swayed by the statements of expert witnesses. One physician insisted that the body exists only to support the brain and that "the brain *is* the individual" (Kennedy 1973:39, emphasis added). The donor's brother was particularly upset because the hospital had allegedly made little effort to locate Tucker's relatives and had treated his body as unclaimed. After the surgeons had been informed by the hospital administration and the police that the next of kin could not be traced, the procurement had gone ahead without the family's permission and with no evidence that Tucker wished to be an organ donor. In court, Tucker's brother testified that he had telephoned the hospital three times but was never informed that his brother was to become an organ donor. He had eventually learned of the transplant from the undertaker.

These cases and one or two others in the United States spurred the medical and legal establishment to create standard criteria for determining brain death (Gaylin 1974; Simmons et al. 1987:25). The Uniform Anatomical Gift Act, which was in place by 1968, was designed to ensure voluntary donation of corpses and body parts for transplantation. But without any standard criteria for determination of brain death, controversies had persisted.

The decision by the Virginia court permitted transplant surgeons and intensivists across the United States to breathe more easily. Critical comments in both the media and professional medical journals about predatory transplant surgery, common during the previous four years, might now subside. *Newsweek,* for example, had published the statement of a public-health official in Washington, D.C., in 1967: "I have a horrible vision of ghouls hovering over an accident victim with long knives unsheathed, waiting to take out his organs as soon as he is pronounced dead" (1967:87). Shortly before the Harvard committee report was made public, an article titled "Transplantation in the Brave New World" appeared in a psychiatric journal. The author, a physician, brings up the role of medicine in Nazi Germany; writes of a future in which suicide-assistance squads roam the streets; and envisions the "arrangement" of accidents. He too creates a nightmare vision of the surgeon poised over a dying person, waiting to pluck out the heart at the earliest opportunity (Davidson 1968). Professional journals were also beginning to look critically at the issue. A 1968 editorial in the *Annals of Internal Medicine* reminded its readers of the fact that brain-dead organ donors would, for the most part, be young people who died traumatically: donors would have neither a timely nor a "good" death (1968).

A week after publication of the Harvard committee report, but without reference to it, James Appel, president of the American Medical Association, argued that society must face up to the ethical and legal questions posed by organ transplants. He commented negatively in *JAMA* on the "blow by blow" description that the public had been given of the first five heart transplants. Like other authors before him, Appel speculated as to why heart transplants caused so much furor when earlier liver and kidney transplants had occasioned no outcry. He concluded that the answer lay in the symbolic significance of the heart (1968).

Another article in the same journal was one of the first to note that transplantation involves the interests of *two* individuals—the donor and the recipient—and therefore "the people, law, and medicine must come into some comfortable and realistic rapprochement on the moral, ethical, legal, humanistic, and economic aspects of this problem" (Arnold, Zimmermann, and Martin 1968).

The American Journal of Cardiology compiled a list of outcomes of the 146 heart transplants performed through August 1969. Only 21 patients survived (among these, 9 had been operated in the previous two months), and details were not known about one other patient in Switzerland. Barnard's second heart transplant patient, Philip Blaiberg, died of organ rejection 592 days after his operation (Haller and Cerruti 1969:562). No judgments were made in this article, but the figures were damning.

In *Seminars in Psychiatry* Alec Paton, writing in 1971, noted that "millions of words have been written about transplantation." Echoing Appel's speculations, he argued that "world-wide reaction to the first heart transplant showed that emotional attitudes are stronger than many scientists would like to acknowledge. To most people, the heart is more than a pump, and the sanctity of the body, especially when dead, is still firmly held." Presumably because of Barnard's flirtation with the media, Paton denounced transplant operations as public spectacles (reminiscent of human dissection in the sixteenth century). Observing that five heart recipients had become psychotic soon after their operations, Paton questioned why so little had been heard about this. He stopped short of outright condemnation of solid organ transplantation, but commented that since Blaiberg's death there had been an "almost complete cessation" of heart transplants (1971:168).

Indeed, seven years later, the sociologists Renée Fox and Judith Swazey noted that "a quasi-moratorium on human heart transplantation still exists throughout the world" (1978:312). In 1976 only 31 operations had been carried out, many fewer than between 1967 and 1971, when the technique was new. After the initial contagious exhilaration had worn off, only three surgeons, including Christiaan Barnard in Cape Town, continued to perform the procedure. The outlook for recipients of liver transplants remained even more dismal than that of heart recipients (Fox and Swazey 1978:316–17). The situation would not improve for organ recipients until the powerful immunosuppressant cyclosporine was put on the market with great fanfare in 1981 (Fox and Swazey 1992).

In summary, it was not until the first heart transplants were performed that concern about transplants became widespread. Media response moved rapidly from adulation to ambivalence; medical reactions in the two years following the first heart transplants were equally mixed, with the majority of doctors pointing out that the procedure remained experimental and the survival rates dismal. Almost no comment was made, save by one or two critical psychiatrists, about the quality of life of the survivors.

Debate about which tests could be relied on to confirm the clinical judgment of death was common in the medical literature during the late 1960s and early 1970s, coupled with a sense of urgency about standardizing procedures for declaring death and procuring organs. Other worries included who would protect physicians from malpractice suits in connection with the new death and organ procurement (Black 1978: 338) and the negative image of doctors that transplant physicians were creating. It became clear that transplant surgeons had a conflict of interest if they were in any way involved with diagnosing the death of donors or promoting the new death, but in the early years this issue slipped by more or less unnoticed.

The ethical and legal issues raised, with only a few exceptions, were those that continue to plague the transplant world today: the shortage of organs, coupled with questions about their standardization, allocation, and distribution (Hogle 1995). An essay by the theologian William May (1973) is virtually unique for this time in expressing doubts about the strategies for organ procurement.

In the United States it was debated whether it was necessary to approach families to obtain consent for donation. Several European countries, where centralized state power was well established, had already institutionalized "presumed consent," so that organs could be procured unless the patient or family opted out ahead of time.

May was concerned about a policy that permitted the routine cutting up of corpses, "even for high-minded social purposes." He argued that we must face up to the "horror" of what was about to take place: "There is a tinge of the inhuman in the humanitarianism of those who believe that the perception of social need easily overrides all other considerations. . . . Even the proponents of routine salvaging have conceded indirectly to the awkward fact of human revulsion" (1973:5). May was categorically opposed to supporters of presumed consent who argued that requiring prior, explicit consent from prospective donors would mean that fewer organs would be procured. In May's opinion, even if this were the case, prior consent was essential. He dismissed objections that it was inappropriate for hospital staff to make "ghoulish" overtures about donation to relatives of the newly dead: it simply would have to be done. May concluded: "The question remains whether a system that overrides rather than faces up to profound reservations is not, in the long run, more ghoulish in its consequences for the social order" (1973:5).

In retrospect May's comments are particularly pertinent. They appeared at a time when donors, who had been disquietingly visible during the first year of heart transplants, disappeared from public view to become nameless ghosts who haunt the transplant world. The ambiguous status of living cadavers created a loophole in the laws regarding consent to medical procedures. Rather than being granted the rights of patients, including the right of informed consent (instituted in the late 1960s), they were assigned the status of corpses. As a result, their organs could be made available for commodification, perhaps even without the prior consent of the patient or the patient's family.[5] Although this issue was settled reasonably quickly, and individual consent is required throughout North America before donation can take place, other troubling issues were not so easily resolved. It would be another ten years before guidelines for determining brain death were systematized and the new death was legally recognized.

5. In Europe, presumed consent laws are in use in Austria, Belgium, Bulgaria, Cyprus, Denmark, Finland, France, Greece, Hungary, Italy, Luxembourg, Portugal, Spain, Sweden, and several Swiss cantons. These laws, some of which have since been modified since their enactment, have strong and weak forms. In the exclusive or "strong" form, if the deceased has not opted out, then organs can be taken without obtaining family consent. With the "weak," inclusive form, the family must be consulted. In practice the law everywhere is flexible, and it is claimed that the wishes of the family are not overruled.

I was observing in the ICU of a tertiary care hospital in Montreal when news came that a middle-aged man, run over by a garbage truck, had been rushed into the trauma unit, where he was undergoing the usual assessment. The damage looked serious; he was unconscious, and his head had apparently suffered a major blow. It was possible that the man was brain-dead already.

About an hour and a half later, this patient was wheeled into the ICU with his vital signs stabilized and a CAT scan completed. He remained unconscious. As the orderly maneuvered the patient into the assigned space, an intern picked up the patient charts. "Looks like this is going to be a good donor," he said. "Should we call in the transplant coordinator?" A senior intensivist, on the phone at the time, overheard this comment and immediately said, "Not so fast. Slow down." After hanging up, the intensivist looked at the chart for himself and briefly observed the busy nurses as they set to work checking the lines and tubes sustaining the patient.

He turned to the intern and repeated once again, "Not so fast."

When I left the unit an hour or two later, the patient was stable, but the condition of his brain remained in doubt. A week later I was told that this man was out of the ICU and in an ordinary ward where he was breathing on his own and doing well. A full recovery was expected.

There is no possibility that the impulse of the intern would have been followed up prematurely or a transplant coordinator called in to start inquiring about procurement. This episode is nevertheless a cautionary tale. The tendency of the inexperienced today, whether they be green-horn doctors or certain among the stunned relatives, is to move quickly to thinking about donation; to salvage hope from disaster. Clinical experience is the buffer, ensuring that care of the patient comes before an interest in his or her organs.[1]

1. There are, of course, some parts of the world where medical integrity with respect to organ procurement is at times in doubt (Cohen, ms; Scheper-Hughes 2000).

Making the New Death Uniform

Contesting the New Death

Prior to 1968 physicians in North America and Europe had, as a matter of course, quietly turned off the ventilators of patients whose condition they firmly believed was irreversible and would soon result in conventional death. Intensive care units were in effect "a private domain, whatever the formal definition of death, and doctors exercised their discretion" (Rothman 1991:160). In performing such acts, physicians were participating in a long-standing but discreet medical tradition.[1] As the number of artificial ventilators accumulated in ICUs, intensivists had to deal increasingly with unconscious patients with severe head trauma whose condition was, in their estimation, irreversible. Although many died precipitously, others lingered on for days, and doctors had to decide whether to remove such individuals from life support. Nevertheless, the practice of unplugging the ventilator remained informal, and more or less concealed, in large part because neither the media nor the public evinced much interest in the practice.

1. My late father-in-law, a general practitioner in England, reminisced once about a house call he had made to a very sick patient suffering from unendurable pain. Knowing nothing more could possibly be done, he had quietly administered an overdose of morphine. Both the patient and his wife had told my father-in-law several times that their suffering was unendurable and had asked if the patient could be "let go." After administering the morphine and descending the stairs from the bedroom, my father-in-law told the patient's wife, "Your husband will sleep well tonight." Informal stories such as these are abundant but have been of little public concern until the past twenty years or so.

This situation changed radically once efforts began to systematize and institutionalize the concept of brain death, notably following the publication of the Harvard Ad Hoc Committee report in 1968. Two definitions of death were now recognized, but the conflicting definitions—the "traditional" failure of the cardiopulmonary system, and the new "brain death"—soon were debated in court. In the spotlight of legal, media, and public examination, physicians sought to refine and justify their practices of managing death.

Shortly before the publication of the Harvard committee report, the Texas transplant surgeon Denton Cooley and his team were confronted with legal difficulties similar to those in the Virginia cases. Cooley wanted to transplant the heart of a welder who had suffered severe brain injury in a brawl. The medical examiner, who was investigating the case for homicide, was concerned that the legal requirements for autopsy should not be violated if the heart were removed from the body. Informed that the patient had already been pronounced dead on the basis of a brain scan and that the heart was only functioning with the aid of a heart-lung machine, the medical examiner promised that no legal action would be taken against the transplant team. The procurement went ahead, and an autopsy was performed on the donor's body the next day (*Newsweek* 1968c).

This case and others, including those in Virginia, hinged on the new concept initially known as "brain death syndrome" (a term used interchangeably with "irreversible coma") and challenged the right of physicians in ICUs to declare brain death unilaterally without legal support. However, because every case was decided in their favor, physicians were effectively given a green light.

A Disorder of Criteria

Throughout the 1970s articles appeared in major American medical journals arguing that the clinical tests used to diagnose brain death were reliable and replicable (Mohandas and Chou 1971; Black 1978; Grenvik et al. 1978). Peter Black's two-part article in the *New England Journal of Medicine* (1978) acknowledges, however, that there is no official consensus in the United States on the criteria for the diagnosis.[2] This article

2. The term *criteria* is used in articles such as the one published in the *New England Journal of Medicine* in 1978 to indicate the set of signs by which a medical condition can be established. For example, fixed and dilated pupils are one criterion of death. The test for this criterion is simple: shining a bright light into the patient's eyes, which would

cites thirty different sets of criteria laid out by various advisory groups, including those of the Harvard group and the Royal College of Physicians and Surgeons of the United Kingdom.[3]

Black, a neurologist, surprisingly concludes that "whole-brain damage from which survival has never been seen can be diagnosed by many different sets of criteria," and that the criteria chosen may depend ultimately on the methods considered most reliable (Black 1978:338). He

---

normally cause the pupils to contract. The absence of legal criteria in the United States was in contrast to the situation in Argentina, Australia, Greece, and Finland, where consensus had been reached and relevant laws passed, and in Canada, France, Great Britain, and Czechoslovakia, where criteria had been agreed on and legal changes were, in most cases, pending.

3. The Conference of Royal Colleges and Faculties of the United Kingdom, greatly influenced by the highly articulate neurologist Christopher Pallis, recommended that death of the brainstem or *lower* brain constitutes the end of life (1976). Their position was: "In so far as the brain cannot function as a whole without a functioning brainstem it follows that, once reliable criteria for loss of brainstem function have been met, the patient can be diagnosed as dead" (Lamb 1985:49). Brain-stem function is diagnosed clinically, without complex technology, and the British, along with many doctors in other countries, rarely make use of the EEG or other machine-made images or printouts to confirm their diagnoses. Such machines are expensive and uncommon, and some doctors doubt their accuracy. Moreover, an EEG informs clinicians only about upper brain activity; it provides no information about the state of the lower brain. The commitment of the President's Commission to the whole-brain formulation was, it seems, an extra-cautious measure that in the end created confusion, both in theory and in clinical practice. Clinicians know that limited cellular activity often persists in the upper brain for perhaps a day or two, even when brain death has been diagnosed. Such activity is revealed by the EEG tests and cerebral blood-flow tests, such as magnetic resonance imaging, frequently employed in North America, and it raises concern and doubts among both clinicians and family members. Pallis maintains a distinction between "death of the whole brain," as specified by the President's Commission, and "death of the brain as a whole," which, he argues, can be established if it is clear that the lower brain has ceased to function. Thus, for Pallis and his colleagues, the whole-brain formulation does not provide any information that is not already provided by the lower-brain formulation. The President's Commission noted that a diagnosis of brain-stem death is actually a prognosis that "a point of no return has been reached in the process of dying," whereas whole-brain death is a diagnosis that indicates that all functions of the brain have been irreversibly damaged (President's Commission 1981:28). Some U.S. doctors have argued that the reliability of the brain-stem diagnosis is in doubt, and British doctors have emphasized that EEG tracings are not always reliable. In practice, the difference between these two approaches is negligible, except that in North America the diagnosis may be delayed while confirming tests are done. An EEG showing a flat line is helpful in confirming what clinical tests have already shown, namely that whole-brain death has occurred. But a readout showing some activity inserts doubt about the accuracy of clinical judgment, doubt that must be eliminated by more tests and further waiting. The President's Commission argued that the same basic criteria apply in Great Britain and the United States in that the brain must be permanently and irreversibly damaged (28). The neurologist James Bernat argues, however, that brain-stem death and whole-brain death share the same definition but differ in their criteria. Bernat believes that it might be possible, using the brain-stem formulation and its accompanying bedside diagnostic test, to misdiagnose patients in the "locked-in-syndrome." Such patients are fully conscious but completely unable to breathe independently, feel, or communicate in any way (1992).

notes that as of 1977, eighteen states had passed brain-death legislation, showing "noteworthy adaptation of the laws to medical and social belief" (399). The author argues forcefully that a clear distinction must be maintained between brain death and other conditions. Widespread recognition of this new diagnosis among the public could be slowed down, he argues, by concerns about "pulling the plug" prematurely, or by confusion of the irreversible, terminal state of brain death with other conditions.[4]

During the 1970s neurologists, independent of transplant surgeons, attempted to standardize the new death. Their articles were almost without exception limited to the physical condition of patients dying of brain trauma—to signs and tests, and their significance as criteria for diagnosing the new death. Little or no mention is made of organ transplants. A breach opened up between intensive care specialists and neurologists on the one hand and transplant surgeons on the other, a division that survives today. Neurologists distanced themselves from what they saw as the showy, somewhat dubious specialty of transplant surgery.[5]

Peter Black evinces some concern about the tainting of his profession when he cites a study from a "reanimation center" in Europe (Bessert et al. 1970) in which organs were procured from only 9 of 1,069 possible donors. To Black, this study and others like it indicate the great pressure that transplant surgeons might exert on ICU staff to increase the number of donated organs for transplant. He notes that the development of strict criteria for brain death is important, irrespective of organ procurement goals, and that the attending physician (the intensivist or neurologist) may find his or her goals quite at odds with those of the transplant surgeon (1978).

Other articles made it clear that not all observers were comfortable with the new death, for varying reasons, and physicians were among the dissenters. One article in the *Lancet* argues, for example, that the "doctor's dilemma" in connection with brain death arises only when patients

4. An article in *Critical Care Medicine* (Grenvik et al. 1978) noted that, contrary to the recommendation of the Harvard committee report, a second set of diagnostic tests for brain death was not deemed necessary by all the advisory groups. When repeat tests were advised, the recommended intervals between the first and second sets of tests ranged from thirty minutes to twenty-four hours. Nor was there agreement about when to certify death. Some of the groups stated that it should be done when brain death was formally declared; others, when the ventilator was removed and the heart stopped beating.

5. Several physicians commented to me that neurologists and transplant surgeons represent two poles in contemporary medicine, the one being conservative and cautious and the other flamboyant and eager to experiment.

are put on ventilators in the first place and is therefore of the doctor's making. This author affirms that the interests of neurologists are not the same as those of transplant surgeons. He notes that "prolongation of life" when nothing can be done for a patient reflects no credit on the attending doctor. Such patients should never be hooked up to life support in the first place: "It would be unfortunate if the time came when no patient in hospital could decently die without the last rite of modern medicine—a statutory period on the ventilator" (1974).

A 1979 article in the *Journal of Pediatrics,* the first of several similar publications to appear over the next decade, describes how an infant born prematurely made a "full recovery" from a three day brain-stem failure (the equivalent of brain death). The authors of this article called for caution in assuming that there was no hope for newborn infants with severe brain hemorrhages (Pasternak and Volpe 1979). Specialists in pediatric intensive care units continue to show the greatest caution and doubts about the reliability of brain-death diagnoses.

In the *Journal of the American Medical Association,* Paul Byrne and his colleagues, a group of pediatricians, set out their opposition to brain death. They distinguish clearly between cessation of brain function and the death of a person (1979). This distinction, rarely voiced in the medical literature of the 1960s and 1970s, has become increasingly prominent in recent years. Byrne and his coauthors are opposed to the "strict materialism" exhibited by some of their medical colleagues and argue that " 'brain function' is so defined [by them] as to take the place of the immaterial principle or 'soul' of man" (Byrne et al. 1979:1986). They insist that brain death stands in "flat contradiction" to the canons of Christianity, Judaism, Islam, Hinduism, and some other religious affiliations. They also argue that according to the current criteria for brain death, if the condition can be diagnosed in cases where the brain has ceased to function for hours or even days as a result of hypothermia, drug overdose, or other causes, but normal function is restored, then logically such patients must have been "resurrected from the dead." To assume that these cases are aberrations, and that such patients only "seem" to be brain-dead is, they insist, to adopt a concept empirically unable to do the job it is designed to accomplish.

Willard Gaylin, a psychiatrist and past president of the Hastings Center for research into bioethical problems, argued in an article titled "Harvesting the Dead" that the new definition of death "now permits the physician to 'pull the plug' without even committing an act of passive euthanasia" (1974:24).[6] The new cadavers, Gaylin insists, have the legal status of the dead but none of the qualities usually associated with dead bodies. " 'Neomorts' are warm, respire, have a pulse, and excrete, their bodies require nursing, including dietary and grooming attention . . . *and could probably be maintained so for a period of years*" (emphasis in original). Gaylin suggests that neomorts could be made use of legally to "serve science and mankind in dramatically useful ways." He visualizes "farms of cadavers" that require feeding and maintenance before their eventual harvest (1974:26).[7] Gaylin's prophesy of the various uses to which "neomorts" could be put became reality within the next decade, when they were used as experimental subjects for the testing of new drugs and diagnostic instruments (Dickson 1988; La Puma 1988).

Gaylin's arguments created ripples in medical circles, but they had little effect on the public. It took one widely reported case to stir up a second round of widespread unrest about the new death. As one lawyer ineptly put it, "The tragedy of Karen Ann Quinlan has been thoroughly beaten to death from legal and medical commentators to prime-time television drama" (Savage 1980).

In April 1975, for reasons that have never been made clear, twenty-one-year-old Karen Ann Quinlan ceased breathing for at least two fifteen-minute periods. She was given mouth-to-mouth resuscitation by friends. On arrival at the hospital, her pupils were dilated, and she showed no response to stimuli calculated to cause deep pain. Quinlan was later diagnosed as being in a "persistent vegetative state" (PVS), a term first coined in 1972 (Jennett and Plum). Although her upper brain was critically damaged, her lower brain remained relatively intact, so that after several weeks of complete unresponsiveness she regained sleep-wake cycles and had some reflex responses. As far as could be ascertained, she was completely unconscious and lacked any signs of cognitive activity. Her EEG was abnormal but showed some activity, and blood flow inside the cranium was normal, but Quinlan was kept on a ventilator because her ability to breathe independently, although not destroyed, was impaired.

---

6. *Passive euthanasia* refers to the practice of stopping all medical treatment when the situation is judged hopeless, as opposed to *active euthanasia*, in which something is administered or done to end the patient's life.

7. It is possible that Gaylin's image of "farms of cadavers" influenced the production of the 1978 movie *Coma*, in which the bodies of comatose or brain-dead "patients" are suspended side by side in a huge refrigerated warehouse.

In writing about this case, Savage notes that "the Harvard Committee's 'brain death' criteria may be oversimplified." In any case, in his estimation, Quinlan did not meet them. Rather, she manifested what had come to be known as "cerebral death," that is, having no cognitive function. She also met the criteria for a definition of death briefly in use in the late 1970s, namely "lung death," a concept applied to any patient on a respirator for thirty days or more who showed no improvement in pulmonary function. Quinlan did not, however, meet the traditional criteria for cardiac death. According to Savage, she was a patient who, because her heart was still beating, was alive, but who would never regain consciousness, and who in all probability would die if removed from life support.

Karen's condition worsened, she lost a great deal of weight, and her posture was described as "fetal-like and grotesque." Her father, Joseph Quinlan, asked in 1976 to be made the guardian of "the person and property" of his daughter so that his wish to discontinue treatment could be implemented (355 A2d 647 [1976]). After two months of debate, the New Jersey Supreme Court ruled that life support could be withdrawn from a "terminal, incompetent patient" if both the ethics committee of the hospital and the attending physician agreed that there was no reasonable possibility of Quinlan ever regaining a "cognitive, sapient state" (Pollock 1978:5). Artificial ventilation was stopped, but, to everyone's surprise, Quinlan was able to breathe on her own. After a further nine years of lying unconscious, she was eventually pronounced dead on June 11, 1985, from pneumonia, a disease she had contracted many months before.

The Quinlan case and others like it opened up debate about passive euthanasia and heightened existing tensions between the legal and medical worlds over the condition of patients "in that terrible limbo someplace" between life and death (Pollock 1978). The public, which had lapsed into apathy about technological death after the excitement over the first heart transplants, was now reengaged with the issue. Medicine was under new pressure to clarify, standardize, and justify their decisions about patients on ventilators. Pernick documents the sudden increase of articles in the media and popular literature about thanatology, "death with dignity," and termination of treatment (1999:17). Questions began to be asked forcefully about what exactly is meant by a "person" and a "body," and the relation between them in both life and in death.

Closing the Loopholes

The neurologist who attended Karen Quinlan, Julius Korein, was eager that the debate over death should be clarified so that what he described as ambiguous terminology leading to "gross distortion and misunderstanding" be eliminated (1978:1). He organized a conference in 1977 under the auspices of the New York Academy of Sciences, the proceedings of which were published one year later. He insists that "to continue to maintain the function of the body of a brain dead patient only because the technical means exist is a moral and economic atrocity that has evolved because of a perversion of modern science." Korein would make an exception only to facilitate organ transplants, an endeavor he describes as morally sound. (Korein was cognizant that Quinlan, still alive at this time, was not brain-dead, and would therefore be exempt from his recommendations [1978:33].)

Several papers dealing with legal, ethical, religious, and social issues were included in this conference. The philosopher Robert Veatch raises the question that had heretofore been set aside: whether "the person as a whole should be considered dead when the brain is dead" (1978:308). Veatch argues that four distinct questions should be kept separate: What are the best technical measures of the destruction of the brain? What is it that is so essential to our concept of human life that its loss should lead us to treat the individual as dead? When should our laws and our courts regard a person as dead, and when should a medical professional be authorized to pronounce death?

Veatch sets out four concepts of death: irreversible loss of the soul (a concept little used by those trained in the "world view of Western science," according to Veatch; but see chapter 10); irreversible cessation of the flow of "vital" fluids, of which the blood is the most obvious; irreversible loss of bodily integration, including spontaneous breathing, bodily reflexes, responses to stimuli, and so on; and finally, irreversible loss of consciousness or "a capacity for special interaction." In Veatch's opinion, the second and third concepts are biological reductionism; he personally favors the final one.

The important question, Veatch insists, is "not the choice between heart and brain, but rather which parts of the nervous system are so essential to human function that their irreversible loss would constitute death of the person as a whole" (1978:313). Even though in theory the brain should not exhibit any activity at all to be counted as brain-dead, clusters of brain cells often show some activity even when brain death is diagnosed (as the New York conference verified) and so, Veatch argues, one has to decide that some function above the cellular level must be present for an individual to be counted as alive. Veatch concludes, as have other participants in this debate, that no amount of technical information can ever answer conceptual and policy questions about death.

During the final discussion of the conference a report was given about a patient who had been diagnosed as brain-dead and transferred from an outlying hospital to one in central Pittsburgh for organ procurement. On repeating tests in the tertiary care hospital, it was established that the patient was not brain-dead; he was successfully resuscitated, respiratory support was continued, and plans for organ transplants were hastily abandoned. After only two weeks, the patient was sitting up in a wheelchair, eating, and talking; after another two months, he was discharged from hospital with virtually no after-effects. Those present agreed on the need for the application of ever-stricter criteria for brain death (1978:437).

Toward a Uniform Determination of Death

By 1981 six different types of brain-death statute were in existence in the United States (Pallis 1990), and a consistent public policy on the recognition of death was urgently sought. A special President's Commission was set up. In contrast to the Harvard committee, fewer than half its members were physicians. No transplant surgeons were asked to participate. After extensive discussion, the commission proposed a Uniform Determination of Death Act that was immediately supported by the American Medical Association and the American Bar Association. This act was subsequently adopted by the majority of state legislatures. Also in 1981, the Law Reform Commission of Canada published a document that became the basis for amendments to federal statutory law in connection with the recognition of death.

The President's Commission was mandated to "study and recommend ways in which the traditional legal standards can be updated in order to provide clear and principled guidance for determining whether such [artificially maintained] bodies are alive or dead" (1981:3). It set out to write an unambiguous definition of death to be incorporated, for the first time, into federal law (Annas 1988). The commission stated that it was necessary to improve what they characterized as "obsolete" diagnostic criteria in the Harvard committee statement. This strategy was opposed by a number of physicians, philosophers, and theologians who argued that the law should not have the final word on death.

The commission was explicit that its task of making a "determination of death" was quite separate from the question of allowing someone to die, although both arise from "common roots in society" (President's Commission 1981:4). It heard testimony from numerous experts, including neurologists and neurosurgeons, who argued that the legal definition of death should incorporate irreversible loss of whole-brain function.[8] The Commission also reviewed the views of leaders of the "right to life" movement, who insisted that a "clear line" must be drawn between the living and the dead, but who agreed that they could support "total brain death" (11). Even so, although the report gave emphasis to "total and irreversible brain cessation," it stressed that the commission was concerned with the death of a human being and "not the 'death' of cells tissues and organs." It asserted that policy conclusions and the statute recommendation must "accurately reflect the social meaning of death and not constitute a mere legal fiction" (31).

The commission concluded:

> The living differ from the dead in many ways. The dead do not think, interact, autoregulate or maintain organic identity through time, for example. Not all the living can always do *all* of these activities, however; nor is there one single characteristic (e.g., breathing, yawning, etc.) the loss of which signifies death. Rather, what is missing in the dead is a cluster of attributes, all of which form part of an organism's responsiveness to its internal and external environment.
>
> (36)

8. The President's Commission agreed that irreversible loss of whole-brain function should become a statutory definition of death for the following reasons:

1. Such a law would establish the legality of pronouncing death based on brain criteria;
2. The use of the brain-based standard when the heart-lung standard is not applicable would protect patients against ill-advised, idiosyncratic pronouncements of death;
3. Legal recognition of the brain-based standard would remove the doubt that exists in some states over the use of patients without brain functions as organ donors;
4. A single set of standards for death pronouncements is appropriate for all legal purposes (encompassing inheritance, taxes, and criminal trials, as well as medical treatment); and
5. Maintaining a dead body on artificial support systems consumes scarce medical resources and may unnecessarily deplete the family's emotional and financial resources.

(President's Commission 1981:10)

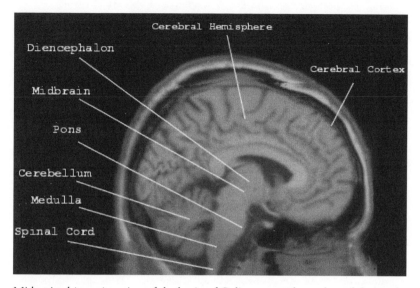

Midsagittal (cross) section of the brain of Colin, a recently graduated doctoral student in neurology. The image is created from a composite of twenty-seven magnetic resonance imaging (MRI) scans. When people speak of the "higher brain" they are referring to the cerebral hemisphere, surrounded by the cerebral cortex. When they speak of the "lower brain" or "brain stem" they have in mind the diencephalon, midbrain, pons, and medulla. Courtesy of the McConnell Brain Imaging Center, Montreal Neurological Institute.

It claimed that the concept of brain death "enjoys near universal acceptance in our society" (36). However, the public was not polled or called on to testify before the commission, and to this day we have no more than anecdotal evidence on which to ground such an assertion. On the other hand, there *is* substantial evidence indicating that a good proportion of the public is opposed to organ donation (Prottas 1994). Whether this is because people do not accept brain death as the end of human life has not been established. Given the confusion over the concept of brain death manifested by the media and the medical and legal professions in the preceding years, near-universal acceptance of brain death among the public in the early 1980s seems highly unlikely. Very few people could have had much of an idea what the term *brain death* signifies, aside from confusing images obtained from science fiction and movies such as *Coma.*

The commission was at pains to establish a set of standards that would be accepted throughout the United States. Despite its mandate to focus on the determination of death in the individual, the commission was clearly aware that its decision would influence organ transplantation. The difficulties of transporting bodies across state lines for the purposes of "treatment" without clear public policy in place were raised as a major stumbling block. It was also emphasized that physicians must know as early as possible along the continuum of dying when a mechanically supported patient's brain ceases to function, in order to care properly for organs designated for transplant.

As with the Harvard committee report, the interests of the organ transplant enterprise determined the direction of these arguments. The commission's report explicitly stated that, even when the patient is on a respirator, internal organs undergo changes that make them less fit for transplant unless they are carefully perfused and certain medications avoided. These comments were made at exactly the time when powerful new immunosuppressant drugs became available and the number of organ transplants was rapidly increasing.

The commission recommended adoption of a concept of "whole-brain death," equated with an "irreversible loss of all brain function." This condition was carefully distinguished from a "persistent vegetative state," as exemplified by Karen Ann Quinlan and the similar case of Nancy Beth Cruzan, whose brain stems continued to function. The earlier Harvard definition of "irreversible coma" left room for doubt, the commission argued, as to whether such patients could be taken for dead. To the commission, these patients count as persons, but patients diagnosed as brain-dead do not: they do not exhibit the "cluster of attributes" required to constitute a person.

Despite the effort to create uniformity, after the act was passed numerous medical professionals, philosophers, and social scientists pointed out ambiguities in its wording. These persisted largely because *two* sets of criteria for determination of death were made legal: both irreversible cessation of circulatory and respiratory functions *and* irreversible cessation of all functions of the entire brain, including the brain stem.

In summarizing this controversy, the philosopher David Lamb argued that ambiguity arose because the commission wished to avoid making a statement that appeared to be a radical departure—a "paradigm shift"—from the conventional recognition of death (1985). Lamb argued that most members of the public would be unlikely to cooperate with donation if they understood that the definition of death itself was being tinkered with, especially since brain death could not be confirmed by external observations. Patients' relatives, unable to confirm the diagnosis with their own eyes, would have to be willing to accept the results of medical tests.

To avoid public concern, the brain-based standard was simply made supplementary to the older standard for death. The commission thereby avoided the contention that brain death was a new creation intimately associated with life-support technology. Lamb supports this latter position, about which he believes the commission should have been more explicit, and claims that the ventilator has permitted us to comprehend that cardiac death is merely a prediction of the permanent nonfunctioning of the organism as a whole. Roland Puccetti, another philosopher, makes this line of argument clear: "Strictly speaking it is not true that men die of heart attacks or drowning or lung cancer. Rather these events cause paralysis or destruction of respiratory or cardiac functions which causes anoxia [a lack of oxygen] in the brain; and it is *this* which in turn causes the death of the brain and the person" (1976:250). Using this formulation, physical death does not take place until the brain, the "critical" system, is no longer capable of integrating vital subsystems: "Given that life is essentially a matter of organization, the moment of death is not the cessation of breathing and circulation, but when breathing and circulation lack neurological integration" (Lamb 1985:26). Lamb insists that there can be no *new* way of being dead, because death must always be linked to an irreversible change in the state of the organism as a whole. He concludes that brain death does not represent a new concept but is, nevertheless, a "radical reformulation of traditional concepts of death" (18). Lamb is explicit that this biological definition is the only accurate and safe way to talk about death. He is concerned that the perceived "organ shortage" will take over, permitting ever more individuals incapacitated in one way or another to be counted as dead.

As the 1968 Harvard group had done, the commission struggled to transform dying, widely regarded as a process, into a moment that could be confirmed scientifically and legally, while at the same time making it appear that nothing had radically altered. Because of their interest in organs for transplant, the commission, like the Harvard committee, sought to establish the earliest possible moment when physical death could be seen as imminent—in other words, the moment when an irreversible process had set in. In a statement much broader than that of the Harvard committee, the commission argued that if it could be agreed that the brain was no longer functioning in an integrated fashion, and that this situation could only deteriorate, then it would "naturally" follow that the "person" no longer existed.

Influential neurologists supported this position: when "neurological disintegration" has been demonstrated, what remains is "no longer a functional or *organic* unity, but merely a *mechanical* complex" (Bernat et al. 1981:391, emphasis in original). Even though many of the cells of the body remain active after this point, it was assumed that few people would dispute this concept of whole-brain death, because the brain, and by extension the "person" located in the brain, were both clearly damaged beyond recovery.

Biological Determinism and Philosophical Essentialism

Although a few outspoken people continued to argue for many years against brain death as the end of life (see, for example, Becker 1975), by the early 1980s virtually all medical professionals and academics writing about the subject in North America recognized the new death. Even so, two dominant, incompatible positions were clearly evident. In one view, death can be assessed solely on the basis of biological measurements; in the second, the death of the person and not of the body is of primary significance. This second type of death, not being directly verifiable, can only be inferred: once an irreversible loss of consciousness is medically established, supporters of this position assume that the person is dead. Some patients have irreversible damage to the whole brain, but many more of them have an intact lower brain and are therefore, by definition, not brain-dead.

The first position, held by physicians and a few philosophers such as Lamb, is that death can be defined as the "permanent cessation of functioning of the organism as a whole," by which is meant the complex interaction of organ systems regulated primarily by the brain. If specific clinical tests indicate that certain criteria have been met, then the patient should be diagnosed as "brain-dead," that is, as having irreversible dysfunction of the whole brain. This reasoning is followed irrespective of whether the patient will become an organ donor. These protagonists disagree whether death of the brain is a process or an event (Bernat et al. 1981; Korein 1978), but there is almost complete support for the idea that permanent cessation of integrated functioning of the biological organism has always been an "implicit" criterion of human death, even before the availability of artificial ventilators (Bernat et al. 1981). Moreover, they claim the brain has "always" been viewed as the center of vital agency, even though, prior to ICU technology, its demise could be assessed only indirectly as an inevitable consequence when the heart stops beating (Korein 1978).

The essence of this view is that the ventilator changes nothing; it merely permits specialists to monitor and manipulate the time of the inevitable biological death. Robert Schwager is adamant, for example, that we are misled by the visual appearance of living cadavers. Because no spontaneous breathing or circulation takes place in such a body without the ventilator, brain death represents no change in the "traditional" concept of death (1978). In making these claims, neurologists and philosophers alike assume that death concerns the organs of the body and is manifestly material. They also assume that verification of death has always been a medical matter. In this they are mistaken.

Karen Gervais, a philosopher, notes that the persistence of disagreement about what *exactly* constitutes death, even among those who argue for death as a measurable biological episode, suggests that extrabiological factors "endowed with significance" are implicated (1986:56). In other words, assumptions about "person" may well be implicated in the creation and implementation of brain-death criteria, no matter how much their role is denied. In formulating the Uniform Determination of Death Act, the commissioners attempted to face up to this dilemma, but were criticized by many for doing so, for muddying the waters.

In the other principal line of argument, the question is when it becomes morally justifiable to consider a person dead. Hans Jonas believes that it is morally wrong to treat brain-dead patients as other than alive. But by the early 1980s a diametrically opposite position, also grounded in moral theory and supported almost exclusively by moral philosophers, was clearly apparent.

Robert Veatch gives us an early taste of these arguments. He posits that "it is an affront to the dignity of the human being to treat him as alive if dead" (1975). The philosophers Michael Green and Daniel Wikler go further. They dismiss as simplistic the moral approaches to brain death taken by most of their colleagues because, they argue, merely attaching a judgment of worthlessness to the condition of brain death does not confirm whether this condition is indeed death. These authors, envisioning arguments about the worth of a brain-dead existence as a slippery slope, insist that a fundamental ontological question must be addressed:

> The notion that the brain dead patient has "ceased to exist as a person" . . . has both a moral and an ontological interpretation. The moral claim is simply that the patient's life now lacks the features that make life more valuable for

people than death. Our ontological claim is that the person who entered the hospital, he whose body is now brain dead, no longer exists (though his body or some of its parts may both exist and live).

(1980:119)

Gervais argues from a more general position:

We have adopted the convention that there is a biologically definable circumstance that constitutes death. We declare an individual dead when that biological condition is determined to have occurred. But we do not choose which biological state constitutes the event of death (which is not just a biological, but also a social, moral and metaphysical event) on the basis of biological reasoning alone. Death is not simply "a matter of scientific fact" . . . The death of a person is different from that of a dog or a cat; every death of a person unravels and reconstitutes a complex net of rights and obligations that usually involve many people. Death is not simply an event in the life of the deceased. . . . Permanent unconsciousness, whatever its basis, represents these changes.

(1986:152)

Green and Wikler sow the seeds of an argument that Gervais elaborates, namely that a permanent lack of consciousness is crucial in establishing death of persons, and therefore that the condition of the upper brain alone can signify death. Lamb stands forcefully against this position, in which, he points out, "personal identity" is made into "the measure of life" (1990:46). He insists that the "essence" of personal identity is an elusive concept and certainly not one on which doctors should rely in making decisions about death. After all, personal identity does not have any specific anatomical location, but is a quality akin to "spirit," "will," or "soul," with religious, legal, and political associations. Above all, Lamb fears that talk about identity and persons opens the door to abuse of patients in an era when pragmatism and utilitarianism hold sway.

Criticisms of the President's Commission report lent momentum during the 1980s to arguments in favor of the concept of upper brain death. Richard Zaner, a bioethicist and the editor of *Death: Beyond Whole-Brain Criteria*, argued that for whole-brain advocates, "it is the biological organism (or, more specifically, the physiological/anatomical nervous system) which is definitive for life and death, not the *person* whose organism (or nervous system) it is" (1988:7). Zaner supports advocates of cerebral, upper-brain-death when he suggests that the President's Commission "put the cart before the horse" by trying to develop a concept of death out of a set of standardized medical tests while evading the central issue of just *who* had died (5). Neither operational criteria nor valid tests can be created, Zaner argues, without a working definition of what it means to die. The team of Edward Bartlett and Stuart Youngner, a philosopher and a psychiatrist, add that such a definition has to be "societal" and not biological, since it is the permanent loss of personhood that should be of central concern, rather than the demise of the physical body (1988).

Cerebral death—an absence of consciousness in a spontaneously breathing body—like whole-brain death, could exist only with the assistance of technomedicine (Kaufman 2000). Although most PVS patients (many of whom might be considered cerebrally dead) do not need the assistance of a ventilator to breathe, intravenous nourishment and tube feeding are essential. Cerebral death confronts us with yet another ambiguous life-form that until recently was imaginable only in science fiction. The determination of cerebral death is made on the basis of an irreversible loss of consciousness.

This kind of argument assumes that "person," "self," and "identity" are constituted and manifested entirely through individual consciousness, in the brain, and, further, that such an idea of person is universal. I disagree. Charles Taylor (1989) has shown how the emergence of a bounded self located in the mind is intimately associated with early modern European history, and anthropological research makes clear considerable geographical variation in the construction of person and self (see Geertz 1973; Heelas and Lock 1981). Even so, commentators arguing in favor of the new deaths persist in their unexamined truth claims.

Historically and cross-culturally, death has been emphasized as a social event: as the death of the person and as a loss experienced by a social unit or units. The physical demise of individuals and their social death do not always coincide closely. Although social and personal death and their memorialization usually take place after physical death, under certain circumstances the situation is reversed. Those who argue for recognition of cerebral death suggest that personal death should be recognized as the end of the road: the fact that the patient's body is alive is irrelevant. Recognition of social death in advance of physical death is most common when individuals are in bondage, servitude, or slavery, are ostracized as polluted, violent, or antisocial, or when they have certain lingering, incapacitating illnesses such as Alzheimer's disease or other dementias (Mulkay and Ernst 1991; Post 1995; Sweeting and Gilhooly 1997). In these situations people are liable to be stripped of the usual complement of moral entitlement, even when clearly alive physically. However, usually we do not go on to bring about their physical death—not yet, that is.

With the assistance of technology we can postpone the physical death of patients whose entire brains are traumatized beyond hope of recovery. If the patient is not to become an organ donor, then usually the process is prolonged only briefly, while brain death is confirmed.[9] When a brain-dead patient is to become an organ donor, then biological dying is postponed for a much longer period, specifically so that the body may be commodified. Here resides a new, technologically manipulated death. To go one step further and equate an irreversible loss of consciousness alone with human death would constitute a radically new departure, one that should not be countenanced without extensive *public* debate. If patients with cerebral death are to become organ donors, then we would be practicing active euthanasia by killing the "person" while preserving the living body as best we can.

Brain-dead patients will, we know for certain, "die" as soon as they are removed from the ventilator. We take comfort from this knowledge when proclaiming them dead even though they look alive. But patients in cerebral death are rarely on ventilators and can usually breathe without assistance. All they need is assistance with feeding—as do a great number of patients who are obviously fully alive. To think of them as dead is entirely counterintuitive, and their condition raises a set of urgent, obdurate problems that we have conveniently ducked. What exactly do we mean by consciousness? Is it located entirely in the brain? Can we determine its irreversibility with certainty? If so, will we be able to reach consensus that an irreversible loss of consciousness alone is the death of a person? Will we then be comfortable having the death of the person routinely count as legal death, so that the physical end can be hastened? Which doctors will be willing to take organs for donation from individuals who may be breathing unaided, even when they have previously given their consent? What should be our response to members of society who do not support cerebral death: do we override their sentiments? What if we find that they are in the majority? How will the economics of long-term care for permanently comatose patients affect these decisions? And how will the so-called shortage of organs for transplant affect our course of action? These troubling questions are addressed in later chapters.

9. This is not the case in Japan, where the ventilator is routinely kept in place even after a diagnosis of brain death (see chapter 11).

Confusion in the Clinic

Over the three decades of the unresolved brain-death debate, intensivists have continued with their daily routine. Small surveys have occasionally been carried out in North America to ascertain what doctors were actually doing and thinking when they attended patients with severe head injuries, some of whom would eventually be declared brain-dead.

In 1970 and 1971, shortly after the Harvard committee report, 1,410 specialists in internal medicine and 650 neurosurgeons were asked whether they would turn off the respirator of a patient who satisfied the Harvard criteria for brain death. There were few differences between these specialists in their responses. Of the entire sample, just over 70 percent reported that they would turn off the ventilator, and slightly less than half reported that they would consult with the family before taking action. The remaining physicians said they would not turn off the respirator because, in their opinion, to do so would be murder (Crane 1976); in other words, these doctors did not accept the concept of brain death.

A couple of years later, a study evaluated the opinions of 100 lay persons, 100 physicians, and 70 first-year medical students about death. The results showed that 46 percent of the physicians, 42 percent of the medical students, and 60 percent of the public did not equate brain death with the end of life. The authors of this article recommended that, among the medical profession at least, it is important to "aim for some unification of thought" in connection with death (Delmonico and Randolph 1973:234).

In 1984, a three-page questionnaire was sent to a random sample of 300 neurologists in the United States and Canada. Of the 112 responses, 94 percent believed that determination of brain death was a meaningful diagnosis. However, among the 54 percent of respondents who actually used this diagnosis in clinical practice between one and five times a year, the criteria used varied considerably (Black and Zervas 1984).[10] More

10. Between 80 and 85 percent of the doctors required an absence of pupillary reflex and corneal reflex, inability to breathe spontaneously when the ventilator was temporarily removed (the apnea test), and an absence of eye movements with head turning (the doll's eyes test). Only 61 percent required an absent cough reflex, 69 percent an absent gag reflex, 59 percent dilated pupils, 56 percent a body temperature of under 90° Fahrenheit, and 43 percent a blood barbiturate level of zero. (Patients admitted to the hospital as hypothermic are excluded and should never be regarded as candidates for a brain-death diagnosis.) Over 65 percent required a flat EEG, but 29 percent required only one reading, and 36 percent required two readings twenty-four hours apart. An absence of deep tendon

than 25 percent thought that no single criterion clearly and conclusively indicated death, and no single clinical finding was cited by every respondent as definitive.[11]

The physicians were apparently unaware of these discrepancies, because 53 percent of them thought that a consensus existed about the criteria for diagnosing brain death. Nevertheless, they disagreed whether national guidelines were needed. Only 38 percent thought that such guidelines would be helpful; 17 percent stated that there should definitely *not* be uniform guidelines, and 51 percent were working in hospitals with no written guidelines. The researchers who conducted the survey concluded that the majority of doctors "seemed to consider the judgment of an individual physician to be accurate" and that a strong preference was shown for physician autonomy in a brain-death diagnosis (172).

The same doctors were asked what they would do when the family of a brain-dead patient did not agree that their relative was dead. Seventy-eight percent said that they would keep the patient on the ventilator, but about a third of them would nevertheless formally declare death. Only 6 percent would stop the ventilator against the family's wishes. The rest were undecided. These findings indicated to the researchers that "there is as much variety in the actions that follow the fulfillment of brain death criteria as there is in the criteria themselves" (173). Despite their wish for autonomy, a good number of physicians apparently recognized the importance of the cooperation of families when making a declaration of brain death. The study does not make clear whether it was concerns about litigation, about organ procurement, ethical and social issues, or whether it was some combination of these factors, that caused the shift in attitude from the earlier studies.

The authors of the 1984 study concluded that the concept of brain death is "novel and radical, although it seems to be a logical extension of previous definitions of death. It is not surprising, therefore, that it leads to ambiguities and contradictions in the behavior of neurologists and neurosurgeons facing its implementation" (Black and Zervas 1984:

---

reflexes was required by only 26 percent. The time interval between the two sets of tests varied between six and twenty-four hours.

11. By the early 1980s, several publications had argued that the diagnosis of brain death in very young children was unreliable, perhaps impossible; nevertheless, 55 percent of the questionnaire respondents used the same criteria for determining brain death in young children as in adults.

174). The existence of ambiguities is perhaps no surprise; but the authors' apparent absence of worry that mistakes might result from the ambiguities is, I think, very surprising indeed.

In 1989 Stuart Youngner and colleagues published what has come to be the most frequently cited research on knowledge among health care professionals about brain death. The report was based on findings from a survey of 195 physicians and nurses in the United States. Eight years after the publication of the Uniform Determination of Death Act, only 35 percent of these respondents correctly identified the established legal and medical criteria for determining brain death, and 58 percent did not consistently use a coherent concept of death. The sample was mixed with respect to age, ethnicity, and religious beliefs, but these differences did not appear to affect individual responses significantly. Professionals working in intensive care units and directly responsible for declaring brain death gave more consistent answers than did respondents who worked in transplant units.

Ninety-five percent of respondents stated that a patient meeting the criteria for whole-brain death was dead, but they reached this conclusion for a variety of reasons. When asked to comment on a patient in a persistent vegetative state who was breathing independently, 38 percent responded that because there was no activity in the upper brain—because the patient was unconscious—this patient too was brain-dead. When pressed for details, about 60 percent of the respondents made statements to the effect that although brain-dead patients are legally dead, nevertheless caregivers continue to believe that the patient is alive but that their condition is hopeless, or that the patient's quality of life is unacceptable.

On the basis of these findings, Youngner and colleagues argue: "Brain death can suggest all too easily that only the brain has died, but that the patient continues to live"(2209). These authors agree with the British neurologist Christopher Pallis that technical data can never answer purely conceptual questions, and that criteria for determining death must be kept separate from concepts that explain the "meaning of death." They argue that "irreversible loss of all brain function has been widely accepted as a *criterion* for determining death, without a corresponding, widely accepted *concept* explaining exactly why brain dead patients *are* dead." Youngner and colleagues are concerned that if health professionals lack consistency in their own understanding of death, they may not be effective in explaining brain death to the families of dying patients. Further, confusion about the status of the brain-dead must surely cause emotional discomfort when sending patients for organ donation (2210).

The philosopher and lawyer team of Daniel Wikler and Alan Weisbard, in an article titled "Appropriate Confusion over Brain Death," insist that the findings of Youngner and colleagues do *not* suggest that brain death is being misdiagnosed. The problem lies, these authors claim, with the conceptual foundations of the whole-brain definition, not in the diagnostic tools or the legal formulation: "There is no consensus over whether, and especially why, [a diagnosis of brain death] means that [a patient has] died" (1989:2246). Although loss of integrative function of the brain is central to the idea of brain death, the entire intensive care unit temporarily serves as an artificial brain stem. This makes it appear to all concerned—physicians, nurses, families—as though the patient is alive. Comments such as these highlight the insurmountable difficulty that even when a living cadaver is declared legally dead, it remains physically and morally anomalous: a hybrid of life and death, irreversibly without consciousness, but sustained by a breathing machine and a team of experts who monitor virtually every body system.

Clearly plenty of room exists for conceptual confusion, but the possibility of actual mistakes and even malpractice cannot be ruled out. One is left to wonder whether there have been cases when procurement has started before the patient is indeed brain-dead. If organ donation proceeds, it is impossible to show when an error has occurred.

Elusive Clarity

Despite persistent doubts as to what actually constitutes death, how best it should be determined in intensive care units, and what it signifies, the criteria for whole-brain death are characterized as exceedingly robust by those who put them into practice. It is often assumed, despite the lack of evidence, that a consensus, one that includes the public, has been reached about this new death. Clearly, however, the debate remains, in Thomas Kuhn's terms, in a paradigm crisis. Even though "experts" have arrived at "a superficial and fragile consensus" (Youngner 1992:570), disputes persist. James Bernat, a neurologist, argues that active disagreement continues about the "concept, and hence the measurement of death" (1992).

With improved technologies in trauma units, brain-dead individuals who are not summarily made into organ donors, but are left attached to ventilators, increasingly survive for months and even years. Is this a "living death"? Because of the existence of transplant technology, incentives to routinize and justify diagnoses of brain death as the end of life have been enormous. Youngner argues that as a result of this pressure "we have identified a group of severely injured and dying persons who are so 'beyond harm' that we feel justified in killing them in order to obtain their organs. Since we would rather not think that we are killing them, we simply gerrymander the line between life and death [as if such a line existed!] to include them in the latter category" (1996:50).

Despite these disquieting thoughts, nearly everyone who has participated in discussions, whether neurologists, philosophers, or lawyers, believes that human death can today be located in the brain—although not everyone believes that death is *exclusively* situated there. Some argue for death as an event, others for a process; but if organs are to be procured for transplant, then, everyone agrees, a legal moment of death must be recognized. This moment, some argue, is when a diagnosis of whole-brain death is made. Others, notably in the United Kingdom, define that moment as the time when brain-stem death is diagnosed. Both these concepts are legally recognized in many parts of the world.[12] Many involved physicians, together with the relatively few philosophers, lawyers, and others who agree with Lamb's position, argue that death should be understood entirely as a scientifically measurable biological event, one that is legally recognized but nevertheless dissociated from moral or societal implications, aside from occasional unavoidable disputes about the settlement of wills.

Yet others, mostly philosophers, argue for a recognition of upper brain or cerebral death. The majority of these are concerned above all with the death of persons, rather than of brains; but they concur that a person's death is nevertheless located in the brain and is manifested solely by an irreversible lack of consciousness.

Although it is often assumed that the history of brain death has followed a common path in Europe and North America, not all of these countries have responded in the same way. Germany, for example, recently reversed an earlier decision to accept brain death as the end of life (Hogle 1999; Schöne-Seifert 1999). Doubts have persisted in Sweden and Denmark, where the concept of brain death was recognized only in

---

12. Several Japanese physicians unofficially recognize brain-stem death and closely follow the research and writing of Christopher Pallis. However, the official criteria in Japan, the Takeuchi criteria, are based on whole-brain death.

the late 1980s and the early 1990s, respectively (Brante and Hallberg 1991; Rix 1999). In Denmark between 1987 and 1990, more than a thousand publications appeared on brain death, and the Danish public participated in a massive debate in which their opinion was carefully polled (a debate that greatly interested the Japanese). The Danish parliament passed a bill in 1990 recognizing a set of brain-death criteria. However, although brain death is acknowledged as integral to the process of dying in certain patients, it is not considered to be the moment of death, which continues to be recognized as the point when the heart and lungs cease to function. The situation in Japan today resembles quite closely that of Denmark (Rix 1999).

The participants in these debates have been aware that the transplant enterprise depends crucially on the presentation of statements, definitions, and guidelines about death to professional organizations, the media, and the public. If the public believes that experts are tinkering with death in order to harvest organs, then organ donation will drop precipitously (Schöne-Seifert 1999). No matter how much certain commentators work to keep organ transplants out of the debate, and try to establish criteria for brain death independently of the desires of the transplant world, these two domains are irrevocably linked.

Given the muddle that remains as to what exactly an irreversibly damaged brain signifies for person and body, the usual hubris about the universal applicability of categories of knowledge created in the West is singularly inappropriate. Is it reasonable to imagine that everyone will respond to a living cadaver in the same way? Or that the moral status of the brain-dead be pronounced on behalf of citizens, whether by medical diagnosis, legal fiat, or philosophical sophistry? One advantage of the drawn-out Japanese debate about brain death has been extensive public discussion. But this happened largely because the media, certain influential intellectuals, and some members of the public, categorically opposed to having death redefined for them by physicians, spoke out. Of course, a price was paid for their concerns, because people waiting for transplants were left in despair and ready to declare, like Kiuchi Hirofumi, that his country was killing him. The Japanese story is taken up in the next chapter.

TRAGEDY

Claude Leduc was nine years old when he died.[1] He was run over by the next-door neighbor while playing in the driveway leading to his house and the neighbor's garage. It was a Sunday afternoon, and his parents were home. They heard the squeal of the car brakes just outside the house and rushed out to find their son, the second of their three boys, lying on the ground with his leg twisted at an impossible angle. He was unconscious and not breathing spontaneously, but this did not trouble his frantic parents as much as the sight of his contorted leg. An ambulance was called, and Claude was given manual ventilation while he was transported for fifteen minutes through the empty Sunday streets to Children's Hospital. His parents traveled in the ambulance and then watched helplessly as the ICU staff placed Claude on the ventilator and then inserted tubes and lines into him. His father recalls that Claude looked perfectly normal, as though he was lying peacefully sleeping, and he and his wife remained more concerned about Claude's leg than anything else.

Claude's father works in the computer business and is a practicing Roman Catholic. His wife was born in Japan but has lived in Canada for twenty-five years. She was raised as a Christian and sometimes at-

1. The interview was conducted in the Leduc home approximately one year after the death of their child.

tends the local Protestant church. All three of their sons attended a local Catholic school.

After the results of various tests came back, the doctor in charge of the case asked Claude's parents to sit down while he talked with them. He told them that Claude was in grave condition, having received a severe blow to his head, and the situation looked very bad indeed. Several hours later, after more clinical tests, the doctor informed them that Claude was brain-dead and that there was no hope for his recovery. The Leducs were told that the tests would be repeated six hours later as a confirmation, but that the situation was irreversible and hopeless. While they were waiting, dazed, Mr. and Mrs. Leduc made several phone calls to their own parents and to their closest friends. Everyone they talked to said that they should not give up hope, that medicine these days can do amazing things; and they were reminded that sometimes miracles happen. Much as the Leducs wanted to believe in a miracle, and even though it looked as though their child was simply sleeping, they accepted what the doctor told them. In retrospect they are grateful for his frank but gentle manner; the resolution of the physician allowed them to come to terms with the situation even when their own families were chiding them for giving up too easily.

Twenty-four hours after Claude's arrival in the hospital, the second set of tests for brain death was done, and the doctor pronounced Claude dead. He then inquired whether the Leducs would like to consider organ donation. Mr. Leduc replied instantly that he did not want this to happen. Over a year after the death of his son, Mr. Leduc said that even though he is a practicing Catholic, he does not believe in life after death. Nevertheless, organ donation simply did not feel right to him; he had a "gut reaction" that he should not agree to it. His wife thought that it might be a generous thing to do if the lives of other children could be saved, but she resigned herself quickly to the decision of her husband. She says that neither she nor her husband has any regrets.

After the second brain-death diagnosis, the Leducs asked for the ventilator to be left on for a few more hours so that they could stay quietly at their son's side. Then they went home, where their children were still hoping for good news because their grandparents had decided that the children's parents must be the ones to tell them that their brother was dead.

Mr. Leduc says that no one in their family has ever needed an organ transplant, and that perhaps if they had had some exposure to that kind of suffering he might have responded differently. Mrs. Leduc emphasizes that they were unable to think about anything other than Claude and that in their state of shock they could not make any decisions that would create yet more anxiety. Neither she nor her husband has signed their driver's license as a potential donor. Although she herself would never have an organ transplant, she says, she probably would want a transplant if one of her children became very sick. Mrs. Leduc immediately acknowledges that her position is contradictory and inconsistent; what worries her most is that someone must die in order for someone else to have a transplant, and she sounds thoroughly Buddhist when she insists, in English, "One shouldn't crave what other people have."[2]

Mr. Leduc agrees with his wife that transplants are "not natural." He says that we "shouldn't interfere and tinker around so much with human life," and adds: "If it was natural to give organs, we'd be able to unzip ourselves and take them out. It's just not rational. Mixing people up is not right—it's all too emotional and irrational." The Leducs donate as much money as they can afford each year to the hospital where their son died.

The funeral was held at Claude's school. The Leducs thought that this arrangement was best for their own children and for Claude's friends. The family goes to visit his grave sometimes, but they never talk about Claude's death. Mr. Leduc describes the family as private, unemotional, and not outwardly expressive. But they do keep Claude's toys, and although his death is not mentioned, they talk about his life very freely. The Leducs believe now that it was God's will that their son should die young. They do not talk about their next-door neighbor; perhaps he moved away.

In the face of tragedy, not everyone is comfortable with the idea of transcending death through a donation of organs. Who would dare to pronounce this family, and the many others like them, as selfish?

---

2. Susan Long (personal communication, 1999) suggests that the idea of "craving" is very close to the biblical notion of "coveting" and that Mrs. Leduc could be drawing on one or both traditions here. Neither Christian nor Buddhist commentators have, to my knowledge, criticized organ transplants on the grounds of craving or covetousness.

FIVE

Japan and the Brain-Death "Problem"

The Wada Case

In August 1968, the world's thirtieth heart transplant was carried out in Sapporo, Japan. Dr. Wada Jiro[1] transplanted the heart of twenty-year-old Yamaguchi Yoshimasa, who had drowned the previous day, into the body of eighteen-year-old Miyazaki Nobuo, whose heart was swollen "due to various complications" (*Asahi Shinbun* 1968a). Wada, a thoracic surgeon, was responsible both for declaring the donor dead and for the transplant surgery. As with previous heart transplants elsewhere, the event was heralded by the media as a medical triumph and the doctor lauded as a hero, but this adulation was short-lived.

The name of the donor was not revealed at the time of the operation because the donor's father requested anonymity. Neither of Yamaguchi's siblings, in their late teens at the time, supported their parents' hesitant decision to donate. But four days after the operation, the seclusion came to an end when they were photographed meeting the recipient's family. The Yamaguchi parents are reported to have said at this meeting that their son, having had no chance in his short life to do anything for society, was now happy. The recipient's father, Mr. Miyazaki, responded that he could not find words enough to express his thanks, and, if the idea were acceptable to the Yamaguchis, he would like their re-

---

1. Japanese names are given here with the family name first, as is customary.

lationship to become as one of relatives. When asked, Yamaguchi's sister agreed that she was now not opposed to the donation, and that she was able to think of her brother as still alive; but, bursting into tears, she added that she wished the body could have been left alone and not cut about (*Asahi Shinbun* 1968b).

Wada reported that the operation had been a technical success, even though several medical colleagues, including thoracic surgeons, described it as premature and experimental. Noting the poor survival rate for previous transplants, one reporter demanded why Wada had gone ahead when he had earlier stated that transplants should not be done until problems with organ rejection had been resolved. Wada claimed that just before going off to the United States for several months of training earlier in the year, he had changed his mind (*Asahi Shinbun* 1968c).

For the first two months after the transplant, Miyazaki apparently made good progress. His condition then took a turn for the worse; he made a transitory recovery but died eighty-three days after the operation. The cause of death was registered as bronchitis (*Asahi Shinbun* 1968d). In the following days, several articles appeared in Japanese newspapers stating that the surgery had been purely experimental and, more ominously, that there was no evidence that the donor had indeed been brain-dead. No EEG printout was available, nor were there any written records about how the donor's death had been determined. It also appeared that Wada had lied about several details of the procedure (*Asahi Shinbun* 1968d). In December 1968, Wada was charged with intentional homicide and professional negligence resulting in death in connection with the deaths of both donor and recipient. The charges were made by an Osaka M.D. whose specialty is herbal medicine, together with several of his colleagues (Nakajima 1985). Two other plaintiffs later brought further charges (Machino and Akiba 1993).

Miyazaki's original physician, speaking eight months after the transplant, asserted that Miyazaki's condition did not warrant a heart transplant. When Miyazaki was transferred to Wada's care (in the same hospital), this doctor understood that only replacement of one mitral valve was needed. During questioning by the police, Wada claimed that three of Miyazaki's heart valves were defective. However, a month later a pathologist from the same Sapporo hospital confirmed that only one valve was damaged. In June 1969, nearly a year after the surgery, the Sapporo Public Prosecutor's Office finally acted on the charges against Wada. Well over one hundred people were interviewed as part of the

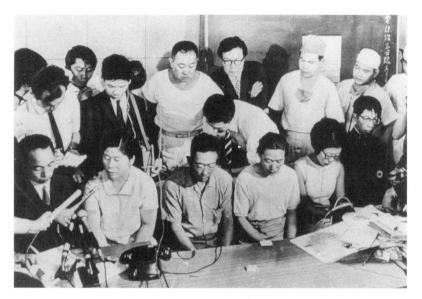

The Wada case. In the front row, the parents of the heart recipient are flanked by the donor's family. Dr. Wada appears in surgical garb in the center of the back row. Reproduced by permission of *Asahi Shinbun*, Tokyo.

formal investigation. Others gave expert testimony, including three doctors who had been requested to examine what was purportedly Miyazaki's own damaged heart.

After the Sapporo and the Supreme Public Prosecutor's offices held a joint session in the fall of 1971, they decided to drop the charges, but a group of thirteen doctors, lawyers, and social commentators, and two former ministers of the Department of Health and Welfare requested that the investigation be continued (a Japanese lawyer later described this group ironically as the "wise men" [Bai 1990:991]). At first the group confined their attention to the ethical matter of human rights, but then they pressed for legal action. After considerable hesitation, the police responded that although many unresolved issues and a "degree of suspicion" remained, they did not have enough evidence to make a conclusive case. Charges were conclusively dropped in August 1972 (Nakajima 1985).

In her 1985 book on brain death (discussed further below), Nakajima Michi, who has a master's degree in law, summarizes the issues in the Wada case that, in her estimation, raised the most suspicion. Why, when Yamaguchi was making a good recovery from drowning, was he suddenly transferred from a small hospital to the Sapporo central hospital? When he was taken from the first hospital, Yamaguchi was breathing independently, and his condition was described as stable. The media and the ambulance driver were told that he needed to be placed in a high-pressure oxygen tent; however, Wada apparently used this device only for about twenty minutes, whereas, if it was to be at all effective, treatment should have been continued for several days.

Nakajima believes Wada started planning the heart transplant as soon as he was informed about the drowning. An unprecedented twenty or more surgeons, all part of Wada's team, surrounded Yamaguchi as he arrived on a stretcher at the Sapporo hospital. A large quantity of blood of Miyazaki's type had already been laid in at the hospital. Nakajima is also concerned, as reporters were, as to when exactly the donor died and how death was determined.

The public furor over the Wada transplant focused on the possible murder of the donor, but the medical profession was more concerned about unprofessional treatment of the recipient, Miyazaki Nobuo. The Sapporo hospital pathologist eventually became convinced that the heart he was given to examine, supposedly Miyazaki's, was either not the original heart or else had been tampered with. The defective valves attached to the heart looked as though they belonged to another heart entirely. It seems clear in retrospect, as Wada's colleagues had intimated, that the recipient was not so ill as to require a heart transplant.

Nakajima asserts that evidence relevant to the case simply disappeared over the two years of the investigation, and, further, that each of the twenty members of the Wada surgical team told exactly the same story to the police, a story that had obviously been rehearsed (see also Nishioka 1989). She criticizes the police for being timid when investigating physicians (Nakajima 1985) and also targets the "protection" that Japanese medical professionals provide for each other (others, too, are very critical of the "predisposition to concealment," *inpei taishitsu,* shown by physicians; see Nishioka 1989).

It was not until 1988 that the Japanese public learned, from some of the findings of the police investigation, that Wada had indeed lied to the media (*Tokyo Shinbun* 1988b). In 1991, a transplant surgeon testifying before a government committee confirmed that after the removal of the recipient's own heart, one of its valves had been replaced by a valve from another heart to exaggerate the degree of deterioration of Miyazaki's heart (*Asahi Shinbun* 1991a).

The Wada case is considered today as a scandal, a barbarous piece of medical experimentation carried out by a doctor who, significantly to some, had received a good portion of his training in America, and who practices medicine in the "wild west" of Japan, the northern island of Hokkaido. Wada is also said to have an aggressive personality, one that is not characteristically Japanese. The case set off a train of events that made it impossible to do organ transplants making use of brain-dead donors without serious fear of legal reprisals. It is therefore perhaps not surprising that it took nearly three decades for brain death to be legally recognized in Japan, and then only under strictly specified conditions; nor that thirty-one years passed before a second heart transplant was carried out, in March 1999.

Before the Wada transplant, two livers had been transplanted at Chiba University in the 1960s; neither of the patients survived, and until 1999 no further transplants using livers or hearts from brain-dead donors were carried out, with one possible exception in 1993 when a liver may have been taken from a brain-dead donor (Nakajima 1994). The transplantation of kidneys, nearly two-thirds of which are procured from living related donors (a practice itself not without ethical concerns), has not been impeded; kidneys are also taken from cadaver donors right after the heart stops beating.[2] The number of kidney transplants is very low compared with that in North America. In 2000, 13,175 patients were on transplant waiting lists and 200,000 were on dialysis, the highest per-capita ratio in the world (Nihon Ishoku Gakkai: 2000).

Since 1989, Japan has pioneered transplants in which a segment of a parent's liver is transplanted into a child (over two hundred such procedures have been done without death of a donor).[3] In 1998 the world's first living-donor lung transplant was carried out in Japan. This procedure requires two donors, in this instance one parent and one sibling. Japanese transplant surgeons often claim that they have been driven to these innovative techniques because of the impasse over brain death. Even after passage of the Organ Transplant Bill in 1997, no donation from brain-dead donors occurred for over a year (Watts 1998a).

2. Relatively few kidney transplants have been transplanted from cadavers anywhere in the world. The results of such transplants are not as good as when kidneys are obtained from brain-dead bodies or living donors.

3. Since the inception of the technique in 1989, 127 children have received segments of liver procured from a parent. These children have a better four-year survival rate than do patients in other countries who have received livers transplanted from brain-dead donors (Ota et al. 1995). In 1999, 218 living related liver donations were carried out in the United States (United Network for Organ Sharing 2000a).

Despite fears of repercussions, doctors have quietly carried out approximately two hundred kidney transplants making use of brain-dead donors (heart and liver transplants would have been too showy and risky). In 1991, a team of physicians appeared defiantly lined up in a newspaper photograph, having decided to go public about a kidney transplant that they had conducted months before, using a brain-dead donor (*Mainichi Daily News* 1991a). In the mid-1990s this practice came to a halt when the Japanese parliament engaged in a debate about brain death; transplant surgeons did not want to risk public furor when use of brain-dead bodies for organ donation might shortly be legalized. However, they had to wait another three years.

It appears that donor families were not always informed that their relatives were brain-dead when donations were made, and that some families may have assumed that the donor's heart had stopped beating before the organs were removed. For example, in another case in 1991, a patient was declared brain-dead by a medical team and his kidneys procured for donation, but it was later revealed that although the family had given consent, they did not realize that their relative was brain-dead and that his heart was still beating. One of the involved surgeons commented, "It didn't even occur to me to tell the family that I was removing the organs after their relative was pronounced brain-dead; they were eager to donate his kidneys, and the chances of success are higher with fresh organs, so I went ahead" (*Mainichi Daily News* 1991b).

From Scandals to Impasse

The Wada case confirmed deeply held suspicions that many Japanese people already held about tertiary care medicine. Until well into the twentieth century, the practice of medicine in Japan, thoroughly and respectably grounded in Confucian ethics, was acclaimed as a benevolent art *(i wa jin jutsu nari)*. In modern Japan the word for benevolence *(jin)* has been turned, through a clever play on words, into that used for money *(kin)*, so that medicine is now ridiculed as a money-making art *(i wa kin jutsu nari)*. In a society where until recently it has occasionally been possible to buy a place in medical school, where cheating on national licensing examinations has been exposed, where doctors (legitimately) make a considerable portion of their income from prescribing medication, and are sometimes implicated in bribery and corruption scandals, the Japanese public, along with some doctors, puts little faith in the profession as a whole. They may respect and trust their own family doctors, but they distrust hospital-based medicine, with its long waits for consultations with doctors that last only a few minutes.

The lawyer Bai Kōichi, writing right after the Wada case about legal aspects of brain death, expresses concerns similar to those aired in Europe and North America: whether two definitions of death can be justified, whether it is appropriate to legislate what constitutes death, and whether physicians should have the sole authority to determine death. But Bai further argues that any definition of death cannot be "developed or modified arbitrarily by the legal profession, or adopted independently by the medical profession, for it must be based on a concept of death acceptable to the public" (1970:39). Even when related arguments are raised in North America, it is usually simply assumed that the public is in agreement with the new death (Black 1978).

Astutely, Bai recognizes that "the body may for a while show features of both life and death" after "death of the brain." He suggests that this time could be called the "alpha period," a time that lies "between life and death, but belonging fully to neither." In Bai's opinion, a legal agreement could be hammered out specifically to cover the removal of organs during the alpha period, provided that potential donors have given prior assent and close relatives agree. Bai is sensitive to the fact that all existing law in connection with life and death depends on a dichotomous distinction. He insists that such a distinction is in effect, arbitrary, although he recognizes its utility in law; but he believes that some flexibility is in order when it comes to the new technological death (1970:41).

In 1974 criteria for brain death were set out in a report by a committee of the Japan Electroencephaly Association, a committee formed right after the Wada case that clearly took its time doing its work. The Wada case having faded from public memory, the report received little public attention; nor did many other publications on brain death appear in the 1970s (Bai 1990).

In 1979 a law was passed in Japan governing the transplantation of corneas and kidneys. Transplants were covered for the first time by the national health insurance system, and a National Center for Kidney Transplantation was established (Bai and Hirabayashi 1984). In 1980 a law was passed that permitted organ procurement only by authorized organ banks, and the sale of organs was prohibited.

The situation changed dramatically in the 1980s, primarily because medical professionals pushed the government to clarify its position on organ transplants from brain-dead donors. The move was spurred by knowledge that the Uniform Determination of Death Act had passed in the United States, allowing organ transplants to become routine in that country, along with the availability of improved immunosuppressants. Japanese lawyers were also worried about the effect of brain death on inheritance claims (*Yomiuri Shinbun* 1984). And public unrest was re-fueled by another controversial transplant case.

In 1984 organs for use in a kidney and pancreas transplant were procured from a forty-one-year-old woman declared brain-dead at Tsu-kuba University. She had reportedly told her husband prior to her illness that she wished to donate her heart but no other organs. Four months later the Tokyo University–based Patient's Rights Committee took the transplant surgeon to court. The recipient, a diabetic, died ten months after transplant surgery, and a second charge was brought in connection with his death.

Confusion arose in this case because the donor was reported as men-tally impaired when hospitalized, because of earlier brain hemorrhages, and although her husband stated that she was willing to donate her heart, the physician apparently interpreted this to mean that her inten-tion was to donate all her organs (Nakajima 1985). Partly in response to this much-publicized case, the Life Ethics Problem Study Parlimen-tarians League, composed of twenty-eight Diet members and forty-five other professionals, was established. This group endorsed the need for legislation about brain death, but achieved little else. Early in 1988 the Public Prosecutors' Office decided to "freeze," or table, the Tsukuba case, reportedly because it had been impossible to reach consensus about what constitutes human death. Although brain death had been recog-nized in the West and the medical world was calling for its recognition in Japan, a public poll conducted by the Prime Minister's Office in 1987 showed that only 24 percent of respondents thought brain death was the end of life. The Japan Federation of Bar Associations reiterated a common argument that until there was public consensus on the matter, brain death should not be legally recognized (*Mainichi Shinbun* 1988).

In 1983 a Brain Death Study Group, composed of neurosurgeons and anesthesiologists, was formed at the initiative of the Ministry of Health and Welfare and chaired by the neurosurgeon Takeuchi Kazuo. The group's report, which was published by the ministry in 1985, includes the definition of whole-brain death and the criteria for its diagnosis that became the standard in Japan (Kōseishō 1985; Takeuchi et al. 1987). Known as the Takeuchi criteria, these guidelines are very similar to those of the American Uniform Determination of Death Act.[4] Takeuchi claimed, however, that they were stricter: for example, more than two specialists usually confirm the diagnosis, an EEG is routinely used, and brain death is not recognized in children aged six and under (1990). Full details of this report were reported in the media (*Mainichi Daily News* 1985a).

The report recommends that organs can be procured from brain-dead bodies provided that patients have made their wishes known in advance; however, family members may overrule the wishes of the patient. The report is explicit, again in contrast to the situation in North America, that "human death cannot be judged by brain death," and it makes no claims to legal authority. Thus, whether organs could indeed be procured from brain-dead bodies remained ambiguous.

Despite this, brain death has been routinely diagnosed in Japan all along, and in 1987 it was estimated that 70 percent of the larger hospitals and university centers made such diagnoses. However, patients are almost invariably maintained on ventilators after a confirmation of brain death, "because relatives cannot accept the reality and medical personnel fear legal repercussions if they insist on discontinuing cardiopulmonary care" (Takeuchi et al. 1987).

Despite the report and its support by some official groups, disagreement persisted among the representatives of various medical specialties and among individual physicians.[5] The Japan Society of Psychiatrists and Neurologists, for example, expressed a fear that the equation of brain death with human death would place the handicapped, mentally impaired, and disadvantaged at risk for premature determination of death out of a greedy desire to harvest their organs. This group also argued that it is difficult to establish when exactly brain function is irreversibly lost, and they went on to criticize their own profession for never having "faced up" to the Wada case (*Asahi Shinbun* 1991c; Yamauchi 1990).

Much more recently it has become clear that the president of the

4. The Japanese criteria for whole-brain death are as follows: (a) deep coma; (b) cessation of spontaneous breathing; (c) fixed and enlarged pupils; (d) loss of brain-stem reflexes; (e) flat brain waves; (f) all the above conditions must continue for at least six hours. Children under six are not subject to the criteria. Two physicians with no vested interest in the retrieval of the patient's organs, in addition to the patient's attending physician, are required to make the diagnosis.

5. The Ministry report spurred other groups to take a formal position on the matter. In January 1988, for example, after two years of meetings, the Brain Death and Organ Transplantation Committee on Bioethics of the Japan Medical Association voted unanimously to accept brain death as human death.

Association of Emergency Medicine doctors, Otsuka Toshifumi, a charismatic man who fought for recognition for emergency medicine in Japan, was unhappy because leading transplant surgeons never approached him personally, following Japanese protocol, to ask for the cooperation of emergency medicine doctors in procuring organs. Given the compromising and legally questionable situation in which ICU doctors were put when they assisted with the procurement of organs prior to 1997, it is not surprising that Otsuka refused to support the transplant enterprise. The relatively few kidney transplants making use of brain-dead donors prior to 1997 were accomplished by more or less clandestine arrangements made through personal contacts between individual emergency medicine doctors and transplant surgeons. Recipients were selected by the doctors involved.

Even after the Japan Medical Association expressed its support for recognition of brain death, the highly visible Tokyo University–based Patients' Rights Committee, headed by a flamboyant specialist in internal medicine, Honda Katsunori, persisted with its activities. It brought a case against a doctor who is also a Buddhist priest; he turned off the respirator of a comatose woman and arranged for the removal of kidneys and corneas in accordance with a living will and with the consent of the family (*Yomiuri Shinbun* 1992). His religious authority did not protect him from the anger of activists opposed to the recognition of brain death.

Public Persuasions

Articles and books about brain death and organ transplants proliferated during the 1980s, and public opinion was systematically and repeatedly surveyed. A 1984 book, *Inochi Saisentan: Nōshi to zōki ishoku* (The leading edge of life), takes the line that numerous problems must be overcome if transplant technology is to succeed, but it does not in the end oppose transplants (Yomiuri Shinbun Henshūbu 1984). It cites a poll on clinical practice in the ICUs of 90 hospitals. The results show that procedures and decision making about brain death are not standardized, even after the publication of official guidelines; the book includes the observation, frequently echoed in the Japanese literature, that "nonstandardized judgments" about brain death can "cause misunderstanding among Japanese citizens" (40). From the outset, it has been emphasized that the public should be fully apprised of the procurement and transplant endeavor, including the diagnosis of brain death.

The book gives a detailed account of an organization in Osaka that was exposed for acting as a broker for Japanese patients wishing to travel abroad to obtain organs. It opposes at length the commodification of organs, points out the urgent need for educating the Japanese public about donation, and discusses the reservations of certain medical professionals about living related donors. Manabe Hisao, the head of the Japan Transplant Association and a contributor to the book, pointed out that certain Western commentators had described living related donations as "barbaric" and commented that his association wanted to move away from such transplants, provided that the current impasse in Japan over brain-dead donors could be broken.

The book presents the case of a sixty-year-old brain-dead patient who had made it clear that he wanted to donate his heart. Because the doctors feared that they would be "open to criticism for experimentation on a human subject," no effort was made to meet his wishes (74). Such examples are designed expressly to add fuel to the fires of debate about brain death.

The book also reveals the existence of a "Thank You Fund" worth thirty million yen (approximately a quarter of a million dollars), established by a leading transplant surgeon at a major Tokyo hospital, originally out of his own pocket, to provide payments to the families of organ donors. This fund was enlarged by contributions from other doctors, and also, no doubt, by grateful recipients. Payments are described as *kōden,* the expression used for the monetary condolence gifts from friends and associates of a deceased individual to the family. The surgeon who set up this system points out that there are no "social rules" about compensation of donors, implying that one cannot expect donor families to hand over precious commodities such as human organs and receive nothing in return. However, other doctors raised their voices in opposition to this practice as soon as it became public (125).

The final section of the book asserts that in Japan the number of brain-dead patients is much lower than in the United States because of the lower incidence of gunshot wounds and serious traffic accidents. Even if brain death were recognized, organs would still be scarce (223).

A second book, highly critical of the new death, was published in 1986 by the Tokyo University–based Patients' Rights Committee. This collection, based on a symposium attended by well-known Japanese cultural commentators, rehearses arguments commonly mounted by those opposed to the recognition of brain death. It stresses the importance of a national consensus on recognition of brain death (on this point both sides agree). It casts some doctors as "dictators" who are likely to force families to agree to turning off the ventilators of patients pronounced brain-dead. It also claims that the Japanese government wants brain death legalized to reduce medical expenses (see also Ohi et al. 1986). The authors then move on to social and cultural issues, including the human rights of the brain-dead. They claim that organ transplants are "unnatural," and that rejection of organs by recipients' bodies is proof of this. In the United States, they argue, the concepts of body and "soul" are different from those in Japan: whereas for Westerners the soul exists in the mind, in Japan it is dispersed throughout the body. The boundary between life and death is "fuzzy for Japanese," and the dead continue to exist near and among the living. If brain death is recognized as the end of life, they note, then patients in a persistent vegetative state (PVS) will soon also be considered as good-as-dead.

Watanabe Toyō, a religious scholar well versed in Christian theology, has also written a book opposed to recognition of brain death. He argues that death cannot be understood solely in terms of medicine, and he points out that in a "culture of animism" such as that of Japan, where the life principle is diffused both inside and outside the body, it is difficult to accept the "mechanistic view of the human body" that is necessary for an acceptance of brain death and organ transplants (Watanabe 1988).

Umeda Toshirō, a former science editor for the *Asahi Shinbun,* a newspaper comparable in stature to the *New York Times,* takes up the question of organ sales. He comments on a case in which an Osaka businessman paid 19 million yen to a broker to travel to the Philippines to receive a kidney procured from a prison inmate. Umeda does not seek to censure the businessman or to argue that organ sales are immoral, but he asks why on earth, given the wealth and technological expertise of Japan, anyone should be driven to such extremes (Umeda 1989). He blames the Japanese medical establishment for the impasse.

Umeda also notes that although the ethics committees established during the 1980s in many Japanese teaching hospitals were ostensibly modeled after those in America, in reality they are composed almost entirely of professors and clinicians employed by the hospitals. Moreover, their deliberations take place behind closed doors (154). Umeda believes that this mode of conduct has contributed to the lack of public trust. This situation remains essentially unchanged, with one or two notable exceptions, such as the ethics committee of Kitasato University hospital in Kanagawa prefecture, which is composed of nurses, social

workers, and lay people in addition to doctors (although when I attended a meeting of this committee, three of the four doctors present
slept through most of the proceedings).

Among more than a hundred books about brain death and organ
transplants written for the general public, Nakajima Michi's has become
a classic. Nakajima became involved with this subject because of the
death of her husband. Her principal theme is that the new technological
death "cannot be seen" (*mienai shi*). She describes brain death as an
event in which the family, distracted by the technology, is not fully involved emotionally. This situation precludes them from making intuitive
judgments and appropriate responses to the condition of the patient.
She notes that the diffidence of physicians reinforces families' difficulties
in coming to terms with death: doctors usually say, "It *seems* as though
the patient is brain-dead," or "I *think* they are brain-dead," rather than
making clear, definitive statements (Nakajima 1985:12).

Deeply concerned about the objectification of brain-dead bodies, Nakajima writes about the "cannibalism" of organs and is skeptical about
the standard of care for patients with severe head trauma. She is the
only commentator on brain death to have systematically observed clinical practice in ICUs. She emphasizes the obvious grief of families when
the ventilator is turned off, taking their tears as evidence that relatives
can accept the fact of death only when they have visible proof, in the
form of some outward change in the body. (A Japanese transplant surgeon notes that families of brain-dead patients are shown the results of
EEGs to try to convince them that death has indeed occurred, a practice
also sometimes followed in the United States and in Canada [Nihon
Ishoku Gakkai 1991]).

Nakajima reports three cases that she witnessed in which families had
agreed to donate the kidneys of comatose patients, but all the patients
eventually recovered sufficiently to leave the ICU (Nakajima 1985:258).
In her conclusion Nakajima modifies her position and, like the lawyer
Bai Kōichi before her, suggests that the law might be "softened" so that
individuals can be allowed to donate organs without legalizing brain
death as the end of human life.

The brain-death debate in Japan takes place against a backdrop of
what is believed to be happening in the West, which usually means
America. At times the information that circulates is, quite simply,
wrong. Writing in a respectable nursing journal, Amano Keichi states,
for example, that American families who donate organs of brain-dead
relatives receive enormous sums of money in exchange for their "gift."

Amano argues that in America, "where money is everything," a poor black woman in Harlem would think nothing of donating the organs of her child killed in a road accident (1987). Reports of American doctors on the point of retrieving organs when the patient "comes back to life" have also appeared in Japanese publications, heightening public anxiety in Japan (Yomiuri Shinbun Henshūbu 1984:42).

Fueling the Public Imagination

Adding to the mass of reading material on the subject, several novels about brain death appeared during the 1970s and 1980s. Among them was *Shiroi Utage* (White banquet), written by Watanabe Junichi, which originally appeared under another title in 1969. The author was a lecturer at the same hospital as Wada Jiro in Sapporo, and his book is a fictitious account of the Wada affair, including details about the deception. A second novel, *Ikiteiru Shinzō* (Living heart), appeared in 1990 and was televised; this one chronicles a wife's battle to follow through on her dead husband's desire to have his heart donated, against the wishes of his parents and other relatives, leading to the second (fictional) heart transplant performed in Japan. (The second actual transplant took place nearly a decade after the novel was published). The narrative makes much of the fact that the donor, his wife, and their children are Christians who go to church every Sunday and are not therefore "typically" Japanese. This fictional procedure is clearly portrayed as ethical, and the extended family is finally brought into complete agreement when the situation is explained to them fully and clearly. A murder charge is nevertheless leveled at the doctor, and the family is terrified of being accused of conspiracy. At the end of the novel the donor's wife marries the transplant surgeon, and the recipient of the heart arrives unexpectedly at the airport to see the couple off on their honeymoon. The wife, Chōko, is ecstatic to find out that her deceased husband's heart is living in a healthy body (Kaga 1991).

Children are not sheltered from the brain death problem; on the contrary, considerable efforts are made to educate them. *Manga* (comics) have enormous popularity in Japan; their influence on the young is arguably as great as that of television. Science fiction, magical realism, shape-shifting, cyborgs, brain death, persistent vegetative state, and organ transplants have all been featured repeatedly in this medium. The best-selling Black Jack series, created by Tezuka Osamu and read by millions of young Japanese, has vividly depicted the living deaths of

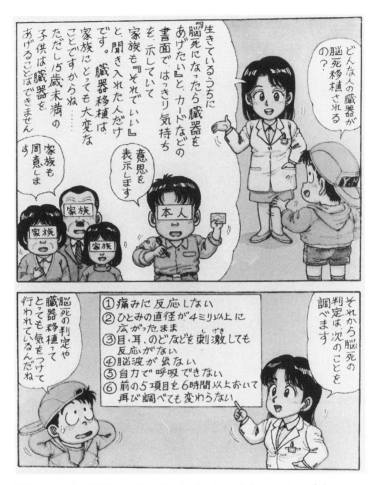

Education for children about brain death and the signing of donor
cards. Illustration by Matsuo Takayoshi from Studio Spice, Tokyo.
This cartoon strip appeared in the children's section of the Yomiuri
newspaper in 1999. Reproduced by permission of the artist.

brain-dead and PVS patients and the moral dilemmas they pose, and the
children's page in major newspapers put out cartoon pages educating
young readers about brain death.

Endless newspaper articles have also appeared on the subject. Editorials have argued that the rights of dying patients must never be compromised (*Yomiuri Shinbun* 1986, 1987) and that the "distance" between heart death and brain death cannot be overcome by "cold
scientific logic." Any changes in conventions about death must wait,

therefore, for the development of public consensus (*Nihon Keizai Shinbun* 1985a; *Mainichi Shinbun* 1985). They demand that medical reports about brain death and other bioethical matters be written in everyday language (*Nihon Keizai Shinbun* 1985b). Articles emphasize that there is no need to implement in practice all the advances made in scientific technologies, nor to follow trends set in other countries (*Tokyo Shinbun* 1985). They criticize the arrogance of doctors (*Asahi Shinbun* 1989a) and argue that doctors must win back the trust of patients before they can expect any cooperation over organ transplants (*Asahi Shinbun* 1987; *Tokyo Shinbun* 1988a); because brain death is "invisible" and "difficult for the family to recognize," trust is imperative (*Yomiuri Shinbun* 1988a).

Chronic Brain Death

Information about brain death does not always travel a one-way path from the United States to Japan. Some American neurologists have watched keenly what takes place in Japanese ICUs. Because ventilators have not usually been turned off after a brain-death diagnosis, lengthy observations of brain-dead patients have been possible in Japan. Japanese intensivists have been able to experiment with the perfusion fluids that keep living cadavers in "stable" condition. By changing the doses of various compounds, one study was able to extend the mean survival time of sixteen brain-dead patients for over three weeks. This 1986 study (Yoshioka et al.) produced high praise from several American neurologists, causing one to state that the idea that brain death leads inevitably to somatic death is exaggerated: "The rationale for accepting brain death must be something other than the fact that the body inevitably dies soon after the brain is dead" (Black 1986). This insight proved prophetic and is now central in the reemerging debate about brain death in North America (see chapter 14).

Results of the above 1986 study became public knowledge in Japan, and the long survival times of one or two of the patients—well over a month—have been cited in the media and in popular books, causing peaks in public anxiety (Tachibana 1988). Nishioka notes one case in which the patient survived for more than one hundred days (1989). Those opposed to the recognition of brain death use these findings to argue that brain-dead patients must be thought of as very much alive and as having patient rights. They insist that the debate is not simply about a few hours' difference between brain death and cardiac death.

Fears were also raised about brain-dead bodies being used as experimental subjects, and such practices going on in France at the time were highlighted as unconscionable (Nishioka 1989).

Many people I have talked to in Japan believe that if it had not been for the Wada case, recognition of brain death would have slipped quietly into routine practice. This case certainly caused immense damage to the public image of medicine and angered many people, but thirty years is a long time for one case of medical malpractice, however repugnant, to keep a nation at an impasse. Reaction to the Wada case is better understood as a symptom of a larger and more diffuse unease over brain death. A brief consideration of Japanese attitudes to science and technology over the past one hundred years gives some perspective on the Wada case and public reactions to it.

AGGRESSIVE HARVESTING

In 1993, twenty-five years after the first two liver transplants using brain-dead donors were conducted, without success, in Japan, a third effort was made in Fukuoka city, in Kyūshū, at the university hospital. The liver had been procured from a patient who died in an emergency medicine center outside Osaka. The patient's wishes about donation were not known, but once he was declared brain-dead the story was leaked to the media amid a flurry of speculation about procuring organs for transplant. It was later reported that the donor's sister had been asked to consider organ donation. She telephoned her eighty-one-year-old mother, who apparently said, "That's OK with me" (*kamahen*). Having heard that their mother agreed, the other siblings also consented.

The donor's sister signed the consent form permitting donation of seven organs and tissues, but the mother apparently had no idea that she was agreeing to donation of so many organs, and she was particularly upset about the removal of the corneas and skin (*Asahi Shinbun* 1994h). Later when asked, she claimed that she had become confused and her "mind went blank"; she had said the first thing that came into her head. She added that she could no longer bear to look at her son as he lay dying in the hospital, and so she had gone home. "I felt as if he were begging to have the ventilator stopped," she said, "and I thought his sister would fall ill if she had to stay and nurse him any longer" (*Asahi Shinbun* 1993c).[1]

---

1. In many Japanese hospitals family members provide all the basic care for patients.

It was also reported that the Kyūshū physicians, flown to Osaka in haste (under pressure from local government and the police and perhaps also from the deterioration of the patient's condition), had decided to remove the liver not while the patient was brain-dead, but immediately after the heart stopped beating. The surgeons were said to have waited one minute following cardiac arrest to harvest the liver and have it transported to Kyūshū, four hundred miles away. There it was transplanted into a patient who, readers were told, was not immunologically compatible with the donor (*Asahi Shinbun* 1993b). On the day of the transplant it was reported that before his heart stopped beating, the donor had been given an injection to keep the liver in good condition. Since this intervention was not in the interests of the patient, it provoked criticism, especially from the media (*Nihon Keizai Shinbun* 1993). The medical team was publicly chided for its "aggressive" behavior.

The wife of the recipient, at her own insistence, appeared on television, together with the recipient's sister, to thank the donor and the transplant team. The patient lived for less than three months, and the new liver never did function properly. The lawyer Nakajima Michi, already well-known to the public for her participation in the brain-death debate, asserted in print that this case was as bad as the Wada episode. She claims that the donor's heart was probably still beating when the liver was removed and that the involved physicians simply said otherwise to placate the authorities and the public (1994).

A citizen's group based in Osaka had murder charges brought against the involved doctors almost one year after the transplant. After the passing of the Organ Transplant Law, the case was dropped in 1998, together with other outstanding court cases and public inquiries connected with the management of brain-dead patients in Japan.

SIX

Technology as Other

Japanese Modernity and Technology

Modernity is typically associated with progress, rationalization, and secularization. By these yardsticks Japan has been quintessentially modern for some time now, although several scholars claim that today the country is better characterized as an exemplar of postmodernity (Miyoshi and Harootunian 1989). Regardless of these appellations, it is clear that many influential people in Japan remain resolutely concerned about "tradition," a past that is self-consciously identified with a specific history and culture, so much so that claims to Japanese uniqueness are by no means unheard of. Contemporary Japanese attitudes toward technology, science, and modern medicine are linked to a widespread ambivalence about modernization in general. What is more, Japanese attitudes toward modernization cannot be understood in isolation from interpretations of the relationship of Japan to the West—to Europe and North America. The current debate about body technologies in Japan— the feasibility of tinkering with the margins between culture and nature, and the very creation of those margins—takes place in light of received wisdom about the Other, the West. At the same time, nostalgia about the loss of an "authentic" Japanese past contributes prominently to the debate.

As with the concept of "culture" in English, the corresponding Japanese terms have had different meanings attributed to them throughout history. *Bunka* and *bunmei* (in modern Japanese usage, "culture" and "civilization," respectively) first appeared in the classical period in Ja-

pan, often as oppositions to *bu* (the military); scholarly learning and the
written word were set off from the "world of the sword" (Morris-Suzuki
1995). From the thirteenth century, the Buddhist-inspired idea of self-
knowledge through deliberate cultivation of *kokoro*—the human spirit—
has been an explicit source of cultural authenticity. Paradoxically, cultivation of *kokoro* has intimate ties with the military world of the samurai (Najita 1989).

At various junctures in Japanese history, different movements have
called for a return to the "real" and "essential," pre-Buddhist Japanese
past and to a cultivation of Japanese knowledge and virtue, over-
shadowed by doubtful influences from the Asian mainland and more
recently from Europe and America. Central to these nativistic movements is an idea of an animistically based, emotionally appropriate relationship with nature, one grounded in "true feelings" (Harootunian
1988:369).

By the early nineteenth century the idea of a Japanese nation had
taken root, and science and technology were recognized as crucial to its
development. Although indigenous developments were seen as vital,
technology from the outside—from the West—was eagerly sought after.
Throughout the late nineteenth century this quest for mastery of Western
science and technology "was grounded in [a] sense of cultural certitude"
(Najita 1989), a sensibility that the "core" or the bass note (*koso*) of
Japanese culture and its special affiliation with the natural world would
remain unaffected by technological intrusions. Technology, aligned with
the Other, was placed in opposition to culture and epitomized by the
platitudes *wakon yōsai* (Japanese spirit and Western technology), and
tōyō dōtoku, seiyō gijutsu (Eastern morality, Western technology). Najita and other historians of Japan have shown how this confidence in
the endurance of culture was gradually eroded. In the twentieth century,
particularly after World War II, internal tension erupted over Japan's
increasing technological sophistication and internationalization (Najita
1989). Fears multiplied about the collapse of the nation's cultural heritage and self-colonization by means of technology, and one reaction was
a reassertion of cultural essentialism and of the importance of authentic
feelings (Harootunian 1989).

Eminent Japanese thinkers grappled with the problem of how Eastern
thought might overcome the dualities of a modernity grounded in Western thinking. Tessa Morris-Suzuki has argued that the idea of a "modern" Japanese culture first crystallized in the 1920s (1995). This "invented tradition" (Hobsbawm and Ranger 1983), fostered by the state,

was envisioned as a coherent whole in which, by definition, all Japanese citizens participated: a self-conscious creation, exclusive of outsiders and constructed in opposition to the Other of the West.

With defeat in war, a movement swelled to throw out the old and tainted and to grasp modernity, Western-style, even more firmly. However, in the 1960s a reaction set in. Initially stimulated by resentment of the Allied Army of Occupation, and later of American forces still present in Japan, this sentiment was also fueled by the ubiquitous Westernization of daily life, accompanied by deeply ingrained and widely reported feelings that the essence of Japanese moral life was being dissolved. Somewhat similar fears are apparent in North America and Europe in assertions that ethnic minorities, immigrants, and refugees are disruptive of social and moral order.

Perhaps the dominant theme in the Japanese cultural debate over the past forty years has been the extent to which it is possible or appropriate to continue to cultivate uniqueness. Conservative reconstructions of history by intellectuals suggest that Japanese have from mythological times been "naturally" bonded as a moral, social, and linguistic unit (Kosaku 1992). The majority of Japanese oppose the extreme form of this rhetoric, which slips into racism and xenophobia; but such discourse, at times explicitly supported by the government (Pyle 1987; Gluck 1993) and inflamed by trade wars, whaling and international peacekeeping disputes, and the recent economic recession in Asia, cannot be dismissed entirely (Cummings 1993; Kalland and Moeran 1992).

The specters of individualism, utilitarianism, and super-rationalism—values closely associated with the West—push some Japanese toward a rhetoric of difference, even though they are not always enamored of its nationalistic and essentialist associations. Cultivation of an idyllic recollection of rural Japan reveals anxiety and a sense of loss (Ivy 1995; Tamanoi 1998). However, appellations such as "tradition," "cultural heritage," and "religion" smack of a premodern sentimentality, and even of superstition, to many people, and most astute commentators view the search for authenticity with cynicism.

Even so, in contrast to the United States, and even to Canada—a nation exquisitely sensitive to cultural pluralism from its founding— Japan is deeply aware of "culture" as a political force that unifies the country but separates it from the outside. For example, from a Japanese perspective, the uses to which brain-dead bodies are systematically put, such as organ donation, are largely products of American pragmatism, a cultural force that encourages a utilitarian attitude toward commodification of the brain-dead. Japanese arguments for and against recognition of the new death are inevitably colored by the awareness of this outside influence.

Cultivating Doubt

Among the best-known opponents of the recognition of brain death is Tachibana Takashi, an award-winning journalist for the *Yomiuri Shinbun*, the largest national newspaper in Japan. In a series of well-illustrated, best-selling books (with over four hundred thousand copies sold), as well as numerous articles and television programs, Tachibana has made it his mission to inform the Japanese public about brain death. Tachibana has maintained that he is not opposed in principle to organ transplants or to the recognition of brain death as the end of life. He does not create a debate about ontology but focuses on questions of medical accuracy and on the life that remains in a brain-dead body. If it could be conclusively proved that brain death is the end of life, then Tachibana would be satisfied.

Tachibana was one of the first observers, neurological specialists included, to note that residual physiological and endocrinological activities persist in brain cells even when the brain has no integrated function (Tachibana 1991, 1992). In his opinion, for this reason, if for no other, a living cadaver cannot be regarded as dead. This opinion is shared by a minority of medical specialists in Japan and elsewhere. Early in his research, Tachibana reached a radical conclusion: in Japan, people may want to move toward a recognition of brain-dead bodies as *socially* dead.

He acknowledges that cultural differences influence ideas about the departure of the soul from the body, and that such ideas probably work in Japan to inhibit a recognition of brain death. In his opinion, however, this type of resistance is "an expression of childishness" (1994:295). Much more important, he argues, are questions of accuracy and honesty. Tachibana has systematically documented cases involving misdiagnosis and error and given them considerable public exposure.

In December 1990, Japanese national television (NHK) transmitted a three-hour prime-time program produced by Tachibana. The first half was devoted to a film, made largely in America, about the harvesting and distribution of organs. The second half presented a round-table discussion among six Japanese "experts," three for and three against the acceptance of brain death. This program had millions of viewers. When I showed portions of it to a small audience of Americans, several were truly shocked, never having considered until then where organs for transplant come from.

To the accompaniment of sentimental music, the film introduces viewers to a beguiling Japanese child who was born from a brain-dead mother. This child, we are told, symbolizes a new life started from what is thought of by some as a dead body. The audience is then taken to North Carolina, where a young man, badly damaged in a road accident, is pronounced brain-dead and transported to another hospital for organ procurement. His heart is about to be removed when he "comes back to life." He lives for another six days before finally being declared dead. This portion of the program ends with a close-up of a large, ornamental cross outside the hospital, and a pan of a nearby graveyard, filled with crosses, with the hospital in the background. An association is being made between the Christian culture of America and recognition of brain death.

In the next scene, an American doctor states that not only is it difficult to diagnose brain death, but that a clear legal definition is not possible. This doctor suggests that if the guidelines are too lenient, then cases may be misdiagnosed, but with too stringent a diagnosis, many organs "go to waste." Willard Gaylin, the psychiatrist formerly associated with the Hastings Center in New York, introduces his concept of "neomorts." Gaylin describes his "excitement" on realizing that neomorts could be used for testing new drugs, for medical students to dissect instead of the bodies of "poor people," and for "recycling body parts into other people." Earlier in the program, Gaylin vividly describes the way in which neomorts are still warm and breathing but nevertheless legally dead.

Another American doctor states that in his opinion not only the brain-dead, but also people in a persistent vegetative state (*shokubutsu ningen*), will soon be recognized as legally dead. The camera then moves to a Japanese ward full of patients in this condition. Viewers see how some of these patients respond to human communication with subtle movement. We are informed that in a similar institution, thirteen out of thirty patients had made significant recovery after intensive treatment, sometimes to the point of being able to speak again.

Together, these scenes and others like them, including several filmed in Europe, give the impression that brain death is not easily diagnosed. Brain-dead patients are in some sense "living"; and a continuum exists between brain death and other conditions, so that no easy, Western-style dichotomy can be made between the living and the dead. Yet if one waits patiently for proof in the form of whole-body death, vital organs, including the heart, liver, and lungs, will no longer be fit for transplantation.

Viewers are taken into a surgical unit in Florida, where they see in graphic detail, and accompanied by a disturbing, funereal soundtrack, the dismemberment of a young woman, whose long blonde hair is displayed through the drapes. The audience is told that seventeen kinds of organs are taken from this woman, including the heart and large sections of bone, joint, and muscle tissue. We are shown several cartons of dismembered body parts, stored in dry ice, being wheeled out for transplants across the United States. Viewers learn that as a result of this seven-hour "operation," parts of this twenty-one-year-old will "continue to live in seventy other people." We are then shown what is left of the body being sewn up by the junior staff, ready for removal to the morgue.[1]

Viewers are also told about Brazilian children taken to Europe for slaughter and sale of their body parts, and we are shown a line of people in India waiting to sell one of their kidneys, for which they will reportedly receive the equivalent of five years' income (see Cohen, ms., and Scheper-Hughes 2000 for information on such practices).

At the end of the film a professor at Tohoku University in northern Japan describes how, when transplanting brain cells between mice, he could restore some of the brain function that had been destroyed in the recipient mice.[2] This experiment indicates, viewers are told, that a brain-dead person could one day perhaps be restored to normal function. The program emphasizes that because brain death cannot be readily defined, the debate is inevitably linked to ethics and religion—although what these ethics might be is not made clear. An implicit contrast is set up between America and Japan. In America, land of Christianity, altruistic giving is part of the cultural tradition, and decisions about life and death are reached pragmatically; but mistakes are sometimes made about the diagnosis of death. In Japan, which is assumed to be closer to nature, dichotomies do not operate, and people are less willing than in America to tinker with extrahuman forces.

1. After watching this video numerous times, I am convinced that this televised procurement has been cut and spliced from procedures involving more than one organ donor. The donor's raised arm, shown toward the end of the film, appears to be that of a man and not of the young woman originally shown. It would in any case be extremely unusual to remove so many organs from one donor.

2. Experiments of this kind have been repeated, and related work is now being carried out on humans.

In the heated round-table discussion that follows, a lawyer and two doctors create a narrow definition of brain death as an irreversible stoppage of brain functioning that can be rationally, systematically, and accurately deduced. These protagonists for recognition of the new death argue that decisions must be based on universal scientific standards. One of the opponents on the panel counters (presumably misquoting the study by Youngner et al.) that in America only thirty-five percent of doctors can make an accurate diagnosis of brain death.

The experts in support of the new death insist that "emotional" arguments (by which they apparently mean references to values) should be kept out of the discussion, and that in America the donation of organs has been set up on a "rational" basis in which people can freely decline to participate. These experts become emotional themselves, however, when they demand why the life of a patient needing a transplant should not be considered as valuable as the life of a brain-dead patient.

In contrast, the three opposing speakers repeatedly state that the "religious background" to the problem must be considered; that emotional matters and scientific theory should not be kept apart but integrated; that an examination of the "truth" must be accompanied by "feelings" as well as logic, and that the "social concept" of death must be considered. One of these speakers is the conservative philosopher Umehara Takeshi. Characteristically, he makes several deliberately inflammatory statements. He points out that "Japanese people" dislike transplants because they do not like "unnatural" things; that they have never in the past accepted "extreme" Chinese customs, such as foot binding and the eunuch system; and, in a similar vein, that contemporary Japanese "hate" homosexuality and the use of drugs. He then lays blame for the sorry state of the West at the feet of René Descartes, who focused attention on the brain as the center of the living person.

One or two attempts were made during the 1990s to create more nuanced arguments that nevertheless consider cultural variables. The philosopher Morioka Masashiro suggests, for example (in a book that sold twenty thousand copies), that attention should be shifted away from the criteria for standardization of brain death, and toward the brain-dead person in a nexus of distinctly Japanese human relations, both familial and medical (Morioka 1989). Having likened the ICU, with its central observation area and continuous monitoring, to the disciplinary panopticon of Jeremy Bentham, written about by Michel Foucault, Morioka argues that the decision as to whether brain death signals the end of all responsibility for continuing medical care should rest with the family of the patient, not the medical staff.

Morioka seeks to redefine brain death as a social rather than a clinical matter. He has insisted that one should think of brain-dead persons (*nōshi no hito*), not brain-dead corpses (*nōshi tai*) as was often the case prior to the publication of his book. He points out that brain death is described in the media as a problem because, like pollution, the aging society, integration of foreign labor, and bullying in Japanese schools, the issue has profound, sometimes contradictory, social ramifications, and he supports the airing of these issues in public.

In 1992 a second special on prime-time television, also produced by Tachibana, covered several of the brain-death cases that ended up in court. Interviews with dissatisfied relatives of brain-dead patients are included, and a transplant surgeon gives his point of view, with Naka-jima Michi providing opposition. Viewers are taken to a Taipei prison, where a thirty-one-year-old prisoner on death row expresses his wish to donate his organs at death. The prisoner says that he has not thought about things too deeply during his life, but that what he is now doing is a "good, zen kind of action." Most viewers, who would have read in the media that Japanese in need of transplants had on occasion gone to Taiwan to get them, would no doubt have felt uneasy watching this program.

Mobilizing Tradition

When the 1989 film *Jesus of Montréal*, directed by Denis Arcand, was shown in Japan in 1990, it angered citizens' rights groups that oppose the recognition of brain death. This film, by no means a masterpiece in my opinion, recounts the story of a group of young actors who, even though refused permission, nevertheless perform the story of Christ in St. Joseph's Oratory, a pilgrimage site in Montreal, culminating with the Crucifixion. As police try to stop the performance, the actor who plays Christ is accidentally crushed and killed when the cross topples over. He is rushed to hospital, where he becomes a multiple organ donor. Christ's corneas are donated to a blind woman and his heart to a man pronounced medically dead, reminding viewers of the Gospel accounts of the healing of the blind man and the raising of Lazarus.

For some Japanese viewers, this film glorified the transplant enterprise and confirmed the belief that brain death and organ transplants are related to Christian values and therefore to the West. Ota Kazuo, among the best-known of Japan's transplant surgeons from his regular exposure in the media (not all of it good), was asked to comment. Ota notes the sorry plight of individuals waiting for organs and the stigmatization of patients who go abroad for transplants. The surgeon concludes with a plea: "Let *Jesus of Montréal* not disappear like a dream in a summer night." In contrast, the film *All about My Mother,* directed by Pedro Almodovar, which also deals with organ donation, has been praised by the Japanese press for its sensitivity in dealing with this matter. (One American reviewer noted that the film shows "how tragedies of the flesh can yield renewal and hope despite the pain they leave behind" [Maslin 1999].) Given that ten years elapsed between the releases of these two films, one may surmise that Japanese opposition to organ donation has softened.

Tada Tomio, an internationally recognized immunologist at the University of Tokyo, indicates in a Noh play of his own creation that his views are more complex than Ota Kazuo's. Since the fourteenth century this highly stylized Japanese drama form has been a medium for exploring the relationship between the world of spirits and earthly life. It is a conservative tradition, to say the least: since the Meiji Restoration of 1868, only one new play has entered the canon actually performed in public, and that play commemorated the enthronement of Emperor Hirohito in 1928. When the current emperor ascended the throne, no play was written for him (Sanger 1991, citing Gerry Yokota). Nevertheless, Tada's play, titled *The Well of Ignorance (Mumyō no i),* had its premiere at the National Noh Theater before a standing-room-only crowd in 1991. In the audience was "a fair sprinkling of the country's policy-makers and opinion-molders as well as its medical elite" (Sanger 1991). The play was later shown on national television and performed in other parts of the country, and it went on tour in America. The world of Noh usually has little, if any, effect on the Japanese public; performances are considered effete and rarified. This play, however, received considerable news coverage.

The play follows the usual structure of a Noh drama, with two acts linked by an interlude. There is no central dramatic incident in a Noh play; rather, it is designed to encourage the audience to reflect, along with the central character, who is often a ghost, about matters philosophical and metaphysical. The principal actors use words sparingly, together with a stylized body language, to convey their emotions. Much of the narrative is furnished by a chorus of chanters accompanied by traditional musical instruments.

In the first act, a traveling priest approaches an old, dry well in the middle of a wild moor. He sees a woman approaching the well, murmuring to herself. The priest tries in vain to engage her in conversation; as she starts to draw water from the well, a man suddenly appears and stops her. The figures disappear from sight, leaving the priest pondering what he has witnessed.

In the interlude, the priest seeks out a local villager and asks for an explanation. The villager embarks on a long narrative about a fisherman knocked unconscious in a giant storm and taken for dead. The wealthy father of a young, sick woman summons a famous Chinese-style doctor, who removes the fisherman's heart and transplants it into the woman, saving her life. When the woman hears that a "living man" had been sacrificed for her sake, she suffers terrible guilt. The village well runs dry, and the villagers claim that it has been cursed by the suffering, unhappy spirit of the fisherman.

In the second act, the priest intones prayers for the spirits of both the young woman (who did not live long, despite her new heart) and the fisherman. While he does so, a shadow falls across the well. It is the ghost of the fisherman, who laments that he is prevented from following the usual Buddhist path to a peaceful death. His agitation mounts. As the play moves toward its climax, the chorus recounts the fisherman's dying moments:

> A mighty wave brought me to the shore,
> Unconscious, with my spirit already roaming
> Along the path to the land of the dead,
> Although I was still clinging onto life,
> Doctors came at me with blades and scissors,
> . . . cold as ice,
> Tore open my chest and took out my beating heart,
> Making sounds of snipping and cutting
> That I could hear, but my body was frozen
> And no voice came out when I screamed,
> "Am I living or dead?"

The play concludes with the chorus intoning that the spirit of the fisherman is not permitted to join the company of the ancestral dead. Before disappearing into the darkness of the well, both spirits beg the priest to save them from their endless suffering.

In characteristic Noh form, the ambiguity is left unresolved at the end of the play; the audience is left to seek its own resolutions. In choosing the medium of Noh, and not the contemporary theater, Tada was able to give his play mythological dimensions and to infuse it with mystical and nostalgic associations. The genre permits him to give voice to the brain-dead individual, inevitably missing from the contemporary debate. Although a physician himself, Tada believes that the arguments of the medical profession have been heard too often, together with "legal and socio-economic viewpoints that [do] not take into account the true uneasiness of people who have long felt caught between modern materialism and traditional values" (1994).

When I talked with him Tada insisted that he is not personally opposed to organ transplants; on the contrary, his research in immunology is highly pertinent to their success. (Other authors claim that Tada, because he is an immunologist who has spent his life researching the rejection of the "other" by the immune system, *is* opposed to transplants; see Yōrō 1992a). Tada says he is striving above all for a "sound ethics" and a thorough discussion of the complex facets of the brain-death problem: "Donors and recipients have to compete for limited resources . . . we need to acknowledge the light and shadow of this medical technology" (Tada 1994.)

The story is modeled on a Chinese legend first written down in 300 B.C., in which a beating heart is taken out of a fisherman who has drowned in a storm, and placed into the body of a sick young woman who later dies of a guilty conscience.[3] Gerry Yokota, an American specialist in Noh drama, points out how suitable the form is for a subtle handling of power relationships. The central antagonist, the doctor, never appears on the stage; nor does the young woman's wealthy father. The fisherman, "blinded by torment, is unable to see his true adversary, unable to judge who is responsible, and he vents his wrath on the woman as scapegoat" (1991:443). The Japanese audience knows this ploy well. The masked drama, although it does not portray oppressive realities directly, permits an understanding, from the silences as much as from the action, of what the protagonists themselves cannot fully comprehend. Yokota argues that Noh "thrives on the dynamics of justice and injustice, oppression and liberation—including the oppression of and liberation from tradition" (1991:444).[4]

Tada's play can be read simply as an allegory of the current national angst in Japan about brain death (and he says explicitly that it is modeled

3. *Manyōshū*, book 5.
4. Perhaps Yokota can be charged with imbuing fourteenth-century Japan with a twentieth-century American sensibility; nevertheless, Noh's power to fire up emotions about moral issues can have major political import.

on both Chinese legend and the Wada case). But the tradition of Noh makes the play more than a modern morality story. While raising anxiety about organ transplants, it subtly unifies the audience by drawing on and rekindling their sensitivity to the qualities widely ascribed to Japanese, including shared belief in the power of the past and an anthropomorphic spirit world associated with everyday life.

Both Tachibana's television programs and Tada's play heighten ambiguity about technologically manipulated death and to some degree distinguish Japan from the Other. Additional television programs have worked even more directly to deepen anxieties about the new death. Three or four hospitals in Japan specialize in the treatment of patients in a persistent vegetative state (PVS), and one such hospital has been the subject of a moving documentary. It shows patients who, as the result of intensive therapy involving stimulation of the central nervous system, massage, and immersion in hot baths, have made significant recoveries; some have been fully reintegrated into social life. This program and others like it emphasize how often mistakes are made in diagnosing brain trauma. The undeniable neglect of PVS patients in many medical institutions and difficulties in distinguishing between brain death and PVS are underscored.[5]

In at least one hospital drama, on the popular Fuji television network, the usual images of the rational West and the more humane East are reversed. A cold, overly rational Tokyo doctor wants to stop treatment of a brain-dead patient, but he is foiled by a compassionate, empathetic colleague, concerned above all that the patient's family make the decision when they are ready. The second doctor has just returned from medical training in Kansas. A subplot in the same program involves a doctor involved with a liver transplant case who is bribed by a medical instrument company. This program, like those of Tachibana, is designed to heighten viewers' anxiety about the transplant enterprise.

Yet More Scandal

While a steady stream of publications and television programs on brain death was appearing, the majority of them either opposed to it or very

5. No neurologist in North America with whom I have talked agrees with this last assertion, and nearly, but not quite all, Japanese neurologists take the same position.

cautious, further unsavory incidents were reported. In 1989, for example, a doctor at a national medical school hospital was arrested for defrauding a patient of more than 20 million yen ($18,000). The patient died one day after handing the money over, having being told by the doctor that the large fee was necessary as recompense (*sharei*) to the organ donor (*Asahi Shinbun* 1989b).

It is a long-standing custom in Japan to give doctors substantial presents to ensure good medical care, especially for surgery (a custom more than one Japanese doctor has labeled as bribery when talking to me; see also Campbell and Ikegami 1998). It is not surprising, therefore, that many members of the Japanese public believe that a market for human organs is a real possibility and perhaps already exists in their country. Reports of organ-buying brokerages, and their use by desperate Japanese willing to go to Southeast Asia, China, and India for organs, have made these fears more pervasive. So has the practice by some transplant surgeons of offering money to donor families as funerary gifts. Of concern to most critical commentators is less the moral appropriateness or otherwise of selling body parts than a worry that commercialization introduces a fundamental imbalance into a health care system grounded in a principle of equal access for all.

In 1990 yet another brain-death scandal unfolded. In full view of the nation on prime-time television (which I happened also to be watching), police entered Osaka University Hospital to warn surgeons against removing the liver of a fifty-one-year-old man. This patient had provided in his will that his organs could be made available for transplants, and approval had also been obtained from his family. After being hit by a car, he was taken, unconscious, to a nearby hospital and then transferred to the Osaka University Hospital, with the intention of removing his liver and other organs following a pronouncement of brain death made by three independent teams of doctors. The police declared that an autopsy was legally necessary after the car accident; they also reminded the doctors that brain death is not legally recognized in Japan and warned them to wait until the heart had stopped beating.

Television viewers were entertained by the sight of police marching purposefully around hospital corridors and defiant doctors shutting doors against both television cameras and the police. By the time the liver was eventually removed from the patient, after his heart had stopped beating, it had degenerated badly and was unusable, but the kidneys and pancreas were transplanted into waiting patients. It was revealed that the police had intervened in similar cases before. One that has taken on iconic qualities, known simply as the Handai case, took place in 1990 at the same Osaka hospital.

Once the Japan Medical Association had approved of a brain-death diagnosis in 1988, a defiant ethics committee of the medical school of Osaka University (known familiarly as Handai) decided unilaterally to go ahead with transplants from brain-dead donors, even though the legality of such procedures remained doubtful. In 1990, the hospital admitted a forty-year-old businessman who had sustained a very severe head injury in an assault. The patient was declared brain-dead one month after his initial hospitalization, and his wife, when approached by the doctors, told them that she would donate her husband's organs "if they can be of use to others" (*Yomiuri Shinbun* 1990a). Twenty-four hours after the first diagnosis, when brain death was declared for the second time, the death certificate was signed. In keeping with the protocol for assault cases, the physicians telephoned the Osaka police the next day, informing them that the patient was dead and stating that they wanted to procure organs and had the family's consent. The police immediately objected and pointed out that an autopsy was necessary. Ten personnel from police headquarters in Osaka rushed to the hospital and witnessed the removal of the ventilator, whereupon the man's heart stopped beating. It was apparently agreed that removal of the kidneys would not in any way affect the autopsy, and they were removed for transplant at the same time as the autopsy was carried out.

A newspaper report the following day noted that a catheter had been inserted into the patient's femoral artery before his heart had stopped beating so that fluids could be injected to preserve the kidneys. The family registered surprise when they were told later about this procedure. This article also noted that it is illegal in Japan to remove corneas or kidneys from any body that has suffered an "abnormal death" (*Nihon Keizai Shinbun* 1990a). An article by another newspaper claimed that "the enthusiasm" of the hospital had eventually won over the police (*Yomiuri Shinbun* 1990b). The Patient's Rights Committee of Tokyo University once again took action and accused the physician who removed the kidneys of homicide.

In 1992 a book with the title *Four Deaths: The Truth about the Murder of the Brain-Dead Organ Donor at the Osaka University Hospital* was devoted to this case. It claims that two days before brain death was established, the attention of the clinical staff shifted from care of the patient to maintenance of his organs. It also asserts that the will of the donor was not known, that the patient's father had refused to co-operate with the procurement, and that his wife was not informed by the doctors that her husband was brain-dead but was instead given a very confusing statement about his condition. The doctor is reported to have informed the patient's wife that if her husband's care were contin-ued it would be meaningless, very expensive, and no longer covered by the health care system.

The book reveals that when an intensivist testified at the legal hearing in connection with the homicide charge, he stated that brain death was not determined by the national criteria, but rather that the involved clinicians "sensed" that the patient was brain-dead (Kikan Medicaru Toritomento Henshūbū 1992). The ironic title of the book alludes to the fact that in court the involved specialists came up with four different moments, spanning several days, when this patient was determined to be dead.

At this time the *Asahi Shinbun* described the medical world as "irri-tated" with the government's dithering about brain death. Doctors sensed, the newspaper claimed, that their international reputations were withering on the vine. At the annual meeting of the Japan Medical As-sociation held in Kyoto in 1990, which I attended, two plenary sessions and several smaller panels were devoted to brain death and organ trans-plants. The principal presenters were surgeons who had lived and worked in the United States and who had practiced transplant surgery there. Every one of them asserted that Japanese medicine was suffering because of the national uproar over brain death. They all showed slides of themselves standing, usually in surgical garb, beside American trans-plant surgeons and happy, lively organ recipients. This meeting of the JMA was one of the few occasions prior to the late 1990s when attention focused on patients whose lives might have been lengthened by organ transplants (see also Miura 1991; *Newsweek Nihon Han* 1993).

Television documentaries about brain death, PVS, and related con-ditions, the Noh play of Tada Tomio, the *manga* (comics) of Tezuka Osamu and others, general and specialist books, and incessant news-paper reporting have worked in concert to foster anxiety and doubt about the new death. Actions of the transplant community, on the one hand, and the reactions of the police, media, certain lawyers and intel-lectuals, and concerned citizens (including doctors), on the other, have fomented this debate for three decades. The extent and vehemence of

these disputes make it comparable to the abortion debate in America—
although no one in Japan has been murdered for their views.

Even so, many people remain indifferent to the issue because so few
are directly affected. Yet the fact that the debate in Japan has consumed
the time, energy, and emotions of so many people testifies to a widespread concern that they are witnessing a major disruption in their society.

In North America, by contrast, although uncertainty about the new
death was evident during the 1970s, by the 1980s brain death diagnoses
and organ procurement had become routine. What little debate took
place was confined largely to professional circles and focused on issues
of medical and legal certainty. Some philosophical discussion also took
place about the death of persons, but the consequences of the invention
of a new death, either for involved clinicians and families or for society
at large, was barely raised.

The following case study was reported in the *Journal of the American Medical Association* in August 1983:

> On Jan. 25, 1983, a previously healthy 27-year-old woman presented to her local hospital at 22 weeks' gestation with a five-day history of worsening headaches followed by several hours of vomiting and disorientation. Results of physical examination were consistent with a 22-week gestation and were otherwise unremarkable; normal vital signs and no focal neurological deficits were noted. Results of a lumbar puncture were normal except for a slightly elevated opening pressure of 20 cm of water. . . . Four hours after presentation, the patient had a generalized seizure and a respiratory arrest.
>
> After cardiopulmonary resuscitation, ventilatory support was continued in the intensive care unit, where examination revealed no response to painful stimuli, fixed and dilated pupils, papilledema, and absent doll's eye movements. A computed tomographic scan of the head showed marked dilation of the lateral and third ventricles with a mass obstructing the fourth ventricle. . . . The electroencephalogram was again isoelectric[1] two days later. There was no change in the patient's condition, and a diagnosis of brain death was made at that time, using the Harvard criteria. During this period the fetal heart rate pattern remained normal. In accordance with the strongly expressed wishes of the father, a decision was made to provide cardiorespiratory support to the mother in an attempt to maintain the fetus in utero until it reached a viable gestational age.
>
> (Field et al. 1988:816)

1. That is, the EEG tracing was flat.

A massive technological onslaught was undertaken with this patient that continued until the thirty-first week of gestation. The fetal heart rate was monitored at every nursing shift, and serial sonograms were performed. In addition to constant monitoring, feeding, and nursing care, the living cadaver was treated for hypotension, temperature fluctuations, diabetes insipidus, hypothyroidism, and cortisol deficiency. On the twenty-eighth day a major infection took hold, but it was eventually controlled with antibiotics. On the fifty-eighth day a staphylococcus infection developed. While this was being treated, repeated sonograms showed no growth of the fetus over the previous two weeks. A decision was made to deliver the fetus by cesarean section on the sixty-third day of hospitalization. A male infant weighing 1,440 grams (just over 3 pounds) was delivered. The ventilator was turned off, and the heart of the mother stopped beating shortly thereafter. The infant was taken to the neonatal intensive care unit, and at three weeks of age was transferred to a hospital near his home. At eighteen months of age he was doing well.

As part of the ethical discussion that followed the presentation of this case, the authors note:

> A long tradition of fetal rescue exists in Western society. Asklepios was "cut out alive from the womb of his dead mother by Apollo." During the reign of King Numa Pompilius of Rome in the seventh century B.C., the *Lex Regia* was established, mandating the abdominal delivery of a term fetus in the event of the death of its mother. Six hundred years later, during the time of the Roman emperors, this became known as *Lex Cesarea*, the origination of the term *cesarean* delivery. . . . Current available technology has made postmortem somatic support of a mother possible to effect the "rescue" of her very premature fetus. Could the existence of this technology lead to the requirement that it be applied in all cases of maternal death?
>
> (Field et al. 1988: 821)

There is no mention in this ethical discussion of how the nurses and other involved ICU attendants felt about caring intensively for sixty-three days for a brain-dead body and its fetus. Nor is there any discussion about whether the father visited his wife during this time. The chronic ambiguity created by keeping a living cadaver suspended in a hybrid state for over two months is suppressed in favor of a discussion about how the feat was accomplished and whether it should be routinized because the technology is available. In the United States, as contrasted with Japan, the social repercussions of this case go unremarked.

Prevailing against Inertia

An Interim Resolution
to the Brain-Death Debate

A Move to Closure

During the 1990s, the dispute over brain death in Japan came to a head; it reached a partial resolution when the Organ Transplant Law was passed in 1997. In an atmosphere of continuing confrontation, distrust, and public uncertainty, the Japanese government finally decided to exert some leadership in the brain-death debate, and in 1989 the Provisional Commission for the Study on Brain Death and Organ Transplantation (*Rinji nōshi oyobi zōki ishoku chōsa kai*) was formed. This committee was composed of fifteen members, including lawyers, a university president, the vice governor of Tokyo, a newspaper editor, several businessmen, an expert in health policy, a member of the Science and Technology Council of Japan, and a writer. Five key advisers were also associated with the committee, but no practicing clinicians were asked to participate. The group was charged to make a report to the prime minister's office by 1991. According to the media, its formation signaled that the government was ready to recognize brain death legally as death.

From its first meeting in March 1990, the commission met every month until it produced its final report, behind schedule, in January 1992. Its activities included eleven sessions with presentations by invited experts, including the physician Takeuchi Kazuo, after whom the Japanese brain-death criteria are named, and several writers and cultural critics. The committee undertook three "domestic inspection tours" to the emergency departments of several hospitals and held six public hearings in different parts of the country. It also organized two questionnaires, one sent to one thousand "authorities," including medical professionals, and a second sent to three thousand members of the public. Among the authorities, more than 65 percent supported a recognition of brain death as the end of life. Among the public, only 44.6 percent were of this opinion, but 72 percent stated that they had an interest in organ transplants and brain death. The committee concluded that, given more time, public opposition would surely dissipate, but in the meantime no pressure should be placed on families to have a ventilator turned off in the ICU.

The commission also undertook an "overseas inspection tour."[1] One of its explicit mandates was to visit Europe, America, Australia, and Thailand to study policies and attitudes toward brain death and organ transplants. This commission was requested, in effect, to recommend solutions for Japan in light of close scrutiny of the Other. Such inspection tours in connection with other aspects of Japanese modernization and globalization were quite common during the latter part of the twentieth century.

Of the countries the group visited, Denmark captured the most attention in Japan because brain death had been legally recognized there just a few months before the tour. Until then Danish patients had been obliged to go abroad, usually to Germany, for transplants. Prior to the recognition of brain death in Denmark, there had been over two hundred public hearings and extensive government publicity on the subject (*Nihon Keizai Shinbun* 1990b). Observations there led some of the Japanese delegates to state that, despite numerous publications, there still had not been enough public discussion at home. The committee was impressed with the public trust in doctors in other countries, particularly in Europe, a situation that they contrasted positively with that of Japan (*Nihon Keizai Shinbun* 1990b).

The committee remained deeply divided, and a minority report had to be appended to the final report, even though the group was expected to reach consensus. The majority position was that the existing criteria

---

1. This activity calls to mind the Iwakura Mission of more than 100 years ago, in which, immediately following the end of 250 years of self-imposed isolation, a group of cultural ambassadors from Japan was sent to various European countries and the United States. Their task was to examine the democratic processes, the school system, the armed forces, the legal and medical systems, and the treatment of women in various countries.

for recognition of brain death, the Takeuchi criteria, as set out by the Ministry of Health and Welfare, were appropriate, and that brain death represents the " 'death of a person' *medically*": that is, individual biological death (*kotaishi*). The report points out that it is not appropriate to conflate this medical death with the social and legal death of a person (*hito no shi*), but that clearly in Japan the public increasingly has accepted that brain death does indeed mean the death of the person in *every* sense (Provisional Commission 1992:5, emphasis added). The report concluded that organ transplants using brain-dead donors "should be authorized under certain circumstances" (1992:iii), but that no doctor should be obliged to turn off a ventilator once brain death is declared because this requirement would "grossly offend the doubters' feelings" (1992:5).

Dissenting committee members and advisers (four in all) were not opposed to organ transplants in principle. Their main objection was that the equation of brain death with human death (*ningen no shi*) is illogical, and, moreover, the only reason to do so is to justify procuring organs from the brain-dead. The dissenters represented the majority argument as follows:

> Death is a medical and biological issue, but at the same time a social and legal as well as a philosophical and religious issue. It is proper to give priority to the medical and biological view in determining death, however. Hence, one must acknowledge "brain death" as the "death of a person" according to the latest medical and biological knowledge, which says that a human being is to be comprehended as an organically integrated entity, and the organ that ensures organic integrity is the brain. Thus when the brain dies, the person loses organic integrity, and therefore "brain death" is the "death of a person."
>
> (Provisional Commission 1992:17)

The dissenters insist that to accept brain death as the end of human life is to depart from what in Japan are known as the "three-symptom criteria of death" (no pulse, no breathing, and pupil dilation—that is, cardiopulmonary death). These criteria represent death as it is intuitively understood by almost everyone and can be directly observed, whereas determining the "invisible death" of the brain is a "secret rite" performed behind closed doors (here the dissenters follow the 1985 criticisms of Nakajima Michi). They argue that if brain death could be shown to be "an unshakable understanding of the truth," then no one would hesitate to accept it. Clearly this is not the case, the opposition

says, and moreover the Japanese committee seems to be bent on following "like sheep" the conclusions of the 1981 President's Commission in
the United States.

The dissenters also criticize an unquestioned "rationalism" that implies that the "core" of human life lies in the "faculty of reason," located
in the brain; a mechanistic view of the human body with replaceable
parts; and a view that "whatever is done in the West should be brought
as quickly as possible to Japan." The dissenters would prefer that "modern Western culture" be assimilated critically instead of blindly (Provisional Commission 1992:22).

It later became clear that some of the committee's discussions had
been very heated, even "violent," and included verbal attacks. The philosopher Umehara Takeshi stated that when he had expressed his opinion against brain death, a member of the majority faction had shouted,
"Murderer." But, commented Umehara later, "Surely it is they who are
the murderers?" Nakajima Michi added, "If doctors look at brain-dead
people as corpses, how can we protect these patients?" (Umehara and
Nakajima 1992:306). Apparently many individuals who testified before
the committee, including several scientists and doctors, argued against
the acceptance of brain death, but nevertheless a majority of the committee moved to support its recognition (*Nihon Keizai Shinbun* 1992).

Right after the publication of the committee report, the Japan Federation of Bar Associations (*Nihon Bengoshi Rengōkai*) reasserted the
position it took after the Wada case: that unforeseen consequences might
result from recognition of brain death. It reaffirmed that without a public consensus, the federation could not accept brain death (*Asahi Shinbun* 1992b). The Ministry of Justice, the National Police Agency, and
the Supreme Public Prosecutor's Office each announced their continued
resistance to a recognition of brain death (*Asahi Shinbun* 1992a).

Mistrust of the Medical Profession

Throughout this debate, the Patients' Rights Committee, lawyers, the
police, many authors and journalists, and even a good number of the
medical profession publicly contested the authority of transplant surgeons. All of these groups have stated repeatedly that one of their principal causes for concern is a lack of trust in the medical teams who will
make decisions about brain death; they believed that in the rush to retrieve organs, the process of dying would be hastened or even misdiagnosed. Certain opposition groups, notably the Patients' Rights Com-

mittee, together with several lawyers, explicitly criticized what they described as the secrecy and arrogance of the medical profession and pointed out repeatedly that Japanese citizens are vulnerable to exploitation by doctors.

This widespread public expression of lack of trust in the medical profession marks a significant difference between Japan and North America. The Japanese debate bristles with rhetoric openly critical of medicine, especially as practiced in tertiary care hospitals. In addition to the brain-death scandals, notorious incidents include patient deaths from experimental use of drugs, contaminated blood products, and a stream of cases of malpractice and corruption (Leflar 1996). It is well known that the founder of the Japanese Green Cross, still an active member, was involved with wartime atrocities in Manchuria.

From the late 1970s the medical profession in Japan came under increasing criticism for lack of quality control. Peer review was not institutionalized; postgraduate education standards and specialization requirements were lax; and external oversight was poorly developed (Ikegami 1988; Leflar 1996:8). Ethics committees were not customary in all hospitals, and those that existed usually rubber-stamped research and other activities.

Japanese medicine, influenced at the end of the nineteenth century by German military medicine,[2] has been decried as simultaneously feudalistic and paternalistic; it has assumed that frank discussion is not necessary, since tacit understanding exists between doctors and patients because of their shared cultural heritage. Vagueness on the doctor's part is seen as a virtue—a buffering of patient anxiety in the face of unpleasant diagnoses.[3] When drugs are prescribed, patients are not customarily told of possible side effects. Moreover, patients are conditioned to believe that one "puts oneself in the hands of the doctor," deferring to the superior knowledge of the expert. However, in recent decades, although

---

2. Many Japanese doctors early in the twentieth century trained in Germany and returned to become leaders in Japanese medicine. Several influential German doctors, some of them associated with the military, also lived and worked in Japan and had a profound influence on medical practice. Hamano Kenzō suggests that this exchange has contributed to the authoritarian and paternalistic attitude still evident in Japanese medicine (Hamano 1997).

3. Miyaji Naoko, herself a physician, established from interviews that American doctors often do not reveal uncertain or poor prognoses to patients. They claimed that they were respecting the principles of informed consent because patients were signaling, by not asking questions, that they did not want to hear bad news. Full disclosure would take away any hope they might have (Miyaji 1994:810). These practices are similar to those documented in Japan (Long and Long 1982).

many people continue to trust their family doctors, patients have experienced misgivings about hospital-based medicine that media reporting has brought to light. Given the Japanese heritage of paternalism, the idea of autonomous decision making by patients, or even by patients and their families in partnership with doctors, has simply not been part of the cultural or medical tradition in Japan until very recently. In large tertiary care hospitals where commodification of the body is most likely to take place, trust is on very shaky ground because personal relationships with doctors are not established. Even so, because patients' families usually feel indebted to doctors for services rendered, Nakajima assumes they are likely to agree to organ donation if asked directly, whether or not they feel comfortable about it (1985:217).

It was in this climate that the concept of *infōmudo konsento* (informed consent) was created in Japan (Leflar 1996). The first report on the subject by the Japan Medical Association was produced in 1990 by the *Nihon Ishikai Seimei Rinri Kondankai* (Japan Medical Association Bioethics Roundtable). Robert Leflar's research shows that the meaning of informed consent can range in Japan from the idea of a "courteous dialogue" between doctor and patient to a choice of treatments.

Medical practice has come under fire in Japan in recent years, and patients' rights groups have formed to try to force some policy changes. These activities are part of a general movement for reform, spurred by scandals in business, industry, the banks, and government, most of which relate to bribery and influence-peddling. As a result, the idea of transparency (*tōmeisei*)—of open debate and public decision making— now has a firm hold in public consciousness. The medical profession can no longer expect to pursue its former practices (Leflar 1996:63).

This public skepticism was no doubt the reason that the commission on brain death, in an unusual move, held almost all of its meetings in public and why the Japanese public has been polled so frequently on the matter. The idea that there must be public consensus before brain death can be recognized has been repeated like a mantra.

Many of those who oppose recognition of brain death are concerned more about the codification of informed consent in Japanese medical practice than about brain death per se. The debate has become a powerful weapon for medical reform on a much larger scale. As one doctor put it to me, "Recognition of brain death is being held hostage until bigger things are settled" (see also Leflar 1996:66).

Some changes have resulted from this drive for reform. Patients today are more often than not told when they have cancer.[4] In theory, patients can gain access to their own medical records, although only at the physician's discretion; and guidelines for obtaining informed consent are widely circulated among doctors. But the medical profession has by no means capitulated under this onslaught. The definition of informed consent proposed by the Japan Medical Association gives, as Leflar puts it, "ample room for physician discretion in the nature and extent of information to be given the patient." The JMA report states explicitly that various types of information should be given "to the extent that time permits" (Leflar 1996:98), and the entire exercise is grounded not in patient rights but in patient expectations. However, there is now a near-universal acceptance among the medical profession of informed consent, although it may not always be implemented, and even some physicians have challenged their colleagues to change their ways and take a consumerist, rights-oriented approach to patient care (Leflar 1996:101). Informed consent is not required by Japanese law, although this is not altogether surprising given that Japan is not a litigious society.

In contrast to North America, then, in Japan repeated medical scandals, what is assumed to be paternalistic clinical practice, and legal opposition have been important contributing factors in making recognition of brain death a problem.

Moralizing about Tradition

A few years prior to the passing of the transplant law in 1997, Japanese recipients of organ transplants (usually performed in the United States or Australia) testified publicly for the first time. A symposium held before the Fifteenth World Congress of the Transplantation Society in Kyoto in 1994 included testimonies by half a dozen transplant recipients and several parents of young recipients. Other parents, of children who had died while waiting for organs, gave heartbreaking accounts of their travails. Several of them had received anonymous hate mail after going abroad for surgery and had not had the courage to speak out earlier.

Participants had to run a gauntlet of protesters outside the conference center. Among them were representatives of the physically disabled, who

4. Perhaps the imperial surgeon will not be required in the future, as he was in 1988 when the Emperor Showa was dying of cancer, to appear on television and mislead the entire nation about the nature of the emperor's illness.

distributed a pamphlet protesting proposed modifications to the Eugenic Protection Law that would make it easier to obtain abortions. Protesters against recognition of brain death paired their position with that of opponents of abortion, claiming that the proposed Organ Transplant Bill would introduce yet another form of eugenics. This pamphlet and others like it explicitly link the rights of the unborn with rights of the dying and the brain-dead.

Lobbies in Japan that aggressively promote individual rights are not usually well received, and the disabled have had to struggle to be heard. Some of these activists have adopted the position that every fetus has a right to life. In North America this type of argument effectively places them in opposition to dominant feminist arguments. In Japan, not only does it create ripples of apprehension among feminists, but aggressive promotion of the rights of the brain-dead also incites misgivings among large segments of the public, whether they are for or against the recognition of brain death as the end of life. Those on the conservative end of the spectrum, who argue that recognition of brain death would be immoral—a mindless aping of the "West"—find the promotion of individual rights equally unpalatable.

These incidents during the 1990s highlighted the fissures among individuals and groups opposed to the recognition of brain death. It is clear that both the culture of Japanese tradition and the culture of the "West," with its emphasis on individual rights and autonomy, have been put to work in fending off recognition of the new death. This observation raises a reflexive question: Why have arguments about individual rights never been raised in connection with the brain-dead in Europe or North America? Apparently there, the corpselike status of the brain-dead was secure from very early on. Individual rights are today part of international discourse, and the concept has penetrated almost every corner of the globe, but the situations in which such "rights" may be applicable are not self-evident.

Fragmentation of the opposition to brain death may have given certain transplant patients and their relatives the strength to "come out" and face the Japanese public at the Kyoto conference. Others followed suit.[5] At one meeting of several hundred people that I attended in Tokyo,

5. Many *hibakusha* (atomic-bomb victims) apparently experienced guilt because their "needs" were extraordinary and in excess of what could be expected of a fair and equitable health care system. Some patients waiting for transplants, and their families, demonstrate similar beliefs and undemanding behavior.

designed to promote recognition of brain death, a representative of the Ministry of Health and Welfare, a member of the Japanese Diet, several physicians, and other "experts" were asked to speak, together with transplant recipients. Many members of the audience were emotionally overcome. Kiuchi Hirofumi was on the platform to express his deep appreciation to the donor of his new heart and to the donor's family. He expressed guilt about obtaining his heart in America while Japanese with similar diseases, but without the financial resources to go abroad, continue to die. "Japan has killed them," he said, "just as I felt Japan was going to kill me. I want everyone to know that a heart transplant is no longer a miracle. Out of a total of thirty people who went abroad for heart transplants, twenty-seven are living productive, active, and healthy lives. I have a friend who is ill now. Please change the law and save him."

Despite such public pleas, about half of the members of the Japanese Association for Philosophical and Ethical Research in Medicine continued to oppose legislation supporting brain death as the end of life. Like disability activists, they expressed concern about the human rights of the brain-dead (*Transplant News* 1994). No such argument could have been produced by a North American society for bioethics. On the contrary, such reasoning has tended to work towards an expansion of the good-as-dead status to apply to broader classes of patients whose lives are deemed futile (Lock, in press).

Meanwhile, the minister of health and welfare announced in 1994 that his ministry was not opposed to transplant surgery involving brain-dead donors. However, the actions of a team of doctors at Yokohama General Hospital once again produced a strong current of criticism, both within the Japan Medical Association and among the public. These surgeons admitted that early in 1994 they had removed kidneys from four brain-dead patients before their hearts had stopped beating and transplanted them into eight recipients. Yokohama General Hospital is a large urban tertiary care center, but it has no ethics committee and so did not meet the requirements set out by the Ministry of Health and Welfare for an organ transplant center. Moreover, the apnea test, one of the indispensable tests for determining brain death according to the Takeuchi criteria, was not used (*Asahi Shinbun* 1994d). Critics claim that the transplant surgeons were involved with neurologists in making the brain-death diagnoses and in obtaining family consent for transplantation.

Citizens against Brain Death

During the 1990s, together with Patients' Rights Group based at Tokyo University, numerous citizens' groups formed a grass-roots opposition to the recognition of brain death. These groups hold regular meetings and publish national newsletters giving details about murder charges they have brought against doctors, along with details about cases in which brain-dead patients have supposedly come back to life.

Such groups also organize public demonstrations in which physically disabled individuals and nurses, some of whom work in ICUs, often support them (*Asahi Shinbun* 1993c). They participate in media events and submit petitions against the recognition of the new death to various official committees. The letters have hundreds of signatures appended, including those of well-known intellectuals and celebrities.

I have interviewed several members of these groups, who complain repeatedly that in Japan the public is not yet accorded full democratic rights and that the opinions of ordinary people are brushed aside. Here again, they self-consciously mobilize the tradition of the West, embraced as part of Japanese modernization.

I attended a meeting of one of these groups in Kyoto in 1994, right before the international transplant conference. This well-known group was founded by a physician, Yamaguchi Kenichiro, who works with neurologically impaired patients. Participants hold regular "study" sessions on a range of issues bearing on ethics in medicine, and although brain death has recently been given priority, the group is also extremely active on euthanasia, the rights of the disabled, genetic counseling, reproductive technologies, eugenics, Nazi medicine, and, of passionate interest to several members of this group, Unit 731, the wartime site of Japanese experimentation on Chinese prisoners. Group members find common themes in the various bioethics issues that they discuss, and one of their prime fears about recognition of brain death is that patients in this condition will be used as experimental subjects.

At the close of the meeting, at which I gave a presentation about organ transplantation in Montreal, this group climbed onto a bus to go to a demonstration outside the international transplant conference, where they would distribute leaflets in English and Japanese. They wanted the transplant world to be made fully cognizant of what they called "suspicious experiments" in connection with organ procurement in Japan, as well as of the increasing worldwide commercialization of human organs. Further, they wanted to force an acknowledgment of the rights of brain-dead patients. After spending two days with this opposition group, I rather sheepishly made my way past the demonstrators into the entrance hall, only to discover several of the leaders of this group already there, preparing to pose searching questions directly to conference speakers.

Individuals have varied motives for joining these groups. Perhaps the majority are concerned with human rights, human experimentation, informed consent, and ethical issues associated with the new biomedical technologies. Others, however, oppose recognition of brain death simply because they think the idea of procuring organs from the brain-dead is spooky. Teraoka Reiko, who participates in a Tokyo-based opposition group, informed me that she is both "modern" and "premodern." She participates fully, as she puts it, in a technologically sophisticated society; but when her mother died, both she and her children were certain that her mother's spirit remained in the house. She says that if she were to have a transplant, she would feel as though someone else's spirit was residing in her. Should the transplant fail, it would certainly be *tatari*—retribution by the spirit. Teraoka says that no one taught her to feel this way, but that she is an animist, although without any formal religious affiliation.

Reaching Public Consensus

Concurrent with government, professional, and media presentations on the brain-death problem has been the unprecedented search for a public consensus (*kokuminteki gōi*). At least fourteen national surveys on brain death and organ transplants, and numerous other smaller ones, were conducted between 1983 and 1996. Over the years, the number of respondents who recognized brain death as the end of life increased from 29 percent to just over 50 percent, with more men than women answering positively. However, the numbers dropped from 53 percent and 54 percent in two 1996 surveys to 40 percent in 1997 (*Yomiuri Shinbun* 1996b; *Asahi Shinbun* 1996b; *Asahi Shinbun* 1997g). This drop may have been due to fears about the possible spread of AIDS through transplants and a heightened distrust of doctors (*Asahi Shinbun* 1996b). The number of respondents who supported organ transplantation in principle declined from 84 percent to 73 percent.

Almost all these surveys show that many more people approve of organ transplants from brain-dead patients than accept brain death as human death. This apparent paradox can perhaps be reconciled: respondents frequently agree that even if brain death is not officially recognized as the end of life, organ procurement from the brain-dead may be acceptable provided that both the donor and her family have given prior consent (*Mainichi Shinbun* 1991). In other words, respondents do not wish to impede those who want to volunteer as organ donors, but most people would not choose to do so themselves. They demonstrate this by answering that they would not want to be counted as dead if diagnosed as brain-dead.

Even though nothing like a public consensus has been reached, and despite the weight of the negative media campaign, a large number of Japanese appear willing to have brain death recognized. The polls also reveal that the majority are not opposed to organ transplants, although the fact that Japanese have had to travel abroad for transplants and to buy organs has caused a great deal of tension and sometimes overt hostility.

Opposition groups frequently use these polls to bolster their arguments, because of the claim that public consensus must be reached before brain death can be nationally recognized. Nudeshima points out that at least one poll in the 1980s in the United States showed that only just over 50 percent of respondents supported organ donation (Manninen and Evans 1985), and a similar poll conducted in Japan in 1990 gave a result only one percentage point lower (*Yomiuri Shinbun*, cited in Nudeshima 1991a). One is left with the feeling, voiced by many members of the Japanese public, that the exercise of repeatedly surveying the nation is a farce (Morioka 1995): the questions asked are often ambiguous, and the idea of consensus on such an issue is without meaning. Extensive public discussion about this sensitive subject is essential, but opinion polls do not substitute for such a discussion.

The Law Steps In

Although it was assumed that the report of the special commission would clear the way for a bill to be presented to the Japanese Diet, heated public debate continued, and submission of a bill was repeatedly put off, often with the excuse that further public discussion and consensus were needed. Finally, in the spring of 1994, a private member's bill calling for the recognition of brain death as the end of human life and for legalization of the removal of organs from brain-dead patients, with family consent, was submitted to the government by former foreign minister and physician Nakayama Taro, who had been involved from the start in the official deliberations about brain death. The complex bill, of twenty-four sections, did not require that a patient's will (*ishi*) be known, but simply that it be "surmised" (*sontaku suru*) by close relatives. In May 1994 lawyers introduced a second bill, this one opposing the recognition of brain death as the end of life but supporting those who choose to donate organs should they become brain-dead, provided that the patient's prior will was known (*Nihon Keizai Shinbun* 1994a).

Discussion of the bills was also repeatedly postponed, and when parliament was dissolved and a new government elected in autumn 1994, both bills were expected to die (*Asahi Shinbun* 1994c). A group of over 150 general practitioners handed a statement to the Ministry of Health and Welfare stating that they were opposed to the bills because of their vagueness and a lack of public consensus on the issue (*Mainichi Shinbun* 1994).

Despite the continuing impasse, an air of anticipation was present at this time, punctuated by media commentary. The press reported that in Korea, where brain death was not legally recognized at the time, organ transplants had been performed since 1992.[6] It was suggested that the donors were probably Christians but that Korea's Confucian heritage would surely deter the practice (*Asahi Shinbun* 1994a). During the same period, the stress experienced by patients and families going abroad for transplants was well-documented. At one Australian hospital, of 365 liver transplants performed in the first eleven months of 1994, 20 percent had been done on Japanese patients, many of whom had waited for six months or more in Brisbane before having the operation (*Asahi Shinbun* 1994h).

In autumn 1994, the *Asahi Shinbun* commented critically on a series of advertisements that had appeared all over Tokyo from a man who wished to sell a kidney for 2 million yen (then approximately US$21,000). Several people had responded to the advertisement, but in the end the kidney was not sold (1994f). Advertisements also appeared for a Tokyo brokerage company that arranged for kidney transplants in the Philippines (*Nihon Keizai Shinbun* 1994c). For a month in November 1994, hotlines were set up in Tokyo and Osaka to receive complaints from the public regarding the medical treatment of relatives diagnosed as brain-dead. These hotlines were flooded with phone calls from angry and disillusioned citizens, many of which were reported in the media (*Asahi Shinbun* 1994g).

6. Brain death was legally recognized in Korea in 1998 (Watts 1998b).

From late 1994 through 1996, discussion of the bills in the Diet was postponed in favor of attention to the national economy and international politics. A 1996 statement by the Anesthesiology Association of Japan effectively ruled out organ procurement from brain-dead patients when the group stated that they would not cooperate with procurement of organs until a law was passed (*Asahi Shinbun* 1996c). However, in April 1997, activity resumed, including discussion and hearings in the Lower House of the Diet for and against both the bills. Despite the expressed concern of one member of the House that a brain-death law might well lead to *aotagari* (the harvesting of green rice, meaning that patients might be counted dead before their time—*Asahi Shinbun* 1997c), and caution advised by representatives of sixteen Japanese religious groups (*Asahi Shinbun* 1997e), the Lower House passed the first bill by a vote of 320 to 148, with 32 abstentions. The second bill, which would have recognized brain death medically but not legally, was voted down. The voting was unusual in that members of the Diet were permitted a conscience vote, without obligation to support their political party. The one party throughout that had been completely opposed to both bills was the Japan Communist Party.

Amid another flurry of petitions signed by opposition groups who felt the ground slipping away beneath them—petitions that focused on inappropriate government intrusion into the private life of citizens (*Asahi Shinbun* 1997b), inappropriate commodification of the human body, and fears that organ transplants would not be arranged fairly—the bill went forward for discussion before the Upper House. Deadlock in discussion resulted in a third, compromise bill that was finally passed in mid-June. The compromise bill was discussed for only a few hours by the conservative Upper House, an action described by some observers as flagrantly irresponsible (*Nihon Keizai Shinbun* 1997). In this bill, notably, brain death was not recognized explicitly as human death. The Lower House formally approved the decision the same day.

Just before these bills went to the Upper House, several religious sects submitted statements to the House saying that they could not accept the law as it was worded because in their opinion the soul or spirit (*reikon*) does not completely leave the body (*kanzen ridatsu*) until the heart stops beating (*Asahi Shinbun* 1997e). It is possible that these submissions influenced the law as it was finally constituted in the Upper House.

The compromise bill, which became the Organ Transplant Law on October 16, 1997, is closer in some important points to the original proposal that was rejected by the Lower House than to the Nakayama bill that was passed.[7] The law states that organs may be retrieved from a patient diagnosed as brain-dead, provided the patient has previously given written consent and that the family does not overrule the patient's decision. Donors must be at least fifteen years of age (the minimum age at which an individual can leave a valid will [Zepeda 1998]).[8] Caution is advised in assessing the wishes of potential donors who are mentally handicapped. If no advance directives exist, or if the family is opposed to donation, then a brain-dead patient will continue to receive medical care unless or until the family and medical team agree to turn off the ventilator. Physicians are obliged to keep medical records about consent and procurement procedures and to make them available to patients' families for up to five years.

Brain death is equated with death in Japan, therefore, *only* when patients and families wish to donate organs. The law refers to "the body of a brain-dead entity" (*nōshi shita mono no shintai*), but nowhere does it state explicitly that brain death is equivalent to human death. In the end the bill signifies formal recognition of something very like the "alpha period" suggested by Bai Kōichi nearly thirty years earlier, an ambiguous time of living death to which special laws can be applied.

An additional statement was released several weeks after the law was passed clarifying what constitutes a family. These guidelines state that consent should be obtained from all relatives who lived with the deceased, including grandparents and grandchildren, if appropriate. The "collective will" of the family must be determined by the family itself and presented to physicians by the designated family representative, that is, the head of the family or the person in charge of mourning rituals. If dissent is expressed by relatives other than the coresidential family, then caution is advised. In practice, this means that if a distant relative telephones to say that he or she is opposed to donation, even when close family members are in favor, then it is quite likely that the procurement will be stopped. Contrary to the spirit of the law, a 1998 survey shows that nearly 77 percent of respondents think that the written wishes of the patient should be sufficient and that the consent of the family should not be required. The figures are only slightly lower regarding consent

7. See Zepeda 1998 for a comprehensive account of the legal contribution to brain-death disputes and to the eventual passing of the law in Japan.

8. In effect, this edict prevents Japanese children from receiving hearts from brain-dead donors unless they go overseas: the donated organs will be too big. It is sometimes possible to pare a liver down to the appropriate size. Adult kidneys can usually be used in children.

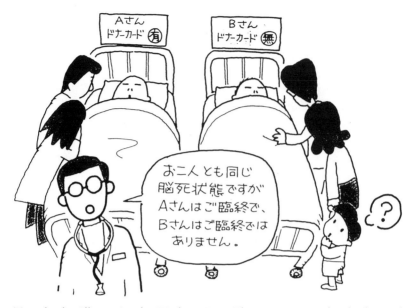

Two deaths. Illustration by Kitahara Isao. The caption says that both people are in the same brain-dead state, but Mr. A, who is willing to be a donor, will get no more treatment, whereas Mr. B, who is not willing to be a donor, will continue to receive treatment. Reproduced from *Iryo '97*, vol. 13, by permission of Medical Friends Co. Ltd., Tokyo.

for donation of corpses for medical purposes (Naikaku Sōri Daijin kanbō kōhōshitsu 1988).

Physicians are not required by law, as they are in most parts of North America, to ask relatives to consider donating a brain-dead patient's organs, nor can they be required by hospital administrators to do so. Initiation of such discussion is left to the family and to forthright doctors. Distribution by the transplant coordination network of over four million donor consent cards has eased this situation somewhat, and several informants, some of them doctors, told me that donor cards should assist families of brain-dead patients enormously in supporting donation. Families know in advance that their relative has expressed a wish to donate, because both the potential donor and a family member must sign the card. Donor cards are readily available in convenience stores and post offices, and people can also indicate their willingness to donate by signing their driver's licenses or filling out the appropriate space on their health care card. It remains to be seen just how effective this massive campaign will be.

The law requires that the time of death must be written down twice on the death certificate for brain-dead patients: once when brain death is confirmed, and again when the heart stops beating. Patients who become brain-dead in effect die twice so that organ procurement can be legalized. Brain death in Japan is thus a socially determined death; for, although it must be rigorously established medically, if the individual or the family does not regard the patient as dead, then the medical diagnosis will not suffice. If organs are removed, this fact too must be noted on the death certificate. The act also stipulates that after a declaration of brain death, the patient's medical expenses will be reimbursed through the health insurance system "for the time being." This means that patients whose families decline to have the ventilator turned off will continue to receive health care coverage. The existing law was subject to revision in the year 2000, but this did not occur. Revisions are now expected in 2003.

The law categorically forbids the buying and selling of organs. Shortly after the bill was passed, it was made known that the cost of organ transplants and the necessary medications would be covered by the national health insurance system. The rudimentary network for coordination of organ procurement and distribution was then consolidated. The country is currently divided into seven districts for this purpose, but as of 2000 there were only eighty "donor coordinators" and ten hospital-affiliated "recipient coordinators." Fifteen coordinators deal with the densely populated Kanto area that includes the Tokyo-Yokohama megalopolis. Tokyo itself has only four donor coordinators and one recipient coordinator. The system is badly underfunded by the Ministry of Health and Welfare, and there are stories of incompetent leadership and coordinator burnout. Its supporters hope that as more organs are donated, funding will increase.

Loose Ends

Immediately after the new law was passed, a national group for the families of traffic accident victims (*zenkoku kōtsū jiko izoku no kai*) set out to abolish it and to promote the use of "nondonor" cards. At the same time a newspaper article proclaimed, "Doctors may be committing unforgivable crimes by performing organ transplants from brain-dead donors, a neurology expert warns." This Tokyo-based neurologist, Furukawa Tetsuo, argues that general anesthesia should be used during procurement of organs because "it still has not been scientifically proved

that brain-dead people are completely unconscious when . . . classified
as brain-dead. It means that brain-dead donors may be experiencing
extreme pain when their organs are being removed by surgeons for use
in others" (*Japan Times* 1997).[9] When I met Furukawa in 1999, he had
recently given a presentation at an international bioethics meeting with
the title "Are the Brain-Dead Really Unconscious?" On the basis of
animal experiments and EEG results using unusual leads (nasopharyn-
geal and intracranial), Furukawa argues that brain activity continues
after brain death, and that in such patients a "primordial" consciousness
may persist. He believes that, although in deep coma, brain-dead patients nevertheless respond in very subtle ways, especially to their mothers, and that the crying sometimes observed in such patients is not a
strictly physiological phenomenon but an expression of emotion.[10]

In March 1998, eight of the outstanding legal cases in which transplant surgeons had been charged with murder, including the Tsukuba
case (by then fourteen years old), were finally dropped on the grounds
of insufficient evidence. Over the years criminal charges have been
brought against more than twenty doctors. Commentators assumed that
dismissal of these cases would at last allow transplants to proceed. However, in May 1998 a hospital attached to Kansai Ikadai University was
ordered by the court to pay 200,000 yen (US$2,000) to a woman whose
daughter had been declared brain-dead and from whom kidneys had
been removed for transplant. A catheter had been inserted into one of
the patient's femoral arteries after brain death was declared and before
her heart stopped beating, to introduce fluids to preserve the kidneys.
This is not an unusual procedure, but the court ruled that the insertion
of the catheter was not part of the treatment of the patient, and therefore
her prior consent was necessary. This ruling suggests clearly that certain
courts in Japan are prepared to pursue charges about the treatment of
brain-dead bodies on the basis that such patients are not legally dead
(*Asahi Shinbun* 1998b).

Also in March 1998, three doctors employed at Naha hospital in
Okinawa were charged with murder by the family of a man whose kidney was removed after his heart stopped beating. The family claims that
the doctors turned down the ventilator even though the patient was not
yet declared brain-dead. The doctors state that they had definitively di-

9. More recently, British anesthetists have declared that they want use made of anesthesia while organs are procured because the involuntary movements of brain-dead bodies when not fully sedated are "disturbing" (Young and Matta 2000).
10. Every other neurologist I have talked to disagrees.

agnosed brain death and that the family understood this and had agreed both to kidney donation and to the turning down of the ventilator, although the medical chart notes that the family had reservations about organ donation. The reporter covering this case says that it underscores the importance of gaining the complete cooperation of families for organ donation (*Asahi Shinbun* 1998b). And so the disputes continue.

No simple ideological or political divisions can be detected between those for and against the acceptance of brain death in Japan, as was made clear when the Diet chose not to vote along party lines. While people of a conservative, traditionalist persuasion are virtually unanimously opposed, they share this position with others who are certainly not in agreement with them politically. This group includes Tachibana Takashi, the journalist and producer of the NHK television programs (whose reporting influenced the downfall of the corrupt former prime minister, Tanaka Kakuei), and a good number of the medical profession, both young and old, including some surgeons. Activists for the handicapped and the mentally ill are also opposed, as are a great number of lawyers, citizens concerned about patients' rights, and the police. Advocates for acceptance include numerous intellectuals and professionals, among them physicians, many of whom have spent time in North America or Europe. They are joined by many others, including patient groups and families and supporters of people who are organ recipients or on transplant waiting lists.

Recognition of brain death as the end of life has in effect been held to ransom for a plethora of reasons, among them a resistance to the power of the medical profession and distrust of hospital-based doctors. Some dissenters claim to want Japan to be more democratic and to develop a more humanly oriented and ethical medical system, one that is free of corruption. Almost no one supports a mindless imitation of the West, especially America. To some, the very idea of this particular technology is repulsive and unnatural.

Breakthrough

Not until the spring of 1999, thirty years after the Wada case and nearly a year and a half after the Organ Transplant Law was passed, were the first transplants from a brain-dead donor carried out. There were, however, fifty-four near misses in the interval. A television documentary elaborates on five of these cases. Even though patients had declared that they wanted to be donors, and in the majority of cases family members supported the donation, the hospital bureaucracies claimed in each case that the donor cards had not been filled out quite correctly. The television program shows just how confusing the cards were at that time and how easy it was to make a mistake. The design of donor cards was since been changed.

On March 1, 1999, the heart, liver, and kidneys procured from a middle-aged woman were transplanted with enormous fanfare into four recipients. This event was marred by remarkable breaches of the privacy of the donor's family and the recipients. Leaked information about a possible donor in Kochi Red Cross Hospital, Shikoku, was first made public on February 25. Within hours about three hundred journalists descended on the hospital, and for the next three days they produced hourly reports on the situation. The donor, whose age and sex were revealed, had been admitted with a brain hemorrhage several days earlier and was declared clinically brain-dead on the day the media made the case public. The family informed the medical team that the patient had signed a donor card and that they agreed to donation. The law requires two sets of tests subsequent to a clinical declaration of brain death, to be conducted by neurospecialists who are not directly involved with the care of the patient. During the first of these legal tests (as they are known), in contrast to the result obtained from the clinical diagnosis, the EEG, in which the machine was set at a very high sensitivity, showed some brain activity (which may well have been simply an artifact of the equipment). The clinical diagnosis was overturned, and the media reported that the comatose patient had been "prematurely" designated as the nation's first organ donor after being "mistakenly" diagnosed as brain-dead (*Japan Times* 1999a).

An emergency medicine doctor responding to these criticisms stated that the second and third set of tests to confirm so-called legal brain death were working well as a check on the process. He added that brain death should never be declared on the basis of a clinical diagnosis alone; all one can say at that stage is that the patient is "as close as it gets to brain death." A lawyer noted with irony that when a friend is brain-dead, one does not know whether to come to the hospital carrying an *omimai* (a present for the sick) or a *kōden* (a funeral gift) (*Yomiuri Shinbun* 1999a).

Hospital administrators and the physicians involved begged the media to leave the donor family in peace. Several editorials noted that other families would be unlikely to agree to donation if they knew their privacy would be violated by paparazzi. After the clinical diagnosis was overturned, the family and the doctors agreed to postpone any decisions for a day or two. The family remained firm in their resolve to donate but demanded that nothing be made public, even when the tests for brain death were repeated. They also asked for permission to take their relative's remains home right after the donation. They added that they were exhausted and wanted a complete news blackout.

The legal tests were completed over the next two days, and the organs were finally procured by the Japan Organ Transplant Network and flown by helicopter to hospitals where anxious recipients were waiting. The entire event was tracked in the media as though, as one cultural critic put it, a war had broken out. Soap operas were interrupted by bulletins about the transplants; evening news programs showed footage of the boxes that contained the organs (Watts 1999). Reporters were permitted, with the consent of the recipient, to watch the heart transplant via closed-circuit television at the Osaka hospital, and the chief surgeon provided commentary about the procedures at each step. This scene, which was carried out in the interests of proving to the public that nothing untoward was happening, was described as a "media carnival" and was reminiscent of the Christiaan Barnard days. Nevertheless, nine citizens' groups submitted a letter to the Ministry of Health and Welfare complaining that secrecy surrounded the entire train of events and particularly the brain-death diagnosis (*Asahi Shinbun* 1999b). The Ministry reacted by refusing to make any official statement about determination of the brain-death diagnosis for two weeks after the event, thus fueling suspicion.

Following the organ procurement, the prime minister told reporters, "I sincerely pray for the repose of the donor's soul, I also pray for the smooth recovery of the recipients" (*Japan Times* 1999b). After an initial partial rejection in the liver recipient, all did well, and the Japanese transplant world breathed an enormous sigh of relief.

As I learned when I went to Tokyo in spring 1999 to talk to neurosurgeons, transplants surgeons, and transplant coordinators about this event, everyone believes that a tug-of-war (*tsunahiki*) took place between the perceived need for the Japanese public to be fully informed and the protection of the privacy of the patients and their families. The media ensured that this tug-of-war was won by those interested in complete disclosure.

Several inconsistencies were exposed: first, the attending emergency medicine doctor who had carried out the original clinical tests did not do them in the exact order as specified by the Takeuchi criteria (which would not normally be a major cause for concern among specialists). Early in the proceedings he included an apnea test, which is not required until brain death is being legally confirmed. The media reported that to do an apnea test the ventilator must be turned off for ten minutes, potentially accelerating the death of brain cells if the patient is not already brain-dead, and this revelation, not surprisingly, caused a flurry of public concern. Second, the donor family made public a letter of protest about the release of information before brain death had been declared. The Japan Organ Transplant Network apologized to the donor family and to the Ministry of Health and Welfare and stated at a press conference that they would in future do everything that they could to protect the privacy of donors.

The 2 million yen (US$20,000) cost of procurement of the organs was also criticized, in particular the use of helicopters to transport the organs. Accusations were made about health care money being swallowed up by the expenses of showy organ transplants. The time it took for the dying donor to be transported to hospital was also questioned, and emergency medical services in Japan were criticized, particularly the ambulance service. The president of the Society for Emergency Medicine took the opportunity to argue for better government support for emergency transport. Several medical professionals commented to me on the bravery of the emergency medicine doctors who had made the procurement possible. To be the first, and to expose one's team to so much media attention, is not to be envied.

The medical specialists with whom I talked believe, despite the criticisms, that brain-death donations are now in principle recognized in Japan, and that after two or three more successful transplants the media will set their sights on other matters. However, many of the doctors also believe that Japanese remain deeply reluctant to donate organs and that the Japan Organ Transplant Network, despite its nationwide campaign, is simply not up to the enormous task of overcoming public inertia.

Several of my Japanese friends and acquaintances commented that it gave them a strange feeling to think about the donor's organs being distributed all over Japan, to end up functioning in four other people. They said they themselves would be very reluctant to donate if they thought their body parts would be dispersed all over the place. More than one person commented on a Japanese television program that had graphically portrayed how in America the donor body, after procurement, is stuffed with packing materials and pieces of pipe in preparation for burial. The authenticity of this information was not questioned.

A national survey, conducted after the first donor had been located but before the transplants were complete, showed that although 30 percent of respondents said they would donate their organs should they be declared brain-dead, only 2.6 percent carried donor cards (*Yomiuri Shinbun* 1999b). A second survey, conducted right after the transplants, found that 6 percent of respondents had signed donor cards and that another 25 percent "would like" to have a donor card. Of these respondents, 66 percent thought it was a good thing that the transplants had taken place (*Mainichi Shinbun* 1999).

The ruling Liberal Democratic Party stated that when the Organ Transplant Law is reviewed, protection of privacy must be given top priority. They expressed concern that donor families may receive hate mail from those who oppose the recognition of brain death, and they worried that people might not fully realize that donation is based on "a gift of love with no compensation" (*Yomiuri Shinbun* 1999c).

Several of the individuals prominent in the brain-death disputes were asked for comments after the first legal procurement. Among them was Wada Jiro, now over seventy years old. He complained that the media has learned nothing since his own attempt at a heart transplant. Nakajima Michi was critical of what she described as a lack of awareness about the regulations of the Organ Transplant Law at the hospital where the brain-death tests were conducted. Nudeshima Jiro told me that he was so disaffected by the Japanese media that he simply refused to talk to them at all. The Japan Federation of Bar Associations remained uncharacteristically quiet.

By the end of 2000 there had been nine successful procurements from ten brain-dead patients. The media hounded the family of the third donor, visiting their house and demanding interviews. The "brain-death problem" is by no means resolved.

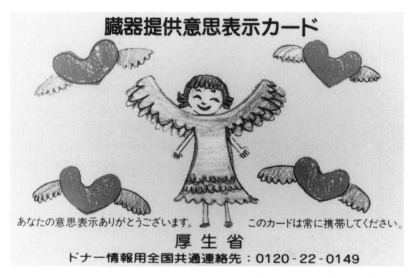

Japanese organ donor card. Angels are not part of Japanese tradition. The iconography on the donor card is decidedly "Western," but appropriately Japanized by being made "cute." Courtesy of Japan Organ Transplant Network, Tokyo.

EIGHT

Social Death and Situated Departures

How alike are the sleeping and the dead.
The image of death cannot be depicted.
The Epic of Gilgamesh, Tablet X,
The Waters of Death

Death and Life were not
Till man made up the whole
Made lock, stock and barrel
Out of his bitter soul.
W. B. Yeats, "The Tower," Part 3

The European and North American literature on medical death in the past hundred years reveals concerns that persist today.[1] Unanimous agreement exists that a diagnosis of death must be conservative. False negatives—treating someone as alive who is actually dead—cause no harm to an individual (provided that this time is not protracted, denying the individual death with dignity). They may result in social costs: resources may be wasted, for treatment and care continue, and a busy ICU in a financially strapped hospital is under constant pressure to free up beds. False positive errors, however, must be ruled out entirely. People must never be misdiagnosed as biologically dead when in fact they are alive: all possibilities of reanimation must be eliminated, and no one should be sent to the morgue before their time. Medical tests to determine death must be absolutely reliable and performed carefully.

A second set of more abstract issues was reactivated with the invention of the new death. Is death an event or a process? Does the vital principle of life reside in a single organ? If so, which one? When does an organism as a whole die, as opposed to its parts? These questions lead to concerns often left unvoiced but nevertheless germane to the care

---

1. I do not discuss the literature on palliative care and euthanasia.

of the dying and dead: What is the relationship between the soul (or mind, or vital essence) and the body? More specifically, when do individuals or persons—as opposed to bodies—die? And how does individual death relate to the moment or process in which the vital essence "leaves" the physical body and ceases to exist? What relationship is there among death as a familial and social event, death of the person, and physical death? Is one form of death given priority over others? And what moral status is assigned to each of these deaths?

Clearly, the condition of "living cadavers" causes confusion, particularly so because we insist categorically that they must be dead if their organs are to be removed; no one considers the possibility, even remotely, of institutionalizing vivisection, although we refer to "vital" organs being removed from the "body." The contradictions created by living cadavers leave room for the production of imaginative discourse. Conceptual maneuvers must be mobilized, whether to enable or to prohibit organ procurement. In the United States and Canada, the dominant discourse has enabled the diagnosis of irreversible loss of consciousness to count as equivalent to the death of the person, thus permitting the utilitarian procurement of organs. In Japan, on the other hand, recognition of brain death was blocked because the dominant discourse in that country insists that an irreversible loss of consciousness is neither biological death nor the death of the person. Recognition of brain death in Japan has come about after years of professional and political rhetorical manipulation, and even now is recognized only conditionally.

When the demise of persons and bodies is made into a measurable biological event, wherever its location in the body, the social significance of death is by default minimized, particularly in ICUs. But perennial concerns cluster around social death, just as they do around biological death, and many of them are particularly relevant to brain death. The form that death takes and its timing color the emotional responses of the living: Had the individual's life run its course, or was death premature and "untimely"? Was the death "good" or "bad"? Was it "natural," or did it involve suffering, violence, trauma, or error? Other issues include the respect and power assigned to corpses, forms of memorialization of the dead, and the extent to which the dead exert an influence on the living.

In short, debate about what exactly constitutes death, its timing and determination, the technological or ritual orchestration of dying, other parties' competing interests in the body, and the emotional and practical responses of the living to the dying are all moral concerns. Such concerns are the products of specific cultural and historical milieus, and they influence the responses by involved families, health care professionals, and society at large, to brain death and organ procurement.

Different meanings attributed to bodies and body parts, the location of vitality in the body and its relationship to the person and society, ideas about continuity after death, and the timing and location of physical death all show that death is far from being uniformly understood. The determination and observance of death illuminate the boundaries constructed between culture and nature, individual and society. Death rituals inevitably confront human mortality, and human groups put culture to work to transcend it and ensure social continuity, even as individual bodies die and decompose.

Even in isolated societies, representations of death and death rites are transformed through innovation and contact with people and ideas from other locations (Woodburn 1982). Even so, some social meanings attributed to death appear to be held in common by peoples everywhere, and if we confine our attention merely to biological death, these social meanings tend to be pushed to one side, or even belittled. A historical and comparative review of the massive literature on death and mortuary practices reveals how stubbornly persistent and uniform are some of the unresolvable ambiguities and disputes about death, a few of which are introduced below. These ambiguities are of particular relevance when a death is thought of as untimely or out of place.

Given that anxiety about death is universal, and that everywhere it means something more than biological failure, it is perhaps surprising that so many families agree to organ donation. One might anticipate that the Japanese resistance to the new death would be the usual response, and that social and familial meanings associated with the dying and the newly dead might override an acceptance of the intrusions into bereavement necessitated by organ procurement.

The Liminality of Dying

The best-known anthropological study of death is a product of the French school founded by Émile Durkheim. Robert Hertz, Durkheim's pupil, researched the symbolism of death through an examination of mortuary practices in Borneo in the first decade of the twentieth century. He concluded that biological death is not experienced as the instantaneous destruction of an individual's life, but rather as a social event. Physical death sets off a series of practices culminating in initiation into a social afterlife as an ancestor. The apprehension associated with death is thus contained through otherworldly continuity (Hertz 1960).

According to Hertz, the corpse is managed as a "natural symbol," redolent with contradictory social meanings. It must be handled with care as much for its moral significance as for its qualities of physical contagion and repulsion. As with other life-cycle transitions, death rites are bounded by rituals of separation followed by a liminal period, an ambiguous state carefully orchestrated by society, and completed through rituals of incorporation into an afterworld or, in secular society, a void (Van Gennep 1960; Turner 1969). This frightening, potentially polluting event is controlled through ritual, but the social order is itself in part reconstituted by means of its performance (Bloch and Parry 1982; Leach 1961). At once and inseparably individual *and* social, death ritual permits a celebration and resolution of the paradox that so exercised Freud, that of the discontinuity of individual lives and the continuity of the social order (Freud 1939; Brown 1961).

Because they are socially transcendent, the dying are made into the "moral architects of the living world" (Comaroff 1984:158). The dead do not simply "watch over" or monitor the world of the living but actually reconstitute everyday life through rituals that strive to negate the decomposition and decay of physical death. One of the most dramatic instances of this negation is furnished by Aghori Hindu ascetics who live on cremation grounds and consume their food out of human skulls. But a belief that new life springs from bare bones following the decomposition of the flesh is by no means limited to ascetics.

The association of death with fecundity is often represented ritually as a gift bestowed on society with the blessing of those in authority. The Christian story of resurrection is a variant on this theme. Society is thus "anchored" not just by political power, but "by some of the deepest emotions, beliefs, and fears of people everywhere" (Bloch and Parry 1982:41). Of course, the "gift" of life is the metaphor most often used to encourage the donation of organs for transplant. Such gifts certainly have the blessing of those in authority, and they very often "save" individual lives, but because organs are objectified as spare body parts and are donated anonymously, both their emotional and social worth are dissipated.

Death and the Social Order

The anthropologist Nadia Seremetakis criticizes Hertz and other scholars who follow his lead because, in her opinion, they focus too narrowly on the internal periodization of the process of death, that is, on the containment of physical death, culminating in burial and the departure of the spirit. She sees these researchers as overly concerned about the management of disorder and pollution and about the return of society to its "normal" integrated, homeostatic condition through mortuary practices. On the basis of her ethnographic work among the Greeks of Inner Mani, Seremetakis argues for "leaky boundaries" between life and death. In her opinion, full social order is never restored. Death, its representation, its discourses, and performance haunt society, and death frequently becomes a site from which the social order is contested. Michael Taussig, for example, writing about the "space of death" in Colombia, describes the coerced transformation of death rituals during colonization as a project of imperialist history, and he documents indigenous resistance to this process. One outcome of colonization, then, may be the politicization of death practices (1987:373).

Japan is a society acutely sensitive to the way in which the social order may be contested through death practices. Ritual suicides by samurai, generals, unrequited lovers, and famous authors are feted as part of Japan's tradition, both inside the country and outside it. Taking one's life to make a statement about the condition of society, or the worth of a cause, or alternatively about a perceived failure of self or another to meet society's expectations, are long-standing practices in Japan. Trauma, whether self-inflicted or accidental, invites reflection, not only about the victim but also about society. Brain death, like suicide, produces profound feelings of disorder in those "left behind."

Good and Bad Death

Sudden and uncontrolled death, and particularly accidental and violent death, death in childbirth, and suicide, raise concerns about the condition of the social order. Death rituals frequently seek to negate the aleatory character of physical death. This negation is often accomplished by masking the discrepancy between the inevitable process of biological death and the social recognition of the end of an individual human life, a process that can be carefully orchestrated. Among the Lugbara of Uganda, for example, a dying man is expected to say his last words to his heir, who then emerges from the hut where they have been closeted together. This moment marks the succession, and even if the sick man lingers, his mortuary rites are then performed as if he were dead (Middleton 1982). Peter Stephenson notes that, in explicit contrast to the "fast (and therefore supposedly 'painless')" death that seems to be commonly desired in North America, among the Hutterites a slow, drawn-out death is considered best. The dying person selects the hymns to be sung and food to be prepared for the ritual to mark his or her death (1983:127). Such examples make it startlingly clear that what is of prime concern is not the moment of physical death but rather the significance of the death to society.

Among the Greeks of Inner Mani, a good death implies an easy separation of the soul from the body. When death is imminent, the mourning of women takes the form of a mimesis of the present disorder and danger, culminating in "screaming the dead," a violent noise completely out of place in everyday life but crucial to a good death. A bad death is accompanied by silence and thus by public shame. Through mourning practices Mani women have appropriated the power to manipulate death, and thus good and bad departures do not depend simply on fate or God but on the disposition of the women (Seremetakis 1991).

Deaths that are badly timed or out of place do not result in the desired regeneration (Thomas 1975:192). For the Merina of central Madagascar there is, apparently, no worse nightmare than that one's body will be lost so that it cannot be placed in the communal tomb; this failure means loss of fertility for the descent group and the complete obliteration of the individual in question (Bloch 1982). Anxiety about dead bodies that are never recovered is very common.

The usual arbitrariness of events leading to brain death—accident, trauma, or violence—make it untimely and therefore bad. No preparation is possible. Because it occurs in an ICU, it is out of place; technology pervades the body. Under such circumstances, it is doubly surprising that so many families agree to donation. Not only must they rapidly confront the reality of what has happened, but they must dismiss all feelings that their brain-dead relative might still be suffering and, further, set aside any discomfort about desecration of the body. The extent of the emotional shift required suggests to me that something other than a charitable impulse is at work, at least for some. Hopes for transcendence, for continuity, and for regaining a modicum of control must surely also play a role.

Robert Jay Lifton, a psychoanalyst who has worked in Japan, insists that a yearning for immortality represents not irrationality or a denial of death, but rather a "compelling and universal inner quest for a continuous symbolic relationship between our finite individual lives and what has gone before and what will come after" (Lifton et al. 1979:7).

This quest, he argues, is part of the special condition of being human, of being aware of history and culture.

Domesticating Death

Anthropologists have evinced less interest in local conceptions about physical death than in the social phenomena surrounding it. When accounting for "causes" of death in other societies, researchers direct attention to the gods, witchcraft, sorcery, or malevolent ancestors. Elaboration of details about these proximate causes usually overtakes any interest in the immediate physical precursors of death, for these, anthropologists assume, do not fall into their domain of inquiry. It is, of course, quite possible that relatively little attention is paid to the physical signs of death in many of the societies that come under anthropological scrutiny, and that researchers are simply and appropriately reflecting local practice. But even so, valuable insights can be gleaned from what little has been written by anthropologists about the actual process of dying.

Many years ago W. H. R. Rivers noted that the people of Eddystone Island in the Solomon Islands make no clear distinction between the living and the dead, as is typical of contemporary thinking in Europe and North America. The terms *toa* and *mate* distinguish between someone who is lively and healthy on the one hand, and someone who is old and weak, seriously ill and dying, or clearly dead, on the other (1926). Similarly, the Lugbara word *dra* is both verb and substantive, meaning both "to die" and "death." Someone who is dead is described as "a person who dies" (Middleton 1982). In rabbinical writing a *goses* is someone who has a hold on life "like that of a flickering candle" and is in the condition of "becoming dead." Rabbis argue among themselves, particularly today, in connection with withdrawal of treatment from terminally ill patients, about the exact time when someone can be definitively thought of as a *goses* (Dorff 1996:174).

Humphreys has argued that whereas the start of the process of dying is usually difficult to determine, and the language noted above apparently reflects this uncertainty, organic death is clearly acknowledged as an irreversible physical process (1981). However, the departure of the soul, person, or spirit is socially constructed and depends on the conception of the relationship between the physical body and the soul or person. In southern medieval Europe, the departure of the soul, in some locations believed to happen from the feet, coincided with the permanent cessation of breathing. In Germanic and Celtic Europe, by contrast, death could not be declared until putrefaction had set in, at which time the soul was believed to separate from the body (Park 1995). In Japan the soul departs when the body becomes cold and starts to stiffen. Comparatively speaking, locating the essence of the individual in the head, and therefore assuming that a nonfunctioning brain is indicative of death, is unusual.

While an individual is "becoming" dead, aside from someone who dies alone or unexpectedly, social and material matters, including inheritance, must be dealt with, the process of grieving takes hold, and memorialization begins, but these activities may commence either before or after the soul has departed and physical death has been established.

Dying is usually thought of as both event and process. Language and ritual can be used to dichotomize the "lively" from those "becoming dead," but the transition from "becoming dead" to "dead" is relatively undifferentiated. Hertz and others were preoccupied with documenting the culturally monitored process of separation of the soul from a dead body. However, the liminal period may commence before biological death sets in. It spans the ambiguous time of biological, spiritual, personal, and social transformations associated with dying and death. Indeed, these transformations may not be complete for many years.

The Body as Classificatory Device

Long-standing disputes about the location of the vital essence in humans are also relevant to differing representations of death. John O'Neill, in his book *Five Bodies,* argues that "modern humans are busy giving a shape to a world that is no longer their own" (1985: 26). By this he means that in contemporary society we do not view the world around us as modeled after our bodies, nor do we recognize the reverse: that is, we do not think of the body as a microcosm of a larger order. It is assumed that we have transcended anthropomorphic thought and live in a rational world neatly compartmentalized into domains where nature and culture, individuals, their bodies, and society are distinct.

In the premodern world, the human body frequently furnishes metaphors for the organization and functioning of society and the cosmos and the spirit world (see, for example, Bastien 1985; Reichel-Dolmatoff

1971; Cunningham 1973). The human body is thus understood as a microcosm, one that, in health, is in harmony with the larger social and cosmological orders. The essence of life is not associated with one particular organ, nor located in the soul, but distributed throughout the entire body, and it often extends into the universe itself (Garcia-Ballester 1995; Granet 1930; Lock 1980).

The importance of maintaining the body in balance and harmony is a deeply entrenched belief in East Asia and is still readily detectable in Japan in school classrooms, martial arts training halls, acupuncture clinics, training programs for business executives, calligraphy classes, and even in blue-collar working life (Kondo 1990; Lock 1980; Rohlen 1974). Although European concepts of anatomy have supplemented the physiologically oriented logic of East Asian medicine, the idea of a life force, *ki*, distributed throughout the body makes intuitive sense to the majority (Lock 1980).

Even when a vital force is conceptualized as dispersed throughout the body, specific organs often take on special significance. Among the Romans, for example, the head contained the soul, but the liver was the seat of the passions. Written and artistic records of the early Christian period reveal that the head became increasingly important, but the heart remained the dominant metaphor for the vital force or affective life (Le Goff 1989). Of course, when Descartes proclaimed that the soul's location was in the pineal gland in the seventeenth century, the heart slipped badly as a contender for sovereign organ. It was soon reconceptualized in medicine as merely a mechanical pump (although its emotional significance is revived each Valentine's Day). The head, container of the mind, soul, brain, or computer that continues to challenge full scientific explanation, is understood today as the control center of the body. The core of individuality has been displaced upward, and when this core is irreversibly damaged, death occurs.

Death in modernity is in theory understood as natural: nothing is watching over us, and we only go around once. Literal belief in transcendence has clearly declined; yet memorialization and ideas about continuity survive, although their form and significance change. Perhaps it is especially important to publicly memorialize untimely deaths given their number and the horror associated with so many of them today. We do this on occasion in connection with genocide, war, and some diseases, notably AIDS; we do it much less in connection with death caused by famine, and with those deaths we label as accidental.

The Scandal of Death

It is true that the proposition "All men are mortal" is
paraded in text-books of logic as an example of a
generalization, but no human being really grasps it,
and our unconscious has as little use now as ever
for the idea of its own mortality.

Sigmund Freud, The "Uncanny"

Received wisdom has it that in the West we deny death, whereas in
Japan, thanks to Buddhism, death may be accepted with resignation or
even celebration. These stereotypes are not completely without foundation, but they obfuscate more than they clarify. If people in Japan
were so easily resigned to death, why should the issue of brain death
cause so much difficulty?

Much has been written about the denial of death in European modernity. Philippe Ariès argues, for example, that death has been "fur-
tively pushed out of the world of familiar things" and associated with
the Other; it has become "unnamable" (1974:106). I digress briefly to
examine this claim, because it appears so convincing to many contemporary philosophers and commentators on the modern condition. A fear
of death might perhaps lead to collusion between medical professionals
and families who cooperate with organ donation. They may hope the
deceased patient will transcend death by "living on" in organ recipients.

Freud, probably more than anyone else, shaped contemporary discourse about the meaning of death. He insisted that although the fact
of biological death cannot be denied, people do not believe in their own
mortality; consequently, the knowledge of death is repressed, and transcendence is internalized to become part of self. Ernest Becker, following
Freud, wrote about "the denial of death" in the early 1970s. He argues
that the "fear of [death] haunts the human animal like nothing else; it
is the mainspring of human activity—activity designed largely to avoid
the fatality of death, to overcome it by denying in some way that it is
the final destiny for man." Even though "primitives" seemingly celebrate
death through affirmative ritual, this is merely a cultural gloss, Becker
claims, over an underlying truth—the ubiquitous fear of death. For
modern "man," no longer given to belief, the fear of death becomes a
prominent part of our "psychological make-up" (1973:ix).

More recently, Zygmunt Bauman offers an elaborate variation on this
argument, insisting "there is hardly a thought more offensive than that
of death; or, rather, of the inevitability of dying; of the transience

of our being-in-the-world" (1992:12). Like other European intellectuals, including Jean Baudrillard, Maurice Merleau-Ponty, Edgar Morin, and Arnold Schopenhauer, he argues that since one cannot experience death and live to talk about it, in the modern world death becomes a scandal, "the ultimate humiliation of reason" (15). For this reason, the argument goes, North America and much of Europe have participated for the better part of a century in a death-defying culture.

Bauman seeks to lay bare the denial of death in contemporary society. He rejects the idea that we can "know death" by proxy, through observing the death of others. Death is therefore reduced simply to an event in the world of objects: "It is *my* death, and my death only, which is not an event of that 'knowable' world of objects. . . . It is my death that cannot be narrated, that is to remain unspeakable" (1992:3). Drawing on Morin, Becker, and Jorge Luis Borges, among others, Bauman asserts that an awareness of mortality is the ultimate source of cultural creativity. His argument turns away from a fear of the future, where death awaits us, and examines instead the constant presence of death in life.

According to Bauman, the paramount task of culture is to seek permanence. However, in contemporary society this enterprise takes the form of "expanding temporal and spatial boundaries of being, with a view to dismantling them altogether" (1992:5). The modern goal becomes one of liberation, by means of culture, from the constraints imposed by nature, and the idea of progress is the linchpin of this ideology. Part of the emancipatory project of modernity is to push back the moment of death, to extend the life span, to "lift the event of death above the level of the mundane, the ordinary, the natural" (5). Death, a biological fact, reemerges as a cultural artifact, humanly constructed. Robert Fulton (1965) argues that we react to modern death as we would to a communicable disease—a condition about which we must be vigilant because in theory it might be avoided even though contagious.

Bauman detects two contradictory strategies deployed simultaneously by contemporary society to combat the void of death. The first, the modern strategy, is to "deconstruct" mortality by battling disease and other threats to life. The containment of death is moved to the center of everyday life: we are enjoined to keep death at bay by dealing appropriately with perceived hazards (see also Lock 1998c). We must exercise, eat correctly, take pills to extend life, and so on. Health becomes a virtue, a means to salvation (Conrad 1994), its cultivation a responsibility of the individual. The social and political origins of inequality, illness, distress, and early mortality are deleted from view.

The second strategy, postmodern in its form, works to deconstruct

immortality entirely, to transform life into an unstoppable, daily rehearsal of the universal mortality of things, to move from the horror of
death to a seeking-out of "death-risks" (see also Morin 1970:73). Risk
and danger are no longer abhorred but become instead the spice of life,
making certain types of accidents (and, incidentally, brain death) more
likely:

> Daily life becomes a perpetual dress rehearsal of death. What is being re-
> hearsed in the first place, is *ephemerality* and *evanescence* of things humans
> may acquire and bonds humans may weave. The impact of such daily re-
> hearsal seems to be similar to one achieved by some preventive inoculations:
> if taken in daily, in partly detoxicated and thus non-deadly doses, the awe-
> some poison seems to lose its venom. Instead it prompts immunity and
> indifference to the toxin in the inoculated organism.
>
> (Bauman 1992:188)

Bauman acknowledges that attitudes toward mortality are diverse,
and he follows Joachim Whaley in recognizing a plethora of emotions
associated with death: fear, sorrow, anger, despair, resentment, resignation, defiance, pity, avarice, triumph, helplessness (1981:9). But Bauman is firm that the task has always been the same: to deal with a
uniquely human awareness of *individual* mortality, a position that in
most societies is subsumed and masked by the need for social continuity.

Thomas Tierney (1997) suggests that Bauman's thesis is prefigured in
the writing of Martin Heidegger in the 1920s. Heidegger insisted that
an authentic experience of death is *concealed* by culture, and, further,
that cultural accounts treat death as something that happens to others
but not to oneself. Death for Heidegger is a "mishap" or a "case,"
providing a constant "tranquilization" against one's own death. He argued that "the dying of Others is seen often enough as a social incon-
venience, if not even a downright tactlessness, against which the public
is to be guarded" (1962:298). Following Freud, no doubt, Heidegger
wrote about a universal "anxiety" in the face of death and postulated
the need for a "freedom toward death," which would be "grounded in
the ability to choose, by and for oneself, what will become of one's life"
(Tierney 1997:62).

Heidegger is very much a prisoner of his time, one in search of a
universal, individualized experience as a basis for transcendence. Here
is the ghost of the Christian story, in which God is transcended by the
individual. In contrast, Bauman sees no possibility for transcendence
and concentrates instead on the unavoidable foreboding in the face of
death: "Death reveals that truth and absurdity are one" (1992:15). Tier-

ney suggests that, for Bauman, the locus of the modern struggle with its enemy of death is clearly the body (not mind, society, or the afterworld). The body is the site of tragedy, the ultimate unresolvable paradox, for it is at once the source of life and of death (1997:59).

The contemporary insistence on an individual pursuit of health is one means to defer mortality (and one that saves governments money if it is successful). But medicine is of course also deeply implicated in this enterprise, and organ transplants offer one means to circumvent the failure of death. Foucault suggests that death denotes today not so much a failure of reason but rather the limits of medical power (1980:138). Death is "evaded" because we moderns have become, thanks to medicine, preoccupied with life. In effect, to medicine all deaths have become "bad" and untimely: each represents a humiliation of the expert. But clearly there are signs, the hospice movement being one, that this position is being challenged. The philosopher Jacques Choron shifts the argument away from a failure of reason and a fear of annihilation and claims instead that the fear is about dying rather than about what happens after death with which we are most concerned (1964:72).

Nostalgia for Transcendence

With modernity, life trajectories are disconnected from representations of cyclical returns and of transcendence; instead they become linear, compressed into a single biological life span. The life course is made into a microcosmic repetition of evolution, a secular cosmology that is used not to mirror society or to celebrate its continuity, nor yet to transcend it, but to dismiss the social order as in effect an elaborate superstructure, a figment of the human imagination. Death is remade entirely as a physical event, one that simply punctuates the end of individual lives. Period. The separation between nature and culture is complete. Thoughts about reanimation and premature burial are dismissed as the stuff of fantasy, science fiction, and the future. According to Freud and his followers, this situation accounts for the angst unique to modernity: we are fully cognizant for the first time that our ideas about mortality and death are fictional constructs.

Nearly a century later Jean Baudrillard goes much further than did Freud and argues that even though biological death is irreversible—"its objective and punctual character is a modern fact of science" (1993:158)—the mortal body of modern man is no more "real" than is the immortal soul (159); both result from a similar abstraction in which an

individual's life is understood as a self-contained unit of soul/mind separate from body with its fixed beginning and end marked by birth and
decay. Try as we might to dissociate life from death, to fantasize that
we can postpone or even eliminate death through individual efforts, we
delude ourselves. Baudrillard insists that, even in modernity, death must
be understood as something other than an individual event.

Walter Benjamin had argued earlier that the struggle becomes one of
reconciling, on the one hand, the representation of death as a "common
denominator" with, on the other hand, the power of death in its indi-
visible uniqueness. Thus, a particular event of death is never simply an
example of the concept of death (1969; see also Schleifer 1993:317;
Bataille 1988). This strategy permits us to engage with death as more
than a measurable, material event. Concerned with the significance of
memory, Benjamin understands death as one of the key "ideas" by
means of which we humans not only bridge the hiatus between the material and its representations, but also attribute history with significance.
History, not as the truth about the past, but as a memorabilia of words
and objects, "creates the chain of tradition which passes a happening
on from generation to generation" (1969:98). A loss of communal memory—the flattening of history—and decontextualization of events are
particularly troubling to Benjamin, and contribute, he argues, to contemporary alienation. Memorialization of past events, both mundane
and spectacular, makes significant contributions to overcoming contemporary alienation and helps to circumvent the idea of death as a scandal.
Transcendence of a sort can be achieved through the work of memory,
but only if the continuity of life is appreciated as a communal endeavor—an argument that makes a great deal of intuitive sense in Japan.

The anthropologist Geoffrey Gorer, writing in the 1950s, emphasized, like so many others, a distinction between an untimely death and
a "good" death. Gorer agrees that during the twentieth century, death
and dying became increasingly "unspeakable." Victorian novels are
filled with elaborate deathbed scenes, and funeral practices of the time
verged on the celebratory. A dramatic decline in public death rites during
the early part of the twentieth century led, Gorer believes, to the rise of
a "pornography of death"—a space in which death was made disgusting
and lewd (1956:59). The subject of death was eliminated from the medical curriculum. In the early 1900s the *Christian Science Monitor* refused
to print the word *death* in its pages. Gorer argues that the inevitable
process of decay has grown as disquieting as "copulation and birth were
a century ago." And he attributes the tendency in part to the medicalization of death.

At the same time, violent death, or at least our consciousness of it, has increased exponentially. Traumatic, untimely, and accidental deaths, many of them "brain" deaths, are indeed a scandal; they shock us, and we cannot deny them because they confront us (from a safe distance) each day in the media (Boltanski 1993). Our voyeuristic participation in violent death through media and films will not abate, Gorer argues, until "natural" death is reinstated in the public consciousness.

Gorer was writing nearly half a century ago. Today public exposure to violent death worldwide is greater than ever. Nevertheless, the link is rarely made explicit in North America between violent (pornographic) deaths and the procurement of organs. Nor are associations usually made between the scandal of death and the commodity status of brain-dead individuals.

Could it be that we in the West are not as "modern" as we imagine ourselves to be, and that our past—notably the Christian past—is a stronger force than we acknowledge? The pervasive metaphor of the "gift of life" in the transplant world suggests a way of transcending bad deaths and restoring order by means of technologically assisted resurrections. In Japan, this metaphor has far less force. More than one Japanese with whom I have talked has commented on this "irrational" aspect of the transplant endeavor.

On the other hand, we should not discount the utilitarian motive in organ procurement: the desire to allay the organ shortage and save lives. Medicalization reinforces the finality of death by establishing biology as the source of truth, and this emphasis on materiality makes the body thinkable as a commodity. The marked bifurcation between life and death, culture and nature (Comaroff 1984) facilitates the necessary objectivity. Death becomes a medical event diagnosed by an absence of the signs and symptoms of life. Treatment beyond this point is futile.

Social and philosophical commentary on death most often relegates physical death to the realm of medicine as well, for during the last century virtually all philosophers and numerous social scientists too have assumed that culture and nature are entirely divorced from one another, although today this position is increasingly questioned. Their writing is concerned with the problem of meaning and not with the body itself: above all with the meaning(s) that can be attributed to death of self and others in a rational, secular society, and with the fear of the void that results. And second, how do we deal with the problem posed by Hamlet—the representation of an event that no one has ever experienced and survived to describe?

This internalized, psychologized fear of death in modern society is assumed to be universal and natural. We believe that with modernity, we have cleared away the detritus of tradition, leaving ourselves to face the unknown, that which cannot be represented, with perpetual despair. And in this climate many of us seek to master the impermanence of the natural body by making use of the ingenious, manipulative technologies of contemporary culture, among which hormone replacement therapy and Viagra are just two examples. Brain-death discourse has certainly been legitimized by positing death as the dualistic Other of life—as an irreversible, final event. Possibilities of movement between the world of the "lively" and the domain of the "becoming dead," and occasional reversals of this process, are excluded from this discussion.

Modernity has exposed the absurdity of our puny efforts to escape the void through cultural elaboration about the hereafter; but there is no security in this discovery. Culture as communal knowledge is diminished, and individual neuroses and anxiety flourish (or so we are informed). This is the milieu in which brain death has been institutionalized as the end of individual life. It is then a short step to install organ donation, the ultimate act of charity, as the "gift of life"—a technological fix to transcend the "scandal" of biological death.

The repression of death in North America and most of Europe might account for the apparent lack of public interest when a new technological death was created by a small group of professionals, the majority of them physicians.[2] It might also explain why we have been so enamored of the idea of saving lives through organ transplants while studiously avoiding reflection on how exactly those organs are procured. On the other hand, if Japanese culture is better able to master a fear of death than is ours, then we must ask again, why has the new death caused such difficulty there? To claim that a universal denial of individual death is characteristic of modernity, or that the idea of death is an offense to rationality, fails to explain the remarkable differences in responses in Japan and North America to brain death.

For all the philosophical talk about the void, many people take refuge in comforting cosmologies. Moreover, not everyone seeks to postpone death, nor actively courts it through blatant risk-taking. Yet, whether our sensibilities are largely premodern, modern, or postmodern, accidental and untimely deaths create disorder. We have found a remarkably

2. But we must also consider those European countries that have been severely troubled by the concept of brain death. A moment's pause reveals why the recent history of Germany makes it impossible to "suppress" death in that country (Hogle 1999).

ingenious way, it seems, to create something of value out of senseless, bad deaths. When life and death are located in the brain, then a dramatic bid can be made to postpone mortality through medical intervention; individual death is transcended in the reanimation of a second dying individual. The culture of the West is at work when authentic experience is confined to individual brains. When the brain is gone the void opens up, swallowing all meaning and value, unless a resurrection can be negotiated.

A rational approach to the medicalized body makes commodification thinkable; a not-so-rational approach is required to support the view that death can be transcended through organ donation. Some donor families and medical professionals clearly buy into this ideology, hidden in the seductive metaphor of the gift of life; others, no doubt, are pragmatists who see no inherent value in a body with no hope for recovery of any kind. For pragmatists, donation is made to society unadorned with any hope of transcendence, and whatever memorialization takes place for the dead person is presumably carried through without anxiety or guilt about what the corpse may have been put through. Rationality, however, is challenged in the face of sudden death and body dismemberment, and feelings of unease sometimes creep back in.

DISCONCERTING MOVEMENTS

From a letter to the *Journal of the American Medical Association:*

This reader . . . was stunned by Dr. Liptak's statement about the "disconcerting" aspects of disconnecting children from ventilators: "They shudder
and gasp and twitch and inevitably lead you to believe that you have made a
mistake and should not have disconnected them." Disconcerting indeed! . . .

Readers of the *Journal* should understand clearly that patients who have
been competently diagnosed to be brain dead neither shudder, nor gasp, nor
twitch when ventilatory support is disconnected. The absence of such responses is, in fact, part of the process of certification of brain death.

It would be reassuring were Dr. Liptak to explain to us that his description
was simply literary license . . . If Dr. Liptak's "brain-dead" patients are indeed responding to disconnection of the ventilator in the manner described,
then it is chillingly clear that they are not, in fact, brain dead.

(Poulton 1986:2028)

Gregory Liptak responded:

Patients who are brain dead often have unusual spontaneous movements
when they are disconnected from their ventilators. Numerous authors have
described these disconcerting phenomena.

Patients who fulfill all the criteria for death, including deep unresponsive
coma, may experience any of the following: goose bumps, shivering, extensor
movements of the arms, rapid flexion of the elbows, elevation of the arms
above the bed, crossing of the hands, reaching of the hands towards the neck,
forced exhalation, and thoracic respiratory-like movements. These complex
sequential movements are felt to be release phenomena from the spinal cord
including the upper cervical cord and do *not* mean that the patient is no
longer brain dead.

(Liptak 1986:2028)

Imagined Continuities

On Becoming an Ancestor

Memory . . . an editorial ministry which reconstructs its past
experience in accordance with the peculiar needs of the
imagination.

> *Jonathan Miller,* McLuhan

In this chapter I examine Japanese attitudes toward their ancestors, in
particular toward their memorialization, and the possible effects of these
customs on responses to the idea of a death located in the brain. Concern
about the memorialization of the dead and the creation of appropriate
links between the living and the dead have been of enormous significance
throughout much of Japanese history, but it was with the formation of
the modern state at the end of the nineteenth century, and again during
the military regime in the early part of the twentieth century, that these
practices first took on national importance.

Cultivating Tradition

Although culture is rarely thought of as a factor in the invention of brain
death and its institutionalization in the United States, Canada, and other
countries of the West, it is often assumed that culture *must* be at work
in Japan. Some Japanese commentators themselves insist that recognition of brain death will violate the moral order of Japanese culture and
society. On the other hand, those in Japan who have wanted brain death
recognized often emphasize, in the words of the government's special
commission, that arguments cannot be found "in traditional Japanese
religious and ethical views that constitute a specific and strong denial of
this view of death [brain death]" (Kantō Chiku Kōchōkai 1992:5). In
other words, the culture of "tradition" should not cause resistance to

the recognition of brain death. Japan has throughout its history been eclectic, a culture of "fusion," in Najita's estimation (1978), in which religious beliefs from several sources have commingled.

Though close, culture and religion are not the same. One thing is clear: it cannot be argued that opposition on the part of religious leaders in Japan has contributed to a resistance to the recognition of brain death or the practice of organ transplants. As Helen Hardacre notes, "Compared with the volume and variety of debate elsewhere [in Japan], the response from Buddhism and Shinto has been almost negligible in spite of the great acrimony and urgent tone of much of the secular discussion" (1994:589).[1]

Stephen Vlastos, a historian, has pointed out that contemporary Japan is widely regarded, both by those born there and by foreigners, as a society "saturated with customs, values, and social relationships that organically link present generations of Japanese to past generations" (1998:1). Moreover, since World War II, Japanese have come to know themselves, and to be known by others, through their cultural traditions. The government has made Japanese "traditions" highly visible and integrated them into the present so that citizens and tourists alike may participate in the past. These reconstructed traditions are bathed in nostalgia—a longing for something precious that has been lost (Ivy 1995; Robertson 1991, 1998). However, many facets of this "found" tradition are, unbeknown to most Japanese, late nineteenth- or early twentieth-century in origin (Vlastos 1998:1).

Vlastos argues that social scientists have conventionally used the idea of tradition in two overlapping forms. In the first, tradition is made discontinuous with and set in opposition to modernity—a thing of the past, old-fashioned, and "smelling of the countryside," as one would say in Japanese. In the second form, the past remains vitally active in the present. In this instance, "rather than representing culture left behind in the transition to modernity, tradition is what modernity *requires* to prevent society from flying apart" (2). Both understandings of tradition are embedded in the competing rhetoric about brain death. Vlastos criticizes these usages as resolutely ahistorical. "Tradition," according to

---

1. One exception has been Sōka Gakkai, Japan's largest lay Buddhist organization, with a membership of over 8.3 million and a powerful political wing. This group stated firmly that transplant surgery is *not* in conflict with the teachings of their organization; on the contrary, they argued early on for the promotion of donor registrars, a donor card, and the establishment of an information network (Ross 1995).

Vlastos—and he is not alone in this view—is not the sum of actual past practices that survive in the present; rather, it "is a modern trope, a prescriptive representation of socially desirable (or sometimes undesirable) institutions and ideas *thought* to have been handed down from generation to generation" (3, emphasis added).

Going beyond the well-known work of Hobsbawm and Ranger (1983), Vlastos argues that tradition is mobilized and constitutive of modern cultural formation and, most important, that the appearance and trajectory of this mobilization reflect society's anxieties and ruptures. Such an approach to tradition does not deny the reality of the past; cultural traditions do not suddenly spring up fully formed, but are created out of material and discursive antecedents. Often, respect for tradition is invoked as a defense against threats to national identity and to moral and social order. The culture of tradition is put to work in the service of a conservative politics as a stabilizing force, and the rhetoric associated with the brain-death problem is illustrative of this process.

Bad Deaths, Unhappy Spirits, and Revenge

In postwar Japan, memorialization of the deceased no longer has national or political significance. But concerns about the respect due to the dead are nevertheless remarkably resilient. Although it is rarely made explicit in public commentary, respect for the ancestors is, I believe, the reason behind many of the opposition arguments. As the director of a nursing school put it to me, "No one talks about the ancestors; they are just there, needing no comment" (Minami Hiroko, personal communication, 1998). Such beliefs are particularly pertinent when Japan, a "harmonious" society with strong human ties, is compared with the "rational," "overly individualistic," "cold" West, where body commodification is thought to be relatively easy.

The idea of ancestors imbued with a power to influence everyday life is, of course, entirely foreign to the dominant tradition in North America. Given that visible evidence of modernity assaults one everywhere in Japan, it is not unreasonable to assume that "traditional" ideas about spirits and the influence of the dead on the living must be obsolete there also. However, just as there is abundant evidence that religious or spiritual beliefs are not in decline in North America, so too in Japan, otherworldly entities, in the form of the ancestors, remain significant. However, for the majority such beliefs are a matter of "custom" and not associated closely with the sacred. The ancestors are, after all, family, and their role is to protect moral order in daily life. Even Japanese who state that they are nonbelievers, when they return to their place of birth, often participate in a few elementary rituals to show respect for the ancestors.

The anthropologist Namihira Emiko, in her cultural account of Japanese attitudes toward death, argues that "traditional" death practices have a firm hold on everyday life in contemporary Japan (Namihira 1988). Her widely read book on the subject was harshly criticized in Japan by those who condemn "superstition" and "old-fashioned" ideas. Several critics have argued that Namihira is presenting ideas held only by people living in remote areas. The same critics insist that cultural analyses of this kind deflect attention from the real reasons behind opposition to brain death, such as unprofessional behavior in the medical world (Nudeshima 1991a).

Namihira illustrates her argument with an analysis of the moving narratives by relatives of victims of the Japan Airlines crash in 1985, in the mountains not far from Tokyo. She concludes that for most respondents the spirit or soul (*reikon*) of the deceased is anthropomorphized and continues to exist, but in a place apart from the everyday world. *Reikon* eat and drink, express emotions, and feel bodily sensations; surviving relatives have an obligation to keep the departed soul or spirit happy and must not give it cause for anger or regret. Great anxiety is created if a dead body cannot be located or identified, because it is believed that *reikon* desire living relatives to transport the body (usually, these days, the ashes after cremation) from the place of death for burial in the place where it formerly lived. If the corpse is not complete (*gotai manzoku),* the spirit remains troubled and restless (36), and if the suffering continues, the *reikon* may cause harm to the living. Many of the relatives of the crash victims were clearly concerned about this possibility.

Similar beliefs are evident elsewhere in daily life in Japan. For example, in 1998 a World War II soldier was finally repatriated from Siberia after fifty-three years. He complained on his return home that his country had made more efforts to recover the bones of dead soldiers from Southeast Asia than to repatriate soldiers still alive in Russia (*New York Times* 1998). Another example comes from a Japanese physician who informed me that when medical students do courses in human anatomy, they are required to gather every piece of the dissected bodies for cremation. If even a tiny part is missing, then it must be found.[2]

In Japan, medical students customarily participate in *kuyō*, a ritual in which they pray that the souls of the bodies they have dissected may depart peacefully from this world. These practices are largely motivated by the potential suffering of the dead individual, for spirits require the same care that one would give a fellow human being. When I have suggested that *kuyō* should perhaps be performed after the procurement of organs, before the body is returned to the family, many physicians supported this idea, and some indicated that such a practice might well increase organ donation. A specialist in Chinese philosophy, Kaji Nobuyuki, made a similar suggestion some years ago (Kaji 1990), but Japanese doctors are not, it seems, aware of Kaji's writing.

Hospitals in Japan have what is known as a *reian shitsu,* a room for the repose of recently departed souls. When a patient dies, the body, robed in a white cotton kimono, is moved to this unadorned room, where the attending doctors and families participate in a ceremony in which they burn incense and say a few prayers. All the doctors with whom I have talked make a point of attending such ceremonies for patients who die while in their care. Physicians believe that their presence in the *reian shitsu* may help the grieving family, but some also participate out of respect for the dead, and to reassure themselves that their clinical care was not in any way inadequate. Once the ceremony is complete, the body is moved to the family home for a wake, or, if the family lives in a small apartment, to a place resembling a funeral parlor.[3] The wake is designed to ensure the safe departure of the spirit. Many people do not believe literally in the soul's departure, and some do not think such rituals necessary, but most are nevertheless at ease in carrying out these customs.

As in most other parts of the world, Japanese distinguish between good and bad deaths. Although most people today reject such ideas, formerly people recognized several classes of spirits, among them *muen-botoke* (buddhas without attachment or affiliation) and *gaki* (hungry ghosts). These spirits are usually those of individuals who died in a state

2. Compared with the stories prevalent until relatively recently in the United Kingdom and North America about medical students playing pranks with parts taken from cadavers laid out for dissection, a mood of respect predominates in Japanese dissection rooms.

3. Funeral establishments in Japanese cities may resemble hotels in their opulence and convenience. The top floor, however, is made over to tatami rooms where families hold wakes. This location ensures that no one will walk over the deceased and facilitates the departure of the soul (Hardacre, personal communication, 2000).

of jealousy, rage, melancholy, or resentment, who are neglected by their descendants, or who have no descendants. They roam the earth in search of food and comfort. Their suffering can and should be appeased through appropriate human intervention, otherwise they will persist as "wild" spirits (aramitama). Such spirits can enter the body of the newly dead; a bladed object, a sword, dagger, sickle, or knife must be placed close to the corpse for protection (Smith 1974:42).

A second, particularly frightening class of wandering spirits are those who die "unnatural" (higōshi) deaths, deaths that according to Buddhist doctrine do not occur because of destiny or karma but are the result of unprecedented disaster (Kimura 1989). All accidental death is inauspicious, but drowning particularly so. Such violent, unanticipated deaths—"bad deaths"—are, of course, the deaths that create potential organ donors. Spirits that arise from bad deaths are dangerous because their anger never ceases; they bear "deep-seated grudges" (onnen). Death outside one's own house, including death in hospital, is one form of unnatural death; death while traveling is also abhorred.

Other forms of unnatural death include death during pregnancy or childbirth (this type of death warrants special funeral rites in at least one Buddhist sect).[4] Death as a result of infanticide (mabiki) or abortion, death in war, suicide, including the double suicide of thwarted lovers, death resulting from capital punishment, and death from certain types of illness are all unnatural. Death at a young age, particularly dying before one's parents or grandparents, and death before marriage and procreation are also "unnatural" (Kimura 1989). The ritual pollution associated with death in the Shinto tradition is especially dangerous in the case of an unnatural death, and the unhappy spirit is likely to stay close to earth and cause misfortune not only to its descendants but also to strangers (Yoshida 1984).

Kabuki and Noh drama are replete with plays about tormented spirits and the tragedy their suffering creates for human life as they act out their grudges (tatari). One of the "new" Japanese religions, founded just after World War II, requires that when an individual's suffering is judged to be caused by an unhappy ancestor, then ties with that ancestor must be severed entirely to release both ancestor and descendant from their suffering. For believers, this drastic move abruptly challenges the usual intergenerational family obligations, thus isolating members of the sect

---

4. I am indebted to Helen Hardacre for this information.

from their families and rendering them more amenable to the demands of the sect's exclusivist leaders (Kerner 1974).

Rituals to appease the suffering of the dead are widely practiced in Japan. Among the most important are *kuyō* carried out for bodies, both human and animal, that have been used in medical education and research (Asquith 1986, 1990). *Kuyō* for the souls of aborted and miscarried fetuses (*mizuko kuyō*) are also widespread. Some Buddhist temples make a great deal of money by officiating at these ceremonies, but the majority oppose such practices as either a cheap vulgarization of Buddhist belief or simply an exploitative endeavor (Hardacre 1997: 207). Despite an abiding fear about the ritual pollution associated with abortion and birth, a few Shinto shrines practice *mizuko kuyō*. Many thousands of Japanese women derive comfort from these practices.

In her research into ideas about good and bad death in contemporary Japan and North America, Susan Long concluded that in Japan death in old age, preferably in one's sleep, or a sudden death (*pokkuri*), resulting from a fatal illness in old age, are thought of as natural. Deaths that do not cause trouble for others—those that avoid a long period of dependence and take place at home, surrounded by the family—are preferable; these are "peaceful" deaths, and, although culturally orchestrated, are also thought of as natural. Death has multiple meanings, Long argues, and bad deaths are opposed explicitly to those understood as natural. Bad deaths involve pain, dependency, and dying in a hospital, especially when supported by medical technology. These deaths, together with accidental and violent deaths, are regarded as neither peaceful nor natural (Long 2000).

The importance assigned to "natural" deaths must surely influence the emotional responses of families at the bedside of brain-dead relatives. Both health care professionals and families may be hesitant to raise the issue of organ donation under these circumstances, because few people can imagine the retrieval of organs from a brain-dead body as a peaceful event.

Becoming an Ancestor

Namihira points out subtle but important distinctions in the Japanese words for dead bodies. The word *shitai* refers to a corpse, but *itai* (with an honorific) is used when family members talk about a deceased relative, or whenever the relationship of the body to living relatives is specified (1988:44). While a corpse remains in the house it is bathed, shaved, dressed, and greeted each day (Becker 1993:130). The concept of *itai* connotes feelings of attachment to a recently deceased relative, and it is the *itai* that makes demands on living descendants (Namihira 1988:46).

Becoming an ancestor is an extended process, and for most families physical death sets in motion a series of rites and ceremonies that culminates in a final memorial service, most commonly on the thirty-third or fiftieth day after death. During this time the spirit loses its intimate, polluting association with the corpse. Eventually it also loses its individual identity and enters the realm of the generalized ancestral spirits, essentially purified and benign (Smith 1974:67). Each spirit passes in time through the various ritual stages, except for those that are neglected or suffer unnatural deaths.

This transition does not depend on the conduct of the individual in life; individual endeavor and personal achievement count for nothing. Attaining ancestorhood depends entirely on the family's loyalty and ritual memorialization of the deceased (Ooms 1967:319). Rituals are the responsibility of household members. A Buddhist priest is usually called in to create a posthumous name for the deceased and to recite sutras, but his participation is peripheral to the death itself.[5] At the time of the funeral, the posthumous name assigned to the deceased is carved by a priest into a memorial tablet (*ihai*) that is placed in the *butsudan* (the family altar, usually kept in the residence of the eldest son). Posthumous names, composed in part of the names assigned to individuals while living, become key elements in the transformation from *reikon* to ancestor, and the memorial tablets attest to the continuity between the living and the dead.

Through these ritual activities, the deceased are memorialized and gradually attain status as ancestors—vital links between this world and the next. It has been argued that the idea of filial piety (*kō*) permits East

---

5. During the Tokugawa period (1603–1868), when the government began to systematically monitor the population, compulsory registry with a Buddhist temple was instituted, in part to rout out Christian converts who could then be disposed of, often violently. The result was that every family was forced to establish a formal relationship with a temple, and Buddhist priests have been involved with the majority of family funerals since that time. However, Buddhist authorities generally deny the existence of spirits of the dead, and they have in the past characterized ancestor worship as mere folk custom. Nevertheless, to most Japanese Buddhism remains closely associated with funerals and with the achievement of ancestorhood, an artifact resulting from historical edict. For most people, association with institutionalized Buddhism is limited exclusively to the times when a family death occurs (Yamaori 1986).

Asians to understand individual lives as part of a family lineage that transcends individual death; the concept of *kō* can be understood, therefore, as a "theory of eternal life" (Kaji 1990:22). But no possibility for *individual* transcendence exists as in Christianity.

Nudeshima Jirō found that fewer than 30 percent of Japanese participated in something approaching a full set of ancestral rites and rituals, but because many more families carry out attenuated versions, overall there is no evidence of a dramatic decline in these rituals (1991a; see also Smith 1974). Nevertheless, loss of ritual knowledge about mortuary practices is the central theme of the highly acclaimed 1984 film *Sōshiki* (Funeral) in which the director, Itami Jūzō, parodies the ineptness of contemporary Japanese in performing rituals. Books to remedy this ignorance, replete with detailed diagrams illustrating correct behavior and clothing at funerals, are on sale in Japanese bookstores.

Even though mortuary practices are attenuated, Keith Brown notes that in Mizuzawa, in the northern part of the main island of Honshū, the ancestors retain a firm hold on residents. Even though farming is often no longer profitable, land is rarely sold because it is passed down through the ancestral line and must be protected. This argument holds even when the farmer knows the family has not always worked the same parcel of land. The idea of the landed estate with its link to the ancestors, rather than its precise location, is what is important (Brown, ms).

Northern Honshū is known as a conservative rural area, but it is by no means atypical. Although in urban areas many families carry out few rituals for the deceased, in other households family members may talk with recently deceased ancestors, whose photographs, together with the memorial tablets, are placed in the *butsudan*. Deceased relatives are regularly offered food, and a place may be set for them at meals. This custom of giving *sonaemono*, ritual offerings, is believed to stabilize the reciprocal arrangement between the deceased and family members (Reading 1991:27). In return for offerings, the family can expect protection. This type of cultural knowledge may not be systematically transmitted to the younger generations any longer, but nevertheless it is promoted by many religious sects (both old and new) and appears regularly in various forms of popular culture.[6] Although not everyone in the extended family may feel strongly about such ritual behavior, and some

---

6. Helen Hardacre, a specialist in Japanese religion, argues that ancestral ritual is one of the most resilient religious observances in Japan and in no way a minority practice (personal communication, 2000).

might prefer to abstain entirely, family members who practice the rituals are generally still supported.

From Ancestor Veneration to Family Memorialization

One facet of "tradition" often mentioned in discussions about Japanese modernity is the relationship of individuals to society. In his book about changing burial rituals in Japan, Nudeshima, like numerous others, notes that people in Japan have in the past been recognized less as individuals than as members of collective entities, with ties that bind them formally and permanently to other individuals. The body is not understood, therefore, as individual property in either life or death, and directions about its disposal and related ritual activities are the prerogative of the family. Even though this family-centered world, monitored by the ancestors, smacks today of the conservative past and has largely been superseded in the postwar years by a late modern, technologically driven society, ideas about generational continuity are not thrown entirely to the winds. Aside from anything else, 60 percent of Japanese reside in extended families for at least part of their lives.

Many Japanese friends and colleagues have indicated to me that they participate in the *bon* ceremony each year and go to visit the graves of deceased relatives. Several surveys have indicated that over 90 percent of respondents visit family graves at least once a year (Kawano, in press; R. Smith 1999). The gravestone is washed, and a few words about family activities may be communicated to the dead. Some people also reflect on family matters while kneeling in front of the *butsudan* at home. An ancestor can continue to age in the minds of his living relatives, who may report to him after the birth of a baby, for example, that he, the ancestor, has become a great-grandfather (R. Smith 1999). These activities are not understood as formalized ancestor worship but simply as activities that indicate family solidarity.[7]

Robert Smith reminds us that the ancestors exist only because the living remember them, and he argues that what takes place today is a simple "memorialism" rather than formal ancestral veneration (Smith 1999). Changes in mortuary practices, including the introduction of personal eulogies (*chōji*) at funerals, reflect this shift. They indicate that

---

7. Ancestor worship now has a negative connotation for most people because of its association with nationalism and a zealous support of the emperor (but see Field 1991). Nevertheless, respect for the dead remains a potent idea to many.

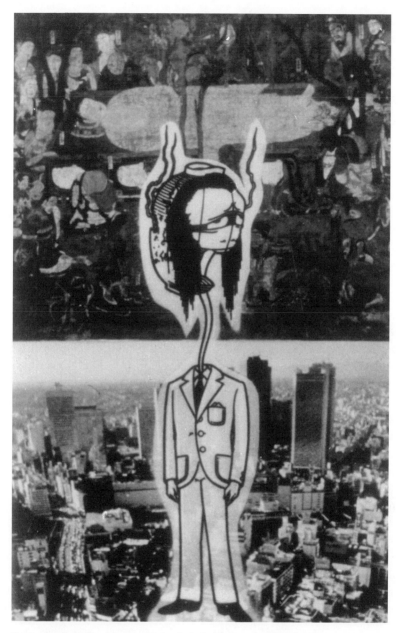

Brain death. A businessman's body is in Tokyo, but his head is in Nirvana.
Reproduced by permission of Osaka Medical Association.

ancestor rituals, together with concerns about succession in the extended household, are in decline, but that commemoration of the deceased as an individual or as part of an extended family remains important (Suzuki 1998).[8] A good number of women today break with tradition by insisting that they will not be buried with their in-laws. This declaration indicates that they no longer believe their principal job in life is to perpetuate their husband's family line, another powerful sign of the wane of the ancestors (Kawano, in press). Recently "natural" burials at places other than designated sites have been made legal, and it is now possible to scatter the ashes after a cremation, often at a location having a special association for the deceased. But, despite these innovations, burial in family plots remains prevalent, and many people feel anxious until they have made and paid for their funeral arrangements.

The idea of *en* (from the Buddhist term *innen,* meaning karmic connection), brings persons, families, objects, and the dead into intimate association. To perpetuate the necessary memorialization and connections, ancestors must be properly buried and their graves regularly tended. In recent years, catering to the increasing number of people who are not, or do not want to be, "connected" to a family after death, several religious organizations have created common burial grounds, where permanent ritual care is carried out on behalf of these unconnected, pitiable souls so that they will not harm the living (Kaneko 1990). Memorialization today is much more informal and individualized than was ancestor veneration, but it nevertheless remains important and is a practice to which, paradoxically, World War II contributed.

The dropping of atomic bombs on Hiroshima and Nagasaki resulted in a massive national memorialization of the victims. It was claimed in the 1980s that in Hiroshima one out of seven people was a *hibakusha,* a survivor of the bomb, and one in three hundred Japanese nationwide were believed to be *hibakusha* (Treat 1995). A vast literature also exists of "little histories" (Gluck 1993) by survivors and their relatives about the bombing and its effects. Much of this memory work, at once political and heart-wrenchingly personal, focuses on those who did not survive—on the massive rupture of continuity. Diaries, novels, and other documents represent a concerted effort to transcend this atrocity even as it is memorialized (Todeschini 1999).

---

8. Brown's data from the north of Japan indicate, as is so often the case, that there is a great deal of regional variation in these matters, and that questions of succession and obligations to the ancestors remain important to some people, especially, perhaps, those who work the land (ms.).

Less dramatically, a good number of groups exist for the writing of personal histories. Very often the narratives focus on the relationship of the writer to a deceased parent or grandparent: someone killed in the war, whom the writer may have known for only a few years before their death, is a favorite subject (Figal 1996). These self-histories (reminiscent of the diaries that form the core of treatment practices for certain types of mental illness in Japan; see Reynolds 1976) are not autobiography, and those who lead the groups insist that a focus on one's own emotions and affairs is inappropriate and shallow. The purpose is to memorialize and to situate oneself in recent Japanese history and as part of a generational family. Mariko Tamanoi argues, however, examining the narratives of rural women in postwar Japanese society, that women often situate themselves in opposition to History writ large (1998)—in opposition, that is, to what the patriarchal family, backed by the ancestors and the emperor, formerly represented for many people.

The idea of the individual as an autonomous entity has made considerable inroads in Japan in postwar years. It is always tempered, however, by powerful forces, among them the education system. Students are taught that they are part of a nation with a long, unbroken history of living in close-knit, harmonious communities. Assertion of individuality in Japan must still overcome the weight of the normative social order. In many families decisions about important matters are still ultimately dealt with by family consensus or by fiat. The male head of the household has the final say, albeit often after family discussion. In the face of extraordinary family trauma, such as the brain death of a relative, it is quite possible that an individual's wishes would be contravened. A 1998 poll shows that 25 percent of respondents would not support the written desire of a family member to become an organ donor, and another 12 percent do not know what they would do (*Asahi Shinbun* 1998c). Even though most people report that they support donation in principle, it would take only one dissenting family member to prevent it.

The rhetoric of continuity, a retelling of the past as it ought to have been (Najita 1978:4), serves to stabilize the dominant, conservative political order. The extended family and in particular its male head, representing not only the living but also previous generations, remain powerful, even though today other forces continually oppose this hegemony. The "foreign" technology of organ procurement and transplants has difficulty becoming established in this environment.

Ancestral Attachments

Boundaries between the social and natural worlds have never been rigidly maintained in Japan, in part *because* ancestors are immortalized as beings who continue to participate in the everyday world. They form a vital bridge between the social and the natural domains. Fleur Wöss concluded that separation of the soul from the body at the moment of death remains central to contemporary Japanese belief about dying (1992). In one survey, only 20 percent responded that they do not believe in the existence of *reikon* (soul or spirit); while 40 percent believe in its continued existence after death, and another 40 percent find themselves unable to answer (*Shōwa 61 Nenban yoron chōsa nenkan* 1987). The same survey shows that among people aged sixteen to twenty-nine, belief in the survival of souls is particularly prevalent (*Shōwa 54 Nenban yoron chōsa nenkan* 1979). Another survey indicated that 23 percent believed that they will become a spirit after death and will return to visit their living relatives once a year at the *bon* festival; 27 percent answered that they would become "nothing" after death and (as so often is the case with survey research in Japan) 42 percent were unable to answer the question (Nagamine 1988:65).

For those who believe in *reikon,* contact with them is usually restricted to a ritualized annual encounter. Fewer than 13 percent believe in the possibility of or wish to seek out contact with spirits at any other time (*Shōwa 55 Nenban yoron chōsa nenkan* 1986). Wöss also cites a 1988 study showing that 77 percent of Japanese teenagers believe in the possibility of wandering and vengeful spirits (a belief no doubt encouraged by interminable reading of comics featuring such themes) (*Yomiuri Shinbun* 1988b). Unfortunately, this survey has not been updated.

A 1979 survey of people of all ages shows that 34 percent believe in ancestral spirits as protective forces, while 59 percent state that they have strong ties to their recently deceased family members (*Shōwa 54 Nenban yoron chōsa nenkan* 1979). Almost two decades later, these sentiments apparently persist: nearly 57 percent of survey respondents believe that they have a strong spiritual tie to their ancestors (Hōsō bunka kenkyūjo Yoron chōsabu 1996). A second survey among people aged fifty to fifty-nine indicates that more than 83 percent think ancestors should be given "proper respect" and that tending the graves of the deceased is one form of respect (Naikaku Sōri Daijin kanbō kōhōshitsu 1998). This same survey indicates that just over 22 percent of respondents believe in life after death, supporting a 1996 survey indicating that

35 percent of people believe in an afterworld (Hōsō bunka kenkyūjo Yoron chōsabu 1996). These latter findings suggest that for the majority, appropriately ritualized memory may be more important than a literal belief in the existence of ancestors.

A 1981 survey shows that more than 60 percent of Japanese consider that when and where one is born and dies are determined by destiny and should not be changed by human intervention (Maruyama et al. 1981). If this finding remains accurate, it must have a profound effect on attitudes toward organ donation and transplants.

Surveys of this kind also make it clear that belief in spirits of the dead is not closely associated with formal religious belief or practices. A 1983 study cited by Namihira showed that of 685 respondents, 66 percent believe that no religious beliefs exist concerning the dead in their part of the country, even though respect for the dead was readily apparent (1988:74–75). These results support the theory that spirits are conceptualized as belonging to "nature" or the wider cosmos, as anthropomorphized forces entirely separate from formal religion (Asquith and Kalland 1997:19).

The philosopher Ōmine Akira argues that this type of thinking represents "quirky local beliefs cherished in our peculiarly unspiritual island country and incomprehensible to most of the world" (1991:69). Ōmine, who is not alone in making this argument, thinks that this "primitive" animism has influenced the practice of Buddhism in Japan. He claims that the "traditional culture and value systems" of other countries, including Buddhist countries such as Thailand, have had the "resilience to confront and absorb the new view of human life opened up by medical science" (68). Animism clearly influences attitudes about the dead in Japan, but, Ōmine argues, these beliefs "simply lack the depth of vision to address a challenge like that of redefining the boundary between life and death" (69). Those who insist that organ transplants and recognition of brain death go against Buddhist doctrine are mistaken, in Ōmine's opinion; their thinking is clouded by animism. For him the rationale for using brain function as the criterion of death is unassailable: it is "what we call consciousness, or the mind, that makes each human being different from every other. And consciousness resides not in the heart or arms or legs but in the brain" (1991:70).

Namihira argues explicitly that the complex beliefs about ancestors continue to inhibit cooperation with organ removal for autopsy and transplants. A questionnaire by a committee set up to encourage the donation of bodies for medical research showed that 66 percent of the

respondents think that cutting into dead bodies is repulsive or cruel
(*kawaisō*) or shows a lack of respect for the dead. Another 40 percent
reported that exposing the body of a recently dead relative to complete
strangers (such as health care professionals) is embarrassing and shows
lack of respect for the deceased (1988).

More people than formerly donate their bodies as anatomical gifts
(Nudeshima 1991b); but if Namihira's 1983 results remain valid, then
the majority of Japanese are still uncomfortable about autopsies and
other medical intrusions into a newly dead body. Fewer people than
previously adhere strongly to a belief in the literal continuity of a soul
or spirit after death. Nevertheless, in interviews I conducted in 1997,
twenty-three of twenty-seven adult Tokyo residents said that the fate of
the body after death, and concern about the well-being of recently deceased relatives, makes them hesitate about both the donation and receiving of organs. None of those interviewed professed to a formal belief
in the idea of ancestor veneration, although about half acknowledged
that respect for their recently deceased parents and grandparents, including ritual observances, remained important to them. Only one or
two people acknowledged an active interest in Buddhism, but more than
half of all informants pointed out that family and social obligations
require that the bodies of deceased family members be treated in accordance with Buddhist-associated ritual.

In sum, social obligations and expectations, perhaps even more than
active spiritual or religious beliefs, appear to motivate respect for recently dead relatives. Memorialization of deceased relatives remains part
of everyday life in both rural and urban Japan. This aspect of the culture
of tradition is likely to discourage some families even from discussing
the possibility of organ donation. Although I can produce little conclusive evidence that these obligations and beliefs directly influence decisions involving brain-dead patients, I have been told several times that
family members often fall into a common Japanese pattern of behavior
while clustered in shock at the bedside: one of "holding back," unwilling
to impose new and foreign ideas on the family as a whole as it starts to
mourn.

Many physicians working in ICUs in Japan believe that they have no
right or obligation to discuss donation with grieving families. A 1998
survey of 362 hospitals officially designated as organ procurement centers revealed that 65 percent of doctors would not take the initiative to
ask families of brain-dead patients about donation even if the patient
had signed a donor card (*Asahi Shinbun* 1998b). Nakajima Michi and

many other commentators have argued that because of sensitivity about indebtedness (*ongaeshi*), many families would feel obligated to donate if their doctors made the request. When Nakajima donated her husband's kidneys, she felt obligated to the doctor for the time and attention he had given her husband. Many doctors, in turn sensitive to this difficulty, are hesitant to broach the subject of organ donation for fear of inadvertently pushing families to do something about which they are reluctant. These attitudes have no doubt contributed to the fact that commodification of the human body for the benefit of science and for unknown strangers has a very short history in Japan.

In North America, where formal religious activity is much more evident than in Japan, the "rational" and the "irrational" also coexist. A belief in angels is apparently widespread among Americans (Gibbs 1993). A study in Oregon (Perkins and Tolle 1992) revealed that a high percentage of people are very uncomfortable about autopsies or other forms of bodily desecration of a recently deceased individual. The same was true in Sweden (Sanner 1994). It is possible, as Nudeshima suggests, that the Japanese public appears to be more resistant to a recognition of brain death and to organ donation than people elsewhere simply because they have been surveyed much more often and with more probing questions and polls. Nudeshima reminds his readers that according to surveys, Japanese are roughly as willing as Americans to donate organs: polls in both countries hover around the 50 percent mark.

According to Nudeshima, the principal reasons for resistance in Japan to recognition of brain death are the obstacles created within the medical profession, in particular its competitive factions, lack of peer review, and lack of quality control. The resulting distrust of doctors ensures that new technologies are perceived with suspicion by the public (1991a). Not all medical technologies are suspect (Ikegami 1988): the new imaging technologies, for example, are embraced wholeheartedly, reproductive and genetic technologies are set to make great inroads in Japan (Lock 1998a), and abortion meets with little resistance. Anxiety about the management of death apparently threatens the social order as most other forms of medical interventions do not.

The scandals associated with organ procurement in Japan and the lack of a system of informed consent have also fueled disputes about brain death, as have media accounts. However, none of these factors fully accounts for the large hiatus between responses to polls in Japan about donation, which are by no means completely negative, and the very small number of procurements, even when no legal restrictions remain. ICU practices in Japan, may account for this discrepancy. It seems that the ancestors often position themselves to watch over what happens in Japanese ICUs.

Technology as a Threat to Culture

Thus far I have limited an examination of "tradition" to concerns about unnatural, traumatic deaths and to the culture of mortuary practices. Nudeshima's senior colleague, Yonemoto Shōhei, a well-known cultural critic in Japan, asserts that modern medicine collided head on with Japanese ideas about life and death "lurking deep within our culture." Yonemoto is not concerned with good and bad deaths, nor with the submersion of individuals in families or the continuity of ancestral lines. Following a line of thinking that resembles Ōmine's, Yonemoto states that, in contrast to "Americans who think of organs as replaceable parts, . . . the Japanese tend to find in every part of a deceased person's body a fragment of that person's mind and spirit" (1985:200). Of the twenty-seven Tokyo residents with whom I talked, more than half were certain that *ki* (the force that accounts for the diffusion of "life" throughout the body) would inevitably be transplanted with a donated organ. A modicum of the "essence" of the donor is conveyed to the organ recipient. Interviews in North America with organ recipients, donors, and even transplant surgeons reveal similar concerns, as chapter 13 makes clear, although there the more contemporary concept of "personality" is usually invoked to explain this transposition, resulting in a highly personalized form of anthropomorphism.

The relation of individuals to the natural world is considered fundamental to the philosophic tradition of East Asia, and the concept of *ki* is crucial to this thinking. Good health, individual well-being, and individual maturity depend on a proper flow of *ki* in the body. *Ki* is manifest everywhere, including in individual bodies; it is individualized but not personalized. That is, *ki* does not take on the specific character of a person, but rather remains in a state of flux, varying with the environment both inside and outside the body.[9]

9. I have found no clear-cut evidence, but it would come as no surprise that the language of East Asian medicine, with its emphasis on *ki*, has undergone some reformulations in light of the insights about homeostatis and interior and exterior milieus made by the nineteenth-century French physiologist Claude Bernard.

Ki, associated originally with Taoism and later, particularly in Japan, with Zen Buddhism, is implicated in many aspects of daily life, including the numerous clinics that use East Asian medicine, schools, the martial arts practiced by many young people, the tea ceremony, and most forms of the indigenous creative arts including calligraphy, all of which have undergone recent revivals over the last thirty years. Its influence has been documented in training programs for bank employees, factory workers, baseball teams and other groups (Kondo 1990; Moeran 1984; Rohlen 1974). Once largely limited to the elite, concepts from the dominant East Asian philosophical tradition have diffused thoroughly into daily life in Japan. They have, of course, been modified, sometimes drastically, but even in rural areas women find time to participate in activities such as poetry writing, the tea ceremony, and flower arrangement, along with English classes and computer studies (Lock 1993). As with mortuary practices, this facet of the culture of tradition, so often disseminated as an unchanged cultural legacy, heightens awareness of a supposed Japanese uniqueness. Such awareness could not be sustained, however, without the otherness of the West.

No substantial research has been done on the subject, but I believe that the East Asian philosophic tradition enables many Japanese to conceptualize the idea of person and the relationship of person to body in a characteristic way. On several occasions, when cajoled somewhat reluctantly into participating in a tea ceremony or into an organized viewing of a Zen garden, I was reminded by my hosts in no uncertain terms that foreigners do not have traditions such as these to calm the body and empty the cluttered mind. Such activities unite mind and body as one, and the correct management of *ki,* including an avoidance of excesses of all kinds, keeps one healthy. What is more, the center of the individual, the core of the person, resides not in the head but in *kokoro.* *Kokoro* is not an anatomical organ but a concept—a crucial part of the collective imagination removed from the foray of daily life. True feelings are located in *kokoro:* this is the source of a stable inner self, but it is not the location of the eminently social concept of "person."

The very diffuseness of *kokoro* gives it enduring strength (Lock 1980; Rohlen 1978), even in the face of the challenge the anatomical sciences have mounted against East Asian philosophical discourse about the body. Psychological discourse, however, even today, has a relatively weak hold in Japan. Psychoanalysis has never really taken root at all, despite extensive exposure to this type of thought from the days of Freud onward. Contemporary psychiatry in Japan makes extensive use of pharmacological interventions, and psychotherapy tends to employ behavioral modification or other forms of cognitive therapy to induce practical changes in a person's daily life. Therapy focuses on how individuals might better adjust to social and family relationships and to everyday reality. The idea of an autonomous, individualized self, essentially synonymous with the "person" in the West, does not sit well in Japan, where "person" is above all reproduced in the public domain, beyond the bounds of the body, as part of a network of ongoing exchange.[10] Personhood is constructed in the space of human relationships. In effect, no single self exists in the public domain, but rather selves are constituted through a variety of subject positions depending on context (Kondo 1990:44). Person, constituted out of multiple situated social selves, remains, perhaps for the majority, a dialogical creation, and decisions about what one does with and what is done to one's body are by no means limited to individual wishes or rights. Moreover, individual self-determination is considered by many as essentially selfish. A key part of the brain death debate has been about whether next of kin can overrule individual wishes about donation of body parts, and the new law acceded to this position.

The "inner," stable self of *kokoro,* in contrast to the more public selves that constitute "person," lies in the depths of the body. It serves as a buffer, secured through tradition, against the ravages of modernity. Although many people find little space for serenity in their busy daily lives, nevertheless *kokoro* remains important. Among the Tokyo residents with whom I talked on this subject, only one-third locate the "center" of their bodies in the brain; most of the others, of varying ages, selected *kokoro* as the site where "self" is centered. The remaining few insisted that there is no "center" that takes priority over anything else. Given the pervasiveness of both *ki* and *kokoro,* for many people "person" does not reside in the brain, nor is it exclusively associated with mind. Such views make it difficult to count brain-dead persons as dead, particularly when a brain-dead body remains so visually alive.

Given that it is a "person" and not a body that is diagnosed as brain-dead, what happens to a brain-dead patient in Japan is inevitably much more than a matter of individual choice. Should organs be transplanted, the procedure is more than a mechanical transfer of body parts. These

10. Dorinne Kondo, in her consideration of discourses of identity in Japan, notes that most anthropological analyses have failed to question Marcel Mauss's fundamental equation of the "self" or the "person" with psychological consciousness—in other words, its formulation as a highly individuated concept (Kondo 1990:35).

facets of the culture of "tradition" contribute to discomfort both with the concept of brain death and with transplant technology.

Despite the media onslaught, many people remain unaffected by the social and moral implications of a recognition of brain death. Many more do not reflect much at all about the ideas of self, and person, or *ki* and *kokoro*. But speakers of Japanese are immersed in a language and an environment in which these concepts are ubiquitous; one cannot communicate without referring repeatedly to them. *Ki* and *kokoro* can and have been mobilized by partisan individuals to elevate anxiety about the new death and the threat they perceive in it to moral order.

Reflections on the Natural

Feelings that brain death does not "fit" with Japanese culture often take the form of a generalized disgust on the part of conservative commentators. These commentators support "tradition" as a force that curbs the destructive threat of modern innovations. In the vast number of magazine articles, books, and newspaper editorials published in Japan on brain death and organ transplants since 1986 (in 1996 alone more than 140 such articles appeared), it is repeatedly asserted that brain death is "unnatural" *(fushizen)*. For example, brain death is reported by one cardiologist to be too "unnatural" to be called "death" (Hirosawa 1992); a psychiatrist describes brain death as going against "natural science" (Kimura 1992). Brain death has been characterized as "contrary to basic human feelings" (see Uozumi 1992). Doctors, philosophers, and others have argued that the idea of "controlling" death goes against nature (Watanabe 1988; Umehara 1992). Organ transplants too have been described as *egetsu nai* (a powerful vernacular expression indicating that something is foul, ugly, or revolting) and *chi ma mire* (bloody) (Fukumoto 1989). Arguments against organ transplants requiring a brain-dead donor appear, therefore, to raise concerns about technological intrusions into the "natural" process of dying in Japan.

In Japanese, several metaphors are pervasively associated with the idea of nature, among which the concept of harmony is perhaps the most common. In classical works of medicine, philosophy, and Confucianism, individuals are exhorted to keep their *ki* in balance and to stay "in harmony" with the natural and social orders. In educational settings of all kinds and in the numerous East Asian medical clinics, the idea of harmony is ubiquitous. This tradition is falsely presented as age-old; an emphasis on harmony can be dated to the military regime of the 1930s (Itō 1998). Buddhist metaphors of transience and impermanence are also closely associated with nature. These metaphors of harmony and of impermanence, likened to the cycles of nature and the seasons, contribute to the idea held both in Japan and elsewhere that Japanese citizens are somehow "closer" to nature than others. It is this rhetoric in particular on which critics of brain death draw.

An ideology of living in harmony with nature—of merging with nature—blurs the boundaries between culture and nature, between what is "artificial" and what is "natural." Although contemplation of nature is a key element in Buddhist practice, notably Zen, nature should nevertheless be enhanced, managed, and tamed to "fit" with cultivated aesthetic tastes: witness Zen gardens and bonsai trees. It is perhaps surprising, then, that brain death and organ transplants should be condemned as unnatural. It is conceivable that exactly the opposite view might have won out: that the manipulation of life and death alters nature for the better. This is the type of argument that colors discourse about abortion in Japan, and which I predict will dominate debate about in vitro fertilization and genetic testing, screening, and therapy as these technologies become routinized (Lock 1998a).[11] Abortion and infanticide have long been used to produce the "correct family" (Cornell 1996), and genetic technologies will no doubt be used in efforts to make "perfect" babies. Manipulation of reproduction does not go against nature, it seems; yet the idea of interfering with death raises the hackles of many outspoken Japanese and makes others feel ill at ease.

We cannot generalize, therefore, about technological imperatives in Japan or elsewhere, nor about aversions to technological innovation, about what is natural and what is not. We must persist in asking instead what it is that is specific to locating death in the brain, organ donation, and the social relations involved in these two endeavors that incites anxiety.

Brain-dead bodies everywhere produce ambiguity, creating space for dispute and anxiety, but clinical practice in ICUs in Japan is informed by the particularly disruptive discourse of the "brain death problem."

11. Although freely available, reproductive technologies in practice are subject to restriction. Surrogacy is not permitted, nor is insemination by a donor other than a close relative of the husband. In vitro fertilization is available primarily, therefore, to permit couples to create "natural" families in which social bonds correspond with biological parenthood. Used this way, this technology reinforces rather than threatens the social order.

Central to these disputes is the idea that death is above all a social event, and almost all public commentary bears on this belief, even when, as in Tachibana's analysis, the focus is diagnostic accuracy. Closely related to a sensitivity about social death are the ideas that persons do not reside in brains and are not confined to individual bodies. Moreover, in many families, persons do not cease to exist at physical death, but continue to interact socially with others as ancestors. Only the most materialistic and resolutely modern of Japanese, of whom there are of course many, would find it an anachronism to think of a person lingering on in an unconscious body after severe head trauma. And even these individuals, confronted with a brain-dead relative, might well have trouble thinking of that person as corpselike and divested of all human qualities.

That the culture of tradition is a powerful force in the brain-death debate does not rule out other sources of controversy. Clearly medical politics and arrogance (also part of contemporary culture) account for a great deal of resistance, among members of the medical profession as well as the public.

Many people can readily agree with criticism of the medical profession. This politicizes the issue even as it marginalizes or explicitly rejects the influence of values and behaviors associated with the past. Many critics who reject cultural influences outright assume that the application of medicine in a modern, technologically advanced society, while it may be corrupt, inequitable, or unethical, is entirely separate from culture. Moreover, a good number of people do not want to be associated in any way with the conservative element that reifies tradition, although they are opposed to the recognition of brain death.

Even so, recognition of brain death as human death has many supporters in Japan, particularly among some sections of the medical world, intellectuals, and patients waiting for organ transplants. Even many critics of the current situation are not in principle opposed to recognition of the new death. Nevertheless, given the inertia of the past thirty years, a powerful conjunction of forces still works against this new technology.

Thus far I have dealt largely with public and professional discourse about the new death. I turn next to clinical practices. One might expect that clinical practice neatly mirrors public, and especially professional, discourse, whether in Japan or North America. But significant disjunctions between the two highlight the ambiguous nature of a living cadaver and show how difficult it is for those who must work closely with this entity to sustain the belief in its complete demise that is necessary for procurements to take place.

MEMORY WORK

Martha's parents had been separated for seven years when she died, aged ten, of a massive brain hemorrhage.[1] She had spent the evening with her father; the two of them had been out to a restaurant, and Martha had gone to bed around nine o'clock, as usual. Her father was awakened in the small hours by the sound of Martha vomiting in the bathroom. He helped her back to bed, but about half an hour later heard more sounds from her room. He thought at first that she was having a nightmare, but by the time he had got out of bed and crossed the hall into his daughter's room, everything was quiet. He found Martha unconscious. As a wave of panic washed over him, he called an ambulance. Then he tried mouth-to-mouth resuscitation. The paramedics administered oxygen and informed Martha's father that the pronounced swelling around her eyes indicated that something serious was probably wrong with her brain. On arrival at the hospital at 4.00 A.M., Martha was rushed straight into the emergency room and then up to the operating theater.

Martha's father, George, telephoned his ex-wife, Francine, who came at once to the hospital. The parents were warned that the surgery could take six hours. George was reasonably hopeful about the outcome because he knew of someone who had recovered after surgery for a brain

---

1. These interviews were conducted approximately one year after Martha's death. Martha's mother invited me to her home, and I met Martha's father in a quiet corner of a public building.

hemorrhage. Francine says that George sat reading *Time* and seemed fairly calm, but she was wracked with fear and could do nothing but sit. Two hours later the surgeon came to find them and told them gently that the situation was hopeless: nothing more could be done, and their daughter was brain-dead. The parents were overwhelmed; as George puts it, "We were comatose ourselves."

Martha was brought back to the ICU, where she was placed in a private room with the tubes, leads, and ventilator still attached to her body. Her parents sat beside her in disbelief. Neither parent recalls clearly what happened over the next few hours. Francine remembers that "another team" came right away and asked them about the possibility of donation. George thinks that this request was not made until the afternoon, perhaps after the brain-death diagnosis was confirmed a second time. Francine recollects that everything was "in a rush, they came right away and asked us to decide. We had a very short time to make up our minds, maybe fifteen or twenty minutes. George was for it right away. I wasn't so keen, in fact I didn't really want to do it. It was all so fast, and I didn't want to lose my daughter yet. The doctor came and talked to both of us, and we had to agree. I sat there thinking, 'I can't have a fight with my ex-husband now, over the body of our daughter.' So I said, 'All right, but not the eyes.' I didn't want her to lose her beautiful eyes."

Francine remembers that through the rest of the day "it was nonstop talking around us as they were testing, testing, taking blood, because they had to do all the compatibility tests. Martha stayed full of tubes— they had to keep her alive, to keep her organs. After a while I couldn't endure it any more. They kept coming and touching her and taking things from her. So I said please give us an hour and leave us in peace. I felt torn—physically torn apart. I didn't really want this to happen, but if I'd said no, everyone would have thought I wasn't being generous. And I'm not like that. Maybe because I'm her mother, I was upset much more than George. I was angry that they kept touching her little body. I just wanted to hold her, hold her peacefully, and I was crying, crying . . ."

George's memory is quite different. He recalls that by coincidence, a few weeks before her death, Martha had watched him checking off the organ donor boxes on his new driver's license. Martha had asked her father what he was doing, and when he explained, she had said at once, "I'd like to do that too." George says this made it much easier for him to decide to donate Martha's organs: "Certainly my daughter would have wanted it. She was a very generous person. It wasn't a tough decision; the tough part was realizing that she wasn't going to survive. But, you know, it's still tough, even when you've decided to donate. You sit there holding the warm hand of your child and you can feel the pulse, and your emotions go back and forth, and you think, OK what is death?

"Because we decided to donate, Martha was on life support longer than usual while everything was made ready. As you know, they have to get a second set of medical opinions about brain death, and then they start taking blood and so on. I was sort of pleased about the extra time. Everyone was very considerate, the hospital staff were great. Very supporting. My wife—ex-wife—and I sat down and talked about the donation calmly with the doctor; she was a woman, as I recall. We made a decision quite quickly. By this time it was the afternoon, and we had until the next day before they took her away. Now, looking back, I have absolutely no regrets. We did the right thing, and there are four other children alive thanks to Martha. I received a letter from one of the mothers whose infant received the liver. I cherish it, and carry it with me all the time, that letter. A seven-month-old baby girl got my daughter's liver, and I'm pleased for her. A year later I sent a little Christmas gift to the kid, but you hear nothing, you know. I had to send the present to the transplant coordinating office. I'd much rather things weren't anonymous, I'd love to meet that little girl. These days I get really angry when I see people who don't love their kids properly. The day before Martha died, I think it was, we were walking near the house, and we saw a father who sort of forced his kid to sit down on a seat beside him—he was rough with the child, and Martha said, 'I'm really lucky to have you as a father.' We were good parents, Francine and I, we lost our only daughter and we lost part of ourselves too—you can't transplant that sort of thing."

Over a year after Martha's death, Francine says, "I'm pleased, I'm finally pleased. If there is a little girl living thanks to Martha's liver, then that's wonderful. But it's taken me a long time. I kept thinking they were hurting her when they were doing all those tests, I was feeling the pain, literally, and I was sure she was feeling it too. The trouble is that you don't really see her die. I suppose I do think a little bit that she is living on in those other kids. But I'm not religious, never have been, although I've become sort of spiritual since Martha died. I'm an artist, and I put more emotion into my work now. Martha was very proud of my paintings, she always encouraged me, so I think now that I must work really hard at it and do something good for her."

TEN

When Bodies Outlive Persons

As a Christian, I believe that there is life after death, and so I understand that this is not the end of life. The soul has a continuation, the soul lives on. Death is only a stage, some would even say a liberation.

Alexander Solzhenitsyn, New Yorker

I always hesitate before using the word "harvest" to describe removal of a donor's organs for transplantation, and yet there is no better term for a process that is so like the gathering of a crop.

Sherwin B. Nuland, New Yorker

Local Routinization and Soft Regulation

Over the past two decades, the diagnosis of whole-brain death has been standardized in intensive care units in many parts of the world. Yet few clinical practitioners ever refer to formal guidelines for determining brain death. Discussions with intensivists reveal that hospital committees either draw up their own criteria (presumably after consulting national guidelines) or, very commonly, intensivists are simply trained by other doctors, without referral to written guidelines. In some regions of North America, the local transplant organization puts out guidelines for determining brain death, and in hospitals where this diagnosis is infrequent, intensivists may refer to this booklet or to plastic pocket cards.

In 1996 and 1997 I interviewed a total of forty intensivists, thirty-two physicians, and eight nurses who work in ICUs about their attitudes and routine practices regarding brain-death diagnoses.[1] These practitioners are employed in hospitals in Canada and the United States, in

1. I have observed in six ICUs, two of them pediatric ICUs (PICUs), all of which are located in hospitals that are part of an urban tertiary health care complex. Unless otherwise

regular ICUs, trauma units, and pediatric ICUs. Not one of them doubts the accuracy of a brain-death diagnosis, *provided* that all the examinations and tests are carried out correctly. The majority believe that, if anything, the criteria for brain death are overly conservative and that some patients may not be declared dead as soon as is warranted. Everyone showed confidence in the current criteria for diagnosing brain death, and several physicians volunteered spontaneously that they were sure that no one was being declared dead while still alive.

In contrast with the discrepancies so evident in previous decades, clinical practices appear to be remarkably uniform today. Even so, debate continues about certain specific diagnostic criteria and as to what *exactly* brain death signifies.

Brain-Death Criteria and Confirmatory Tests

Everyone interviewed agrees that bedside clinical tests for brain death are crucial, replicable, and reliable. No one refers only to printouts or brain scans to make a diagnosis. Whereas technology is said to yield false negatives (that is, the patient appears alive when in fact he or she is brain-dead), good clinical skills do not admit such doubts. Practitioners agree that certain drugs, including central nervous system depressants or muscle relaxants, or a body temperature below 35° C (usually due to drowning), can yield false positives (the patient may appear dead when alive).[2] Under these circumstances it is imperative to wait. The original cause of the trauma should be determined in every case, if at all possible.

Clinical signs of brain death about which there is virtually unanimous agreement are as follows: There should be no response to pain stimuli (such as pinpricks to the hands and feet, hard pressure on the fingernails and toenails, or very hard pressure on the sternum), nor evidence of brain stem reflexes: the pupils should be dilated and not contract in response to light; when the head is moved from side to side, the eyes should stay fixed in a midline position as the head rotates, indicating no

---

noted, the discussion on the management of brain-dead patients refers equally to adults and children. Informants have been given pseudonyms.

2. There are other rather rare conditions that mimic brain death, case studies of which have been reported in medical journals, including Miller Fisher syndrome (a brainstem encephalitis) and Guillain-Barré syndrome (Hughes and McGuire 1997; Ragosta 1993).

control of the eye muscles;[3] the patient should not gag or cough when stimulated, nor respond to cold water being poured into the ear. Some protocols and guidelines suggest that the corneas should be touched with a Q-tip or similar implement to check for a response (*Canadian Medical Association Journal* 1987).

In 1997 an intensivist posted several messages on the Internet site "Defining Death," to say that for him one sure sign of brain death is that the forehead of the patient is cold. An experienced nurse I talked to about this claim replied that this intensivist is "off the wall," not because it is in error to suggest that the heads of brain-dead patients are often disturbingly cold but because this sign could not possibly qualify as a reliable criterion. Apparently there is still room for creative thinking in connection with this diagnosis, and complete unanimity about criteria and tests for brain death does not exist, although there is much more uniformity than there was in the 1970s and 1980s.

In the early days two specialists were required to carry out the battery of tests independently of each other to confirm a brain-death diagnosis. Today this is no longer necessary everywhere in North America, although it provides legal protection should a problem arise. All the intensivists interviewed agreed that the bedside clinical examination for brain death is straightforward. These tests were described as "robust," "simple," and "solid," and, together with the apnea test (which establishes whether the patient can breathe independently of the ventilator), they inform the physician about the condition of the lower brain—the brain stem. If the patient fails to respond to this battery of tests and fails the apnea test, then whole-brain death can provisionally be diagnosed—or even settled on. The patient is then declared dead.

Until relatively recently it has been customary everywhere, when patients are possible organ donors, to repeat the tests after an interval of time. No one I interviewed could think of an occasion when the second tests reversed the findings, provided everything was done correctly. Several physicians recall reversals, but they believed that in those cases the apnea test had not been carried out correctly.

There is, however, enormous variation in the timing of the second set of tests. In many severe trauma cases, the patient is obviously brain-dead on arrival in the unit or shortly thereafter. A patient in this condition shows no response of any kind to pain, nor is there any cough reflex when tubes are inserted into the pharynx to provide oxygen. In

3. The doll's eyes test.

some units, clinical tests and the apnea test are done only once on such patients. In other units the tests are done twice, even though everyone is certain of the diagnosis. Several intensivists, usually following their particular hospital guidelines, wait twelve hours between tests. Today this approach is widely regarded as very conservative, and precautions of this kind inevitably mean that some patients will "crash" (suffer cardiac arrest) and be lost as donors. For other intensivists, the waiting period depends on the condition of the individual patient and may vary from two to twenty-four hours. One of the physicians insisted that the timing is in effect arbitrary. In pediatric units, greater caution is evident in that a longer period of time is usually observed between the two rounds of tests; but in one of the two pediatric units where I conducted interviews, two sets of tests are usually done, and in the other they are rarely carried out. In this second unit, confirmatory nuclear scans (see below) are commonly performed instead; this test is deemed conclusive when it reveals no cerebral blood flow.

Several physicians noted that they decide if and when to do a second set of readings based on the family's response to the first set of tests. Some families, I was told, want to go home after the first tests, already convinced that their relative is dead. On the other hand, if a family is having difficulty in accepting the diagnosis, then the physician may consult with the nurse caring for the patient as to when the family appears prepared to cope with the second set of tests. One intensivist suggested that the second set of readings are in effect done "for the sake of the family."

No one retains any hope for recovery of the patient after a first set of tests diagnoses brain death. However, it is usual to sign the death certificate only after confirmatory tests, leaving space for ambiguity and perhaps, on occasion, false hope. The doctors' confidence in the clinical tests for brain death, and the fact that no one I interviewed has experienced any reversals between the first and second set of tests, when performed correctly, suggest that suitable caution is being applied.[4]

Intensivists differ as to what technologically produced confirmatory results, if any, are used. One indispensable criterion for brain death is

---

4. There is disagreement regarding the assessment of hypothermic patients as to whether the maximum body temperature for warranting extra caution should be 32.2° C or 35° C. (Normal body temperature is 37° C.) Here is a situation in which the interests of the transplant surgeon may not coincide with the objectives of the intensivist. If patients' bodies are warmed up to and kept at or above 35° C, it is more difficult to keep their vital signs stable, and it becomes less likely that their organs will remain suitable for donation.

the inability to breathe spontaneously. This can be demonstrated only by taking the patient off the ventilator, allowing carbon dioxide to accumulate in the blood—thus causing a stimulus to breathe—and seeing what happens. Although everyone agrees that the apnea test is necessary, doctors disagree as to how high the carbon dioxide level should be allowed to rise (risking further injury to the patient and his or her organs), and how long one should wait before deciding the patient is unable to take a breath. In the latter part of 2000 a rancorous exchange took place on the Defining Death website about the risks associated with the apnea test. Because the test has no therapeutic value for the patient, is associated with unpredictability, and, it is claimed, may on occasion kill the patient, great caution is called for. Some physicians refuse to use it.

Particularly with infants, there have been occasions when a patient has started to breathe after a battery of clinical tests have indicated brain death. Among the intensivists I interviewed, five had been involved with cases where there was confusion over the apnea test. One intensivist, then still a resident, had been part of a team that was trying to establish brain death very quickly:

> I suppose we were working under pressure to procure organs for transplant. We did the apnea test for half a minute and the patient didn't breathe. Then we sent the patient to the OR as a donor, and when they stopped the respirator, the patient started breathing. They brought him back to the ICU, and we kept supporting the patient. He finally died about two months later, but it was a complete nightmare. There were no excuses for that, but it was at the time before clear guidelines had been established for brain death—in the early 70s. I always tell my residents about this case, and I always teach people that they must *never* be in a hurry with this diagnosis.

Transplant coordinators are often in a hurry, and they are not above putting pressure on intensivists. Several of the physicians said that they found the apnea test to be particularly stressful. For example, Janet Goodwin, a pediatric intensivist, said: "I hate it, you're standing there with your eyes glued on this child's chest, and after five minutes you start seeing things, imagining you see the chest going up and down. I make sure that the nurses and technicians are looking carefully too, so we can all agree on the result."

Goodwin had recently been involved with a case where voluntary respiration started during the apnea test, even though the first tests all showed that the child was brain-dead. The following day the clinical tests and the apnea test were repeated, and a nuclear scan was done. This time there were no positive responses, but the child was exhibiting one of the most disconcerting signs associated with brain death: frequent spinal reflex movements that caused her body to jerk wildly. These movements, although they do not disprove a brain-death diagnosis, can be devastating for assembled relatives. The doctor commented that if she thinks a brain-death diagnosis is likely, she always warns relatives about what to expect. (None of the interviewed physicians expect relatives to leave the unit when they are carrying out tests for brain death; even so, approximately half stated that families do so voluntarily.)

Another physician, with seven years' experience, recalled the case of a child who had a severe head injury after a traffic accident. The first set of tests indicated brain death, but a little later the child showed signs of breathing independently of the ventilator. A second set of clinical tests confirmed brain death, and shortly thereafter the child's heart stopped functioning, even though she was on a ventilator. This physician believes that certain medications may have made the child appear to be breathing faintly, but another intensivist expressed doubts that this could have been the case.

Doctors also disagree over use of the electroencephalogram (EEG). This dispute has continued for thirty years. Some North American guidelines require use of the EEG, others suggest that it is optional, and others do not recommend it at all. Those interviewed agreed that a flat (isoelectric) EEG indicates that there is no activity in the brain. In a thorough review of the literature, J. R. Hughes found one or two "very rare" cases in which patients recovered after exhibiting what appeared to be a completely flat EEG, but he notes that the records do not mention how long the EEG had been flat. Hughes points out that a major limitation of the EEG is the "inability of the scalp electrodes to record all subcortical activity" (1978:126), so that a flat EEG does not necessarily indicate complete nonfunctioning of the upper brain.

On the other hand, and equally disconcerting, even when clinical tests reveal conclusively that the brain stem is no longer functioning, the EEG often detects slight electrical activity in the cerebral hemispheres. Hughes noted that some researchers describe EEG results as "almost flat," or "almost completely flat," and take this result as corroboration that the patient is brain-dead (127).

False positives with the EEG frequently result from outside electrical interference (external artifacts). One Canadian neurologist asked his wife to prepare a bowl of gelatin (was he not capable of doing this himself?), which he then placed upside down over a plastic model of a head. He attached electrodes from an EEG machine to the gelatin at the sites where they would have been attached to a patient's head; two leads were connected to a respirator and one to an intravenous drip chamber. The resultant EEG tracings looked completely convincing of cerebral activity (Pollock 1978). A few unusual cases have also been reported of genuine cortical activity, including sleep-like activity, showing up on electroencephalograms after patients fulfill the clinical criteria for brain death (Halevy and Brody 1993; Young and Matta 2000).

Other types of confirmatory tests are used at times: among them are various nuclear scans, including MRIs (magnetic resonance imaging), angiography, in which a dye is injected into the patient,[5] and radioisotope studies. These techniques reveal whether there is any blood flow in the brain. Although not used in the United Kingdom, such tests are required in about half the ICUs in America where brain death is diagnosed.[6] Here too, difficulties arise, and many of the interviewed doctors asserted spontaneously that both nuclear scans and EEGs often confuse rather than clarify.

In one instance, where I was a witness to some of the bedside discussion, an infant met all the usual clinical criteria for brain death, and the senior doctor informed the parents that there was no hope for their child, although confirmatory tests would be done. An eager resident, acting within his authority, carried out a nuclear scan (it is unlikely that experienced senior doctors would have ordered this test at this juncture). The scan revealed a small amount of blood flow in the upper brain. The parents were thoroughly disconcerted. The following day, when a second set of clinical tests were done, the brain-death diagnosis of the previous day was confirmed. The attending staff were grateful that the parents seemed to retain faith in the judgment of the doctors and accepted after the second set of tests that their child was dead, but with different parents it might well have been necessary to do a second nuclear scan, thus prolonging the uncertainty.[7]

When commenting on this case, senior intensivists noted scathingly that the inexperience of residents and clinical fellows often causes them to carry out too many tests. In this case, if a nuclear scan was to be done

5. *Angiography* and *arteriography* refer to the same technique.
6. Not all hospitals are equipped to carry out nuclear scans, and in any case the patient must usually be taken to the machine, with all the tubes, lines, and monitoring equipment in place. The best-equipped hospitals now have equipment that can be brought to the patient's bedside, and so this type of test is becoming more common.
7. Confirming brain death in an infant is particularly harrowing not simply because of difficulties in making a diagnosis in a very young child, but because the medical examiner is almost always involved to investigate the possibility of child abuse.

at all, then it should have been done after the two sets of clinical tests, as confirmatory evidence, by which time it is very unlikely that any cerebral activity would have been revealed.

Except where required by hospital guidelines, confirmatory tests are usually done only if doubt exists. As with the apnea test, the presence of the family may influence decisions about if and when to use specific tests. Most people today have been led by the media to believe that a "flat line" means brain death; if the EEG is flat, then families are convinced at once of the death of their relative. If, however, some residual activity appears on the EEG, or else outside interference makes the EEG appear as though the brain is still functioning, then this test creates anxiety among both doctors and families.[8]

A resident informed me that in the hospital where he works, an EEG is used to confirm brain death only when the family demands it, something that had happened several times in his two years' experience. As he put it, "Some families can only be convinced of death when they see a flat line on the monitor." In common with several other physicians, this resident noted that many families are more comfortable with looking at the monitor than looking at the patient. Technology reveals death in a more decisive way than does the body itself.

All the physicians interviewed agreed that a diagnosis of brain death means that treatment of the patient should be stopped. If the patient is a candidate for organ donation, attention is then switched from the patient to the organs (see also Hogle 1999).[9]

In summary, intensivists are unanimous that the clinical criteria for whole-brain death or brain-stem death are infallible if the tests are performed correctly; and they show close to unanimous agreement about the interpretation of test results. Whole-brain death, properly diagnosed, is an irreversible state from which no one, in the experience of the informants, has ever recovered (see also Plum 1999). These doctors are also convinced that although very occasionally discrepancies occur, no one who would have made anything more than a minimal, transitory

8. This type of confusion does not occur in the United Kingdom, where a diagnosis of brain-stem death is used. With such a diagnosis, residual activity in the upper brain is not considered significant.

9. In units where the majority of patients are elderly, or are suffering invasive or degenerative diseases that preclude organ transplantation, the procedure is different. In these cases, which are much more common than cases involving possible donation, doctors are under no pressure to diagnose brain death, except to clarify what care, if any, the patient should continue to receive. Frequently the heart simply stops beating, even when the patient is on the ventilator, and this is considered the moment of death.

recovery has been actively killed by being prematurely disconnected from a ventilator or by undergoing organ retrieval. From observations and discussions in busy, urban ICUs in teaching hospitals where practitioners have experience in dealing with brain death, I am convinced that fatal errors do not happen in these locations. Intensivists have persuaded me that the criteria for a diagnosis of brain death are indeed conservative, and that they are applied in a cautious, defensive way. No one makes the diagnosis alone without other specialists present, and in any case the presence of families usually deters hasty action. However, where intensive care units are poorly equipped, lacking in expertise, or inadequately staffed, the likelihood of error is increased; this is equally true for all countries that participate in the transplant endeavor. It is also the case that undue pressure is sometimes exerted by organ brokers or transplant surgeons. One intensivist in a superbly functioning ICU in the United States told me that he had on occasion been obliged to drive out transplant surgeons who were "trolling" his unit.

Determining the End of Life

Although the physicians I talked to agree that the brain-death diagnosis is robust, they do not believe that patients are biologically dead when sent for organ retrieval. Among the thirty-two physician intensivists interviewed, not one thinks brain death signals the end of biological life, although everyone agreed brain death will lead to complete biological death. As Alan Cohen puts it, "It's not death, but it is an irreversible diagnosis, which I accept." A diagnosis of whole-brain death indicates that the brain has ceased to function as a site for the integration of biological activities in other parts of the body. At the same time, physicians concur that the organs and cells of the body, including small portions of the brain, are alive, thanks to the ventilator. Indeed, if organs are to be transplanted, then circulation and organ function must be kept as close to "normal" as possible. Stuart Youngner and colleagues assert that "maintaining organs for transplantation actually necessitates treating dead patients in many respects as if they were alive" (1985:321).

Intensivists cannot disregard the facts that the brain-dead are warm and usually retain a good color, that digestion, metabolism, and excretion continue, and that the hair and nails continue to grow. A few have observed a brain-dead patient "yawn," and many of them have seen them "cry." Clusters of cells in the brain often exhibit random activity for some time after brain death has been declared, and endocrine and other types of physiological activity continue. It is difficult, therefore, to ignore the signs of life that bombard the senses of individuals caring for the brain dead (Youngner et al. 1985). The term "whole-brain death" is a misnomer, or at the very least misleading. However, Jim Gough argues that "the word brain death may be too artificial because probably the brain isn't completely dead. If you went cell by cell. But on the practical level, the clinical level, this just isn't relevant. Families simply don't care if a few cells are firing or not, what is important to them is that their child is no longer really there. I really don't care what the philosophers say when they argue back and forth."

Most intensivists agree with this position, although they may state it less categorically. They believe that a brain-dead patient not only is irreversibly unconscious but has also completed a second irreversible change, in that the "person" or "spirit" is no longer present in the body. The patient has, therefore, assumed a hybrid status—that of a dead person in a living body. However, rather than dwell on ambiguities or engage in an extended discussion about conceptual ideas concerning death, most clinical practitioners emphasize that the *person* is no longer present.

As Dick Willems (ms.) has pointed out in connection with euthanasia, there is a thrust when dealing with death in the ICU to make biological death coincide with the death of the person. Discomfort exists about the idea of a "person" surviving in a body that is to be counted as dead. On the other hand, many people, including those who argue for the recognition of cerebral death, are equally uncomfortable with the thought of a body kept alive by means of technology when it is clear to them that the "person" is no longer present. Even though the parts of the body do not die simultaneously, and it is unclear what exactly is meant by the death of the person, intensivists attempt to ensure that a diagnosis of brain death and the demise of the person become one and the same thing.

When talking to families, for example, the majority of doctors interviewed make statements such as "The things that make her herself are not there any more," or, "He's not going to recover. Death is inevitable." Charles Robbins, who like many of his colleagues does not like to say that the patient is dead, because he does not believe this is the case, tells the family firmly that the patient is brain-dead, but that there is "absolutely no doubt that things will get worse." Another intensivist, Ravi Kapoor, commented that it is difficult to know what is best to say to the family, because in most cases the doctor does not know their religious beliefs:

I believe that a "humanistic" death happens at the same time as brain death. If I didn't believe this, then I couldn't take care of these patients and permit them to become organ donors. For me the child has gone to heaven or wherever, and I'm dealing with an organism—respectfully, of course, but that child's soul, or whatever you want to call it, is no longer there. I don't know, of course, whether the family believes in souls or not, although sometimes I can make a good guess. So I simply have to say that Johnny is no longer here.

Pablo Mendez thinks of the brain-dead body as a vessel, and informs the family that what is left of their relative is an empty container, because "the person has gone." He believes the "essence" of the patient is no longer present, and this is in effect what he is telling the families of his patients.

A doctor must take control "a bit" when discussing brain death, says Kathleen Wright. Families, she argues, often find it difficult to accept that there is no possibility of recovery, and the doctor cannot afford to appear diffident or equivocating. This is a position that many Japanese intensivists would find troubling. Guy Levec states, "You can't go back to the family and say that their relative is brain-dead; you've *got* to say that they are dead—you could be arrested for messing up on this." He recalls that during his training he described a patient as "basically dead" to his supervisor, who responded abruptly: "He's dead, that's what you mean, basically."

The task for intensivists, then, is to convince the family that even though their relative appears to be sleeping, the person is no longer *essentially* alive; what remains is an organism or vessel that has suffered a mortal blow. In facing up to this unpleasant situation, physicians must come to terms with their own feelings about the diagnosis. This moment is especially poignant because it is also the moment when the question of organ donation is raised. Today, in most parts of North America, if a brain-dead patient is a candidate for donation, physicians are required by law to ask families if they will cooperate.[10] Several intensivists stated that it is clearly inappropriate to approach certain families, especially in cases of family violence or abuse, and they are not always asked; in one American ICU, however, I was told that every family is approached without exception.

Intensivists reported that families often raise the question of organ donation themselves, sometimes even before the first set of tests for brain

10. This is not the case in Quebec, where many of my observations were made.

death are completed. Every doctor tells the family that it is too early to discuss this possibility until at least one set of tests indicates brain death. Elizabeth Rasmussen, for example, insists that a brain-dead patient remains in her mind as a patient to be cared for until the second set of tests is completed, and she cannot possibly consider the patient as a donor until that time. However, the majority of physicians are prepared to listen to family wishes about donation, or to raise the possibility of donation, after the first set of clinical tests indicates brain death. They may even carry out simple screening tests before the first set of brain-death tests, to establish whether the local transplant coordinators might be interested in the patient's organs.

A recent study has shown that nurses are more effective than physicians in talking with families about organ donation. This may be because doctors are too busy and tend to use medical jargon, leaving families confused. This study also found that if families are told that the law requires that they be asked about organ donation, then success rates fall (Meckler 1999).

The move to thinking of the patient as a set of organs is a difficult transition. Interests of transplant surgeons, unwelcome visitors to most ICUs, are put firmly on hold until the ICU staff are satisfied that they are in the presence of a brain-dead body. Neurologists' interests and expertise are clearly at odds with those of transplant surgeons, and even though neither specialty wants to be thought of as inappropriately hastening the death of anyone, neurologists are very resistant to any interest exhibited by transplant surgeons about ICU patients. It is not only the interests of physicians that come into conflict but also, at times, those of parents. In pediatric ICUs, children with head trauma may lie in cubicles close to those waiting for organs. This situation can become highly charged when parents hoping for an organ for their child cast their eyes over the tiny forms around them hooked up to life support.

Doubts among the Certainty

It is clear that intensivists have no doubts about the irreversibility of brain death, but it is also evident that many nevertheless harbor some doubts about the condition of a patient recently declared brain-dead, and it is often the most experienced professionals who exhibit the strongest misgivings. An intensivist I interviewed with over fifteen years' experience admits to worries not unlike those Raymond Hoffenberg experienced when he declared the death of the donor for Christiaan Barnard's second heart transplant. This physician said that he often lies in bed at night after sending a brain-dead body for organ procurement and asks himself, " 'Was that patient *really* dead?' It is irreversible—I know that, and the clinical tests are infallible. My rational mind is sure, but some nagging, irrational doubt seeps in." This doctor, like the majority of intensivists interviewed, takes consolation from the belief that to remain in a persistent vegetative state is much worse than death. If a mistake should be made and a patient diagnosed prematurely, or mistakenly treated as brain-dead, then intensivists assume that brain death would have occurred shortly thereafter, or that the patient would be permanently unconscious. But doubts fester with some people.

Krishna Patel, who moved to North America from India as a child, stated that for him a brain-dead body is "an in-between thing. It's neither a cadaver, nor a person, but then again, there is still somebody's precious child in front of me. The child is legally brain-dead, has no awareness or connection with the world around him, but he's still a child, deserving of respect. I know the child is dead and feels no pain, is no longer suffering, that what's left is essentially a shell. I've done my tests, but there's still a child there." When asked by families, as he often is, if the patient has any consciousness, or feels pain, this intensivist has no difficulty in reassuring them that their child is dead, and is no longer suffering. He notes that it is especially hard for relatives when they take the hand of their child and sometimes, in a reflex, the hand seems to respond and grasps their own.

Janet Goodwin professes to a belief in a spirit or soul that takes leave of the body at death. She believes this happens at the moment when the patient's brain becomes irreversibly damaged. Another experienced intensivist, Joel Singer, insisted at first, as did many of the doctors interviewed, that he has no difficulty with the idea of brain death: "It seems pretty straightforward to me. Do the tests, allow a certain amount of time; a flat EEG and you're dead." Then, ten minutes later, he said, "I guess I equate the death of a person with the death of the spirit because I don't really know about anything else, like a hereafter. I'm not sure anyway, if a hereafter makes a difference or not." When asked what he meant by the word "spirit," he replied: "I guess one would have to take it as meaning that part of a person which is different—sort of not in the physical realm. Outside the physical realm. It's not just the brain, or the mind, but something more than that. I don't really know. But anyway, a brain-dead patient, someone's loved one, won't ever be the person they used to know. Sure their nails can grow and their hair can grow, but that's not the essence."

Yet another senior doctor, Alan Stein, struggling to express his feelings, imbues the physical body with a will: "The body *wants* to die, you can sense that when it becomes difficult to keep the blood pressure stable and so on." Stein, although he accepts that brain death is the end of meaningful life, reveals considerable confusion in talking about the procurement of organs: "We don't want this patient to expire before we can harvest the organs, so it's important to keep them stable and alive, and that's why we keep up the same treatment after brain death." A less experienced intensivist suggested that the "real" death happens when the heart stops: "The patient dies two deaths."

In at least one hospital in California the practice is to complete two sets of clinical tests, then to declare the patient brain-dead; but if the patient is designated an organ donor, the tests for brain death are repeated every few hours until the body is wheeled out of the intensive care unit and into the operating room. When I asked an intensivist in another part of the country what he thought about this practice, his first thought was that there may have been one or more cases in the California hospital in which someone temporarily "came back to life," causing great anxiety. Alternatively, these extra tests may be a precaution against litigation. To my mind, this practice suggests that the involved staff either are not convinced that brain-dead is dead enough to win a dispute should it go to court, or else they have doubts as to whether the patient is indeed in an irreversible condition—although this second possibility seems unlikely.

Clearly the ambiguities and contradictions that Youngner and colleagues detected over a decade ago are still present. One doctor recoiled when I suggested that more public education in connection with brain death might be a good thing. In his opinion, education should take place at the bedside when needed, and not be open to distortion and greater confusion in a public forum, as may have been the case in Japan.

For the majority of the intensivists with whom I talked, brain death signals the beginning of a process of biological death that is hastened with the withdrawal of the ventilator. On the rare occasions when the ventilator is not turned off, the process can continue for days, weeks, or occasionally months and years after the brain is irreversibly damaged.[11] Because there can be no argument about the liveliness of the principal body organs, apart from the brain, a donor is by definition biologically alive, or at least "partially" so, when organ retrieval takes place. Involved physicians must still satisfy themselves that the "person" no longer exists. For all the intensivists except one, absence of person is based on irreversible loss of brain function, which ensures a permanent lack of consciousness, awareness, and sensation. In other words, a sensate, suffering individual has ceased to exist. A few of the physicians express this idea by suggesting that the "soul" or "spirit" has departed; for them this is the moment of death of the person. The majority do not talk about souls but indicate that the person known to the family is no longer present, and will not return. Even these physicians are uncertain as to whether this departure is an event or a process; nevertheless, they are adamant that once brain death is declared, the person is gone.

For only one of the interviewed intensivists does personhood reside in the body as well as the brain. He expresses this notion by stating that his own person is as much embodied in his size nine feet as in his brain. It may not be coincidental that this intensivist was born in the Caribbean to an East Indian family (although his views are very close to those of Hans Jonas, a German, and so perhaps ethnicity is not significant). Nevertheless, the irreversibility of brain death permits this doctor to feel comfortable about encouraging families to donate organs.

Tellingly, among the thirty-two doctors interviewed, only six have signed their donor cards or made other forms of advance directive, and one was unsure whether he had done so. When I pressed for reasons, no one gave me very convincing answers. They said that their families would know what to do, or else that they just didn't feel quite right about it or, alternatively, that they supposed they should get it sorted out.[12]

Nursing the Brain-Dead

All of the eight nurses interviewed think of brain death as a reliable diagnosis and claim that they have no difficulties accepting it. When the first set of clinical tests indicates brain death, these nurses think of their

11. Potential survival time is increasing with improvements in ICU technologies (Shewmon 1998).

12. It would be most interesting to compare these findings with other units, and particularly with the rate of cooperation exhibited by intensivists in other countries.

patients as "pretty much dead," because none of them has ever witnessed a reversal of the diagnosis. However, they do not change their care of or behavior toward patients until after the second set of tests, and even then very little.

Several nurses pointed out that the interval between the tests is a crucial time, during which the family must start to come to terms with the untimely death. Most of the nurses are opposed to discussion of organ donation until after the second set of tests. However, a head nurse, Peter Vincelli, stated that there is often a "kind of 'let's get on with it' tone" among doctors after the first set of tests, and even, at times, among the family—an attitude that would be unimaginable in Japanese ICUs.

While carrying out their work between the two sets of tests, the nurses all continue to talk to their patients and pay close attention to the comfort and cleanliness of the body. Two nurses state that they are acutely aware at this time of the presence of relatives and so deliberately make their behavior around the patient as "normal" as possible. More often than not it is the attending nurse to whom the family puts their urgent questions. In many cases nurses sense that patients are brain-dead before the first set of tests is actually done, for they have been checking the pupils of the eyes and the reflexes regularly. They may have noted that the patient is no longer responding to pain stimuli when tubes are inserted into and taken out of the body. Often it becomes increasingly difficult to keep the body functions under control. The most conclusive sign of approaching brain death is a sudden drop or wild fluctuations in blood pressure.

Catherine Young remarks that if she showed me six patients in the ICU and one of them was brain-dead, I would have no idea which one it was. Patients simply don't look dead, she says, until the heart stops beating; but she also insists that she and her colleagues can often tell when someone is dying, even before measurable clinical signs appear. Young was equally sure that families frequently intuit when the situation has become worse; somehow the patient doesn't look quite the same, and even with the ventilator, the color and texture of the skin change as brain death approaches.

Nurses report that physicians explain very carefully to families about all the tests that they are performing and how to interpret them, but they add that nurses often go over the tests once again with families who, particularly because they are in a state of shock, cannot absorb the information. *Forbes* magazine, reporting on a survey in Boston, states that among families who refused to donate organs, 52 percent said that they had not realized that their brain-dead relative was no longer alive (McMenamin 1996:144). This study does not suggest that intensivists fail to explain things clearly, but rather that devastated families simply cannot take in the information that is being given to them.

After the second set of tests confirms whole-brain death, if the patient will be an organ donor, attention shifts to the condition of individual organs. Fluids are restricted for patients with head injuries to minimize cerebral swelling; however, once the patient is declared brain-dead, high volumes of fluid are administered to "optimize" the function of the vital organs, especially the kidneys. Usually the eyes are taped shut at this juncture to keep the corneas in good condition for transplant.

A nursing supervisor, unconsciously reflecting Japanese ideas, stated that brain death followed by donation is not a "peaceful" death. If the patient is not going to be a donor, lines and tubes are removed quickly, and mourning can commence. Only when the family is ready is the patient sent to the morgue.[13] However, if a patient is to be an organ donor, then the equipment must stay in place; and should cardiac arrest occur, the staff must attempt to resuscitate the body. The small number of donor families interviewed all noted that mourning was impeded by the technological apparatus and that the body was taken away the moment arrangements for donation were complete, sometimes not to be returned to the family for twelve hours or more.

Once the patient has donor status, the majority of nurses regard the body in front of them as no longer fully human: "A brain-dead body can't give you anything back; there's only an envelope of a person left, the machine is doing all the work." Some nurses continue to talk to brain-dead bodies as they "care" for the organs, "out of habit," or "just in case a soul is still there," or "because the soul is probably still in the room," (see also Wolf 1991; Youngner et al. 1985). If the family remains at the bedside, nurses are very alert to their sensibilities. For example, they make the body as accessible as possible by unstrapping the confining arm boards used to keep various lines in place, and they warn the family about spinal reflexes and involuntary hand grasps, reassuring them that these are not signs of life.

Not one of the nurses, even as they reassure families that movement is no indication of life, can think of the body simply as a cadaver. Nurses,

13. One woman told me of her very unpleasant experience in a Canadian hospital after the death of her mother. She wanted to stay with and hold her mother for perhaps half an hour. During this time a doctor repeatedly came into the room and demanded when the body could be wheeled out, because he needed the bed.

as well as families, may experience great discomfort when the brain-dead body is wheeled off to the operating room, still attached to the ventilator and visibly breathing, as though going for surgery. The comments of one little boy as he watched his older brother being taken away for procurement poignantly expose the ambiguity: "That's my brother. He's dead and they're taking him to surgery" (Youngner et al. 1985: 322; see also Crowley, ms.). Even when no organ donation takes place, ambiguity exists: the nurse who turns off the ventilator after a declaration of brain death may feel as though he or she has killed the patient (Crowley, ms).

Like physicians, the majority of nurses think "it is what goes on in your head that makes you a person." Clare Belanger insisted that the idea that nails grow after brain death does not make her uncomfortable. She assumes that death is usually a process, but she also thinks that it can be reduced to an event when sudden, massive trauma is the cause. Confusion is apparent, as among certain physicians, in the way in which some nurses talk about the brain-dead: "Once the patient has been declared brain-dead you still keep them on all of the monitors and the respirator, for two reasons: first of all, the family wants to go in and see the patient *still alive,* and second, soon after, a few minutes after, we'll be asking them to consider organ donation" (emphasis added). A colleague of Belanger insists that brain death is not death, and that patients remain alive until the heart stops beating, which occurs in the operating room if organs are to be procured. Despite these ambiguities, ICU nurses with whom I talked are more conscientious than are physicians about signing donor cards: all but one senior nurse had done so. However, every one of the nurses expressed grave doubts as to whether they would agree to their own child receiving an organ should the question ever arise, at least until the child was five years of age or thereabouts. Nurses agonize over the suffering of small children going through highly invasive procedures, especially when the effort so often appears futile.

Without exception, the interviewed nurses believe that if families want to donate organs, this "gives meaning" to a senseless death, but coming to a decision to donate is not always easy. In the units where I carried out interviews, approximately 50 percent of families agree to procurement. Families usually have several hours to make up their minds, and occasionally they ask to think about it overnight, although this is not always possible.

In the guide for ICU staff produced by Québec Transplant, in a section titled "Surveillance of the Donor," it is noted that "the faster the organs can be procured, the better they will be for transplant; there will be less risk of losing the donor, and a better chance for success with the recipient." The bias of the transplant service is laid bare in this statement, for it is the organs that they actually fear losing, the person of the donor having already died. Several nurses report discomfort when so much emphasis is put on the organs and the functions of the body. Chantal Raymond says, for example:

> It's a strange feeling, having to be so careful with these samples, when we were caring for the patient just a few minutes earlier. It's almost as if you are more caring, and that just doesn't feel right. It's not just all the blood work that one has to do, and checking on the saturation values and so on all the time; we send tests for virology over by taxi, do an echocardiogram to see if they can use the heart, do X rays of the lungs, check on the kidneys. You do hematology, biochemistry, neurology, the lot. We take ten tubes of blood and send them off. And you have to note not just the height and weight of the donor, but the circumference of the abdomen and the thorax too—I don't know what that's for, really, but it's very rigorous. All this takes several hours, and quite often the family is still standing around and watching it all. Someone usually comes from the transplant organization and helps us if they're not too busy, and we can always call them up and check on everything. They get quite impatient, because they've already started making their calls about recipients, and they know who's waiting and who is likely to get the liver and the kidneys and so on, and they have to start getting these patients all lined up, usually in another hospital, for their transplants. There's often quite a bit of pressure.

On one occasion when a transplant coordinator was discussing a procurement with me, she explained how the ICU staff had worked late into the night on an eighteen-year-old potential donor whose blood pressure was unstable. Recipients had been notified and were making their way to several different hospitals. The patient due to get the heart was already under sedation in an operating theater when "the donor crashed." His blood pressure spun out of control, rendering the heart useless, although the other organs were salvageable. It takes little imagination to realize how difficult it must be at times to avoid pressuring families as they ponder their decisions about donation.[14]

In the early days of transplantation, when organ procurement was known as "harvesting" and before a routine had been established, it was

14. I did not feel that it was appropriate to intrude on families when they were being asked about organ donation. Nor do I believe that hospital staff or ethics committees would have permitted me to do so. I was able to talk to several families approximately one year after they had gone through this experience. Several of their responses appear as case studies between chapters.

customary, when a generally healthy patient died during surgery, for the transplant team to be called at once. A Canadian doctor recalls the time when, as a resident in the 1970s, he had spent the entire morning in surgery trying to save the life of a young boy. The boy was eventually declared brain-dead, and the family, without seeing their son, hurriedly consented to organ donation. This doctor recalls what followed as the worst moment of his entire medical career. Together with the nurses, he was required to remain in the operating room and assist the transplant team when they "swarmed in" to harvest organs. He felt such revulsion as he watched the boy being "cannibalized" before his eyes that he had to leave the room to vomit.

Cases such as this were relatively rare, because 95 percent of patients are declared brain-dead in ICUs and not in the operating theater (Bart et al. 1979). However, enough people were disconcerted by this situation that the transition from patient to donor is now clearly demarcated. If a patient is declared brain-dead in the operating theater, the first surgical team is replaced by a completely different transplant team. After procurement of the organs, the transplant surgeons usually go on, with only a brief interlude, to transplant one or more organs into waiting patients. The movement of organs procured from brain-dead bodies into the bodies of recipients causes little or no emotional difficulty, it seems; this, after all, is the giving of life.

Anesthesiologists, some of whom are also intensivists, may find themselves in disturbing circumstances (see also Youngner et al. 1985). Janet Goodwin, who works in a children's hospital, observes:

> Occasionally there is a patient who I've been looking after over the weekend in the ICU, working with closely, hoping that things will improve. The following week I will be having my turn on anesthesiology, and so I don't go to the ICU, and I look up and see them wheeling in the child so we can procure organs from him. The child has taken a turn for the worse and become brain-dead in the day or so after I went off the ICU. For me, this is the most ghastly job that I have to do.

She adds:

> Procurements are not a pretty sight. I always get the hell out of the operating room as soon as I possibly can. As soon as they've got the heart out. Everyone starts to scrabble at that point. It's ghastly, absolutely ghastly. I sort of have to sit down by the machines and just keep checking the dials every couple of minutes so as I don't have to watch what's going on. It's ghoulish, but you just have to try and focus on the fact that those organs are going to do some

good. In a way I *have* to think of them still as patients because they are under my care, and I guess the most important thing is that they are treated with respect, which isn't normally a problem at all. But with procurements there's this conflict between the whole body and the organs. I can't really let myself think of it as a person any more. On the other hand, certainly if I've had contact with them before, and have been caring for them, then it's really hard for me to just accept that that process has ended. There really is a conflict. So I have to think of the body as a vessel, partly because I'm trying to protect myself. It's a really unpleasant emotion, especially because often there's no external trauma, so it's really hard to realize that this young person is dead.

Goodwin mentioned yet another source of ambiguity. She sometimes administers muscle relaxants to organ donors during procurement because they make the surgeons' work easier, and occasionally she uses an anesthetic agent to control the blood pressure that can be so unstable once the brain stem is damaged. She now makes it a practice to announce in the operating room what she is doing, because she has on occasion been confronted by tearful nurses who want to know why a patient who is supposedly dead should need an anesthetic.

Even transplant coordinators, who have minimal or no contact with the donor prior to brain death, express feelings of ambiguity and anthropomorphization. Linda Hogle has shown that the criteria for a "good donor" are not exclusively biological. The life history of the brain-dead donor is also crucial. Obviously heavy smoking and alcohol use render organs useless, but on occasion, even when the donor is apparently "ideal,"—that is, a young male—if his social life has been troubled, then his fitness for donation can be questioned. Hogle found that transplant coordinators often become depressed with their work because, particularly in America, they are dealing so often with what one coordinator termed "the dregs of humanity," by which she meant young people who meet untimely, violent deaths (1995:493).[15] Despite the standardization and routinization of organ procurement, social meanings cannot readily be detached from the body of the donor.

15. In the United States, where 58 percent of organ donors die as a result of external trauma, including gunshot wounds, a social and economic disparity is likely to exist between donor and recipient. American transplant coordinators may develop a perception they are dealing primarily with donors whose lifestyles they do not share and whom they regard as wastrels. The situation is Japan is much closer to that of Canada, where donors are more often victims of intracranial hemorrhage and motor vehicle accidents, and in any case social and economic differentials among Japanese citizens are much narrower. Nevertheless, in Japan deep-rooted concerns exist about inequalities associated with the procurement and distribution of organs.

Medical Opposition to Brain Death

Although a few doctors on the front line exhibit confusion about the concept of brain death, and others admit to emotional turmoil, it is above all the question of certainty that concerns them. Intensivists are satisfied that in practice serious errors are virtually nonexistent. With standardization of criteria, tests for, and diagnosis of brain death, has come security about the concept, seemingly borne out by clinical experience. As a result, discussion about brain death as a concept has not been subjected to systematic medical scrutiny since publication of the Uniform Determination of Death Act (UDDA) in the United States and similar publications in other countries. In recent years, however, this tacit acceptance of brain death as a workable concept, leading to a "robust" diagnosis, has met with some critical opposition.

Paul Byrne and Richard Nilges are physicians actively opposed to brain death. In a recent review article they conclude that the requirement of the UDDA, that "all functions of the entire brain" should have ceased functioning before brain death is declared, is not in fact met in clinical practice, and dying, therefore, *is* confused with death. For these clinicians, "imminent" biological death is not a sufficient criterion for organ donation. Further, they argue that protocols put out by transplant coordinators and transplant surgeons place the donor at risk with their emphasis on a "*rapid* acquisition of *physiologically* sound organs" (1993:4, emphasis in original).

Byrne and Nilges are concerned that small hospitals may not have the facilities or the personnel to conduct tests appropriately. Sometimes, but not always, this difficulty is overcome by repeat tests in tertiary care hospitals. Reviewing the literature on conditions that mimic brain death, they show that the protocols about brain death do not cover all the possibilities, although they acknowledge that these other conditions (for example, brain-stem encephalitis) are very unusual.

These authors recommend use of a larger array of tests for brain-stem reflexes than is recommended by the UDDA. They contend that the function of the reticular formation, which mediates between the lower and upper brain, is poorly understood, and that the tests used for brain death do not assess it. On the basis of their review, these authors claim that they are forced to bring up the "haunting question" of whether the "brain-dead" really have an absence of all brain function. Byrne and Nilges conclude that we should reverse our usual orientation: that we should search not for signs of brain death but for signs of brain life.

They are convinced that if physicians had taken this approach all along, greater efforts would be made to save patients with major brain trauma:

> Gunshot wounds of the brain have not been treated aggressively in the past twenty-five years. Pessimism as to outcome has led to withholding of adequate neurosurgical care (Kaufman:1990). We would suggest that to salvage some benefit out of such tragedies and to salve the consciences of those rendering care, these unfortunate patients (who are usually young and in previous good health) are used as organ donors without being given the benefit of at least an attempt at neurosurgical debridement. The period of lack of improvement in the care of gunshot wounds of the brain almost coincides with the rise of transplant surgery.
>
> (Byrne and Nilges 1993:21)

Twenty years earlier, Diana Crane concluded on the basis of a survey that "physicians are inclined not to treat actively either salvageable or unsalvageable patients who are severely brain damaged. The sanctity of individuality rather than the sanctity of life *per se* appears to be the norm" (1976:21). However, several intensivists whom I interviewed made quite clear their own anxieties about equivocal outcomes from severe brain trauma. These doctors have all witnessed patients who neither deteriorate to brain death nor recover but remain in a persistent vegetative state, as did Karen Ann Quinlan, and they claim that they themselves would rather be dead than in this condition. Aggressive therapy might on occasion lead to something approaching full recovery, but this is extremely unlikely. Most intensivists believe that partial recovery is the best one could hope for. Similarly, many families do not pursue aggressive treatment because they do not want to be the cause of any further suffering for their dying relative, or perhaps because they too are concerned about equivocal outcomes.

Unlike the philosophers discussed earlier, not one of the interviewed intensivists is willing to accept cerebral or upper-brain death alone as equivalent to the end of human life. Apart from any epistemological doubts they may have, intensivists are uncomfortable with such an approach because there are no tests that demonstrate how irreversible is the condition of a traumatized lower brain that retains some function. Everyone knows of the occasional surprising reversal of PVS in which a patient has recovered consciousness and even, at times, returned to a full and active life.

In North America, many of us dread being rendered incapacitated, in particular mentally incapacitated. Although the present research offers no conclusions about the effects of such trepidation on medical practice in ICUs, it may influence the speed of the transition from a patient for whom everything is being done to an organ donor for whom further treatment is futile. With the constraints of space, time, and finances in ICUs, practitioners are increasingly reluctant to undertake interventions seen as futile. The possibility of organ donation permits everyone involved with these tragic cases to feel just a little bit easier in their minds because good can apparently be retrieved from a hopeless situation. It is also possible, as Byrne and Nilges suggest, that we have not put our best efforts into research that would assist with recovery from trauma, largely because we dread that it would be only partially successful. No such accusation can be laid against Japan.

Today a very large number of intensivists and involved families believe that organ donation is the best way to create meaning out of accidental death. A law that requires doctors in most parts of North America to make requests for organs is, it seems, acceptable to the public (although most people probably have not thought about this matter at all). It is firmly believed that individual rights are protected if prior consent is clear. An ideology of individual autonomy prevails even in countries where presumed consent is in operation and where the state is more confident about its powers over dead bodies than is the case in North America, for citizens may opt out of donation. If the letter of the law were followed, then every individual who has consented to donation should automatically become a donor, whether by presumed or prior consent. This is not the case, however. Nowhere in Europe or in North America are family wishes overruled. Physicians are not prepared to wheel away a brain-dead patient for organ procurement when a distraught family begs them not to. In practice, family wishes override those of individuals, just as in Japan, although of course family and individual desires often coincide. However, in North America, most people consider donation the right thing to do, whereas in Japan the dominant ideology has been overwhelmingly that families should not be pressed to think about it. Respect for the living cadaver continues to take priority over the possibility of donation to unknown strangers.

PROCUREMENT ANXIETY

Excuse me if I'm a bit incoherent, I've been up for twenty-four hours straight. You know, by and large I don't have any trouble with procurements. It's never bothered me at all when it's organ procurement from someone of my own age or my parents' age. There are a lot of lawyers and other people out there with balding heads and gray hair and glasses, and so that means there're plenty of donors I've done who look like me. And that doesn't make me feel uncomfortable.

But last night it was a kid, a strapping-looking guy, kind of long and lean, not terribly dissimilar to my own fourteen-year-old son. And you stop and think: "This must never happen to my child. I'm not going to let this happen to my own." I've had this kind of feeling many times in the past, and it's always related to your own kids growing and the stage they're at. So when my kids were two and five, the donors of that age bothered me a lot. Now my kids are eleven and fourteen, a two-year-old doesn't bother me as much. I'm very aware of these feelings of mine, and I have my own ways of dealing with it. I quickly have to move to a position where I tell myself that honoring the kid or the parents is what is important, because there's nothing that could have been done to save the child. I've been agnostic about things for as long as I can remember, but I can't deny my ambivalence about procuring organs from, say, that kid last night. I have to counter my own ambivalences. That could be my kid. So I have to make a pact between me and the donor, the departed donor, and say I'm really going to do my utmost with this transplant. I try to get others to understand too—the med students and potential donors. A child has died, but I can make a difference.

Liver transplant surgeon, United States

One episode has stayed with me as though it was yesterday. We were called down to harvest the kidneys of a young woman in her thirties. This was probably nine or ten years ago. She and her husband and child were driving to Cape Cod for a vacation, and they got a flat tire. So they pulled off to the side of the road and their two-year-old started to dash out onto the express-way, and the pregnant mother ran after him, and in an instant all three of them were killed—except the husband—the mother, the fetus, and the child. And it was one of—you know, when you're doing surgery you want to con-centrate, and it was—I've rarely been so distracted, and even to this day, you know, when someone asks how I feel about the job I'm in, I can't get it out of my mind—it comes back to me at night sometimes. My thoughts keep going back to this man and how, in an instant, his whole life was wiped out. It's certainly made me very introspective. The only thing that kept me going with the procurement was the thought that someone was going to benefit from this, even though it was a tragic event.

Kidney transplant surgeon, United States

I guess we go through different phases in the way that we think about brain death. The first is in medical school, where you question everything and you go over the scientific arguments that explain why we know that someone is brain-dead; then, as a resident, when you deal with patients, you begin to get a closer look at ties between patients and families, so you question it from a bit of a different viewpoint. And then, when you become a staff person, specifically in transplantation, you see things from another aspect altogether. Now you're working for the recipient.

In some places they don't use an anesthetic with the donor patient. We do that, but when you go to a center to take out a liver and they haven't anesthetized the patient, sometimes someone suddenly says, "Hey, the leg moved." This is when we're near the ciliac ganglia that things get very touchy. You remember this sort of thing, and it makes you reassess everything— makes you think about things. Also when I have a donor who's a child it always makes me think twice. It's difficult for me then. I remember taking a liver from a child. I couldn't start the operation. I just couldn't do it.

Then sometimes freak things happen, like, you know the family—that happened to me once. So there are reminders that some issues are never settled, even though I try to repress them. I convince myself that we have taken all the necessary precautionary measures so that no mistakes are made—in a way I hide behind the neurologist—he has to make the big de-cision about the brain-death diagnosis and I trust him completely. But, am I 100 percent sure that we are doing the right thing each time? No. But again, am I ever 100 percent sure that I'm doing the right thing in medicine? No. So I think it's a question of percentages, and I feel that there are enough people who are taking responsibilities, and enough safety checks have been put in place. We've been dealing with brain-dead patients long enough now that we can play the percentages with confidence.

But, you know, I still don't think of the donor as a cadaver. I was with a resident once, we'd done a harvesting, as we call it, a donor retrieval, and we took the organs out, and the resident was tired and wrote down on the chart that "the abdomen was closed and the patient was taken to the recovery room!" That's what we always write after ordinary surgery, of course. It was an honest mistake of a resident who'd been on duty for twenty-five hours in a row. But even so, if it had really been a cadaver in the mind of the resident, then I don't think that mistake would have happened. Of course we always treat a donor body with respect, as though it were a patient. To me it's a patient with no prognosis. Sometimes I hear myself saying to the anesthetist when we've finished the procurement, "OK, you can let him die now." And the anesthetist kind of looks at me, and I catch myself, and then I say, "You're right, the patient is dead. You can discontinue whatever you're doing now."

Liver and kidney transplant surgeon, Canada

It's probably politically correct to think of a brain-dead donor as a kind of patient, but a donor has never been my patient, and never will be. He's not a patient to me. I get offended by newspaper articles and so on that complain about how we don't respect the dead; about how we transplant surgeons mutilate the dead. I don't think of the donor as a patient, I think of the donor as an extension of my patient, and that we're doing things not for him any more, but for people like my patients who desperately need organs.

I don't think you need your heart or your kidney or your liver once you're dead. I think you can have a lot of beliefs about the afterlife if you want, about heaven, or whatever, but I'm sure you don't need those organs. That's got nothing to do with religion. That's biology. It's perfectly possible to be religious and support donation. It just seems so senseless for someone who's dead to go to the grave with all those organs that can help somebody else. It just doesn't make any sense to me.

Heart transplant surgeon, Canada

I'm completely comfortable with brain death because the diagnosis is made by specialists whom I trust completely. At first, in the 70s, not all the neurospecialists accepted the diagnosis, you know. They just felt uncomfortable and insisted that we should use the term "irreversible brain damage" and not brain death. Nowadays most intensivists are very professional about it, but they still don't recruit enough patients from Trauma, so we're always short of organs.

Kidney transplant surgeon, Canada

I remember one time—these patients, you know, they look perfectly all right, they're pink and all that, and we were doing a procurement, and suddenly I felt the guy's arm rise behind me, and this was obviously some sort of neurological reflex, but it is—I mean, deep down, it's pretty spooky. . . .

Yes, I did just call it a patient—because they're still breathing. It's definitely a sort of in-between state. The other striking thing is that once you have the organs out, and you're dissecting them on the back table, the resident is busy sewing him up with huge stitches and then they put him in a bag and cart him away. That's always a bit odd. That always strikes me as odd, something extremely unlike the usual surgical procedure. There I am, giving all my care and attention to the organ. Everybody gives lip service to the care of the patient, but it's really the organs they're caring for.

Still, I'm perfectly comfortable with this. Theoretically, I'm perfectly comfortable. Brain death is actually being brain-dead. I have no questions. I mean, I guess I find these procedures aesthetically unpleasant, but I don't have any moral problems with it. It's a bit like my feelings on abortion. I mean, it's a disgusting procedure, but I don't have a huge ethical problem with it.

Kidney transplant surgeon, United States

I received a good deal of my training in England, and I always make use of anesthetics when procuring kidneys because then the organs are kept in the best possible condition during retrieval. The blood pressure and circulation are properly controlled then. The trouble is that most anesthesiologists in Japan are not keen on donation, and they won't usually give a hand with procurements. Once, the chief anesthesiologist in a hospital where I went to do a procurement refused to let me into the operating room proper, and I had to do the best I could in the room just outside the real OR, which isn't really a completely sterile area. It was really upsetting.

Kidney transplant surgeon, Japan

Yes, I know some surgeons want to use anesthetics during procurement, but I would never do that. I don't need to work with an anesthesiologist. Sometimes we observe movement during a procurement because of the spinal reflexes, but I certainly don't believe that the donor experiences any sensations or pain. They don't feel anything—if I didn't think this, then I could never procure organs from the brain-dead. You know, I personally feel more comfortable about taking organs out of a brain-dead donor than a cadaver donor because by using kidneys taken from a cadaver I put the recipient at greater risk. It's terrible retrieving organs from a patient whose heart has stopped beating. There is an awful rush and enormous pressure, otherwise the kidneys will be no good. Then it's like the TV drama *ER,* and the recipients are definitely going to suffer much more than if it was a brain-dead donor.

Kidney transplant surgeon, Japan

When Persons
Linger in Bodies

Sacrifice

In 1993, four years before the Organ Transplant Law was passed in Japan, Yanagida Kunio, a well-known cultural commentator, found his youngest son, Yojiro, lying on his bed with an electrical cord around his neck, having tried to commit suicide. Yanagida rushed his son to hospital. Within a short time the medical team swarming around the twenty-five-year-old patient had inserted tubes and lines into his body and attached three leads to his chest from the physiological monitor at the head of the bed in order that the functioning of his heart, blood pressure, pulmonary pressure, and central venous pressure could be on display. Yojiro's heartbeat was restored with medical assistance; but his brain had been badly damaged by lack of oxygen.

Yojiro's condition worsened over the next four days. At first, the senior of the four doctors assigned to the case said that at best Yojiro would be in a persistent vegetative state for the rest of his life, but a strong possibility remained that he would become brain-dead. By the third day, the doctor acknowledged that things had taken a turn for the worse, and that Yojiro would almost certainly become brain-dead in the next little while. On the fifth day tests were carried out in front of the family to establish that Yojiro was indeed brain-dead. The tests were repeated on the sixth day, and the diagnosis was confirmed. Even though these results indicated to the neurospecialists that there was no possibility of any recovery, the patient was not declared dead. The attending doctors had already explained carefully before the tests were done that, should brain death be diagnosed, the ventilator would not be turned off until the family requested it. They pointed out that Yojiro's existence would be wholly dependent upon the ventilator, and, even so, his heart rate would gradually decrease and his blood pressure drop so that after a few days, or weeks or months, the heart would cease to function. Death would then be declared (Yanagida 1995).

Reflecting later on his thoughts as his hopes for his son's recovery diminished day by day, Yanagida describes a struggle between his "rational mind" and his "sentimental" feelings, in which loneliness predominated. In an article published in a national weekly a year later, Yanagida recalled that during the first days of the vigil at the bedside, his eldest son had asked the doctor if he could wipe away his brother's tears. The doctor explained that although it *seemed* as though his brother was crying, this was purely a physical phenomenon and should not be taken as an expression of emotion. "We don't know why it happens," he said, "but I assure you, your brother can feel nothing, and makes no responses to the world around him." Yanagida notes that he felt very emotional at this juncture, heightened by the compassion shown by the doctor for the family as a whole.

After this exchange, Yanagida started to think about the possibility of organ donation, stimulated in part by a vivid memory of watching, with his son, Tachibana Takashi's television program on the subject. Yojiro had said at the time that should he become brain-dead, he would not want his life prolonged once it was obvious that there was no hope (1994:154).

Yanagida describes his son's face as "bright and warm" as he held his hand and whispered his name. While he thought about donation, Yanagida felt overwhelmed because he "couldn't bear the idea of someone putting a knife into the body and taking out the heart." He recalls his confusion as he gazed on his son, apparently sleeping peacefully despite the wires snaking around and into him. Then he gazed bleary-eyed at the monitor that continued to tell him, as it had done since it was first switched on, that his son's heart was beating regularly. Yanagida realized that he could not accept the idea that Yojiro's brain was not functioning. What does brain death really signify, he wondered? He pondered the "artificial" death created by science, one in which it is possible to select the final moment rather than wait for fate to determine it.

Yojiro's brother Kenichiro, who sat with his brother a great deal of the time, and helped to wash and shave him and provide other care, confided that he felt every day as though the silent body were communicating with him. He admitted that this was a "strange" feeling, but Yanagida acknowledged that he was experiencing similar sensations. Both of them talked to Yojiro as he lay there, and called his name in an effort to get his attention, particularly after a nurse informed them that "people say that the hearing survives, even in those who are nearly brain-dead."

Yanagida comments on Tachibana Takashi's assertions that in dealing with brain death sentimentality must be ruled out and the situation approached logically and ethically. Yanagida notes that this approach may well be appropriate when creating definitions, criteria, and tests, but that it was impossible to curb the visceral sensations that flooded him as he sat with his son. In the end, it was reflection on these emotional responses that enabled Yanagida to agree to organ donation.

Yojiro, always a sensitive child who did not mix easily with other children, had been subjected to extensive teasing and bullying by his schoolmates. One of his eyes was severely injured when a piece of chalk was hurled at him, and from that time he began to suffer from a characteristic Japanese phobia: a fear of interpersonal relationships (*taijinkyōfushō*). Yojiro gradually withdrew into his own world, and even though he clearly remained close to his father, neither of his parents realized the extent of his misery. He soon dropped out of university but continued his courses by correspondence. Yojiro had been reading *A Hundred Years of Solitude* by Garcia Marquez at the time of his death, and his father believes that this book influenced him profoundly. On the evening that he tried to kill himself, Yojiro told his father that he could not deal with life any longer (1994).

Yojiro had kept a diary and had also written a series of short essays about his feelings of estrangement. On reading the diary while sitting by Yojiro's hospital bed, Yanagida felt a duty to "complete" his son's life as Yojiro would have wished it (1995). The family asked if some of Yojiro's bone marrow could be donated for transplant. The transplant coordinator replied that there were currently no bone-marrow transplant candidates who matched Yojiro's type, but he asked if the family would consider donating kidneys. The family gave permission for perfusion of the kidneys to keep them in good shape while they thought over this request. In the end they agreed, and on the sixth day, after the second diagnosis of brain death, all treatment was stopped, although the ventilator remained in place.

The Yanagidas continued to take part, with the nurses, in the cleaning and care of their son's body. On the ninth day, when Yanagida went by himself to visit his son, he noticed that the heartbeat and blood pressure registering on the monitor were better than they had been the previous day. When he pointed this out to a nurse, she replied that they had been less stable just a short while ago. She agreed when Yanagida questioned her that Yojiro could be responding positively to the presence of his father. Yanagida sat down, took his son's hand and said, "Let's talk together for a while, I'll be with you until the evening" (1995:168).

On the eleventh day, Yanagida and his eldest son took care of Yojiro's body for the last time. The recordings on the monitors by this time were essentially flat. The respirator was turned off in front of the family, and Yojiro's chest stopped moving. At this point death was declared. The body was rushed to the operating room so that Yojiro's kidneys could be transplanted into two recipients the following night.[1] Yanagida felt grateful that he did not have to meet the transplant team. The Yanagidas did not have to reach a decision about donation of the heart, liver, or other solid organs because these were no longer of use once the heart had stopped beating. Yanagida describes his son's donation as a positive sacrifice that would help other people, one that he, Yojiro's father, had found the strength to facilitate.

One of the articles written by Yanagida about the death of his son became a book that sold over half a million copies. Below I elaborate on the responses of Japanese clinicians when asked about brain death. It appears that the experience of the Yanagida family while their son was in intensive care is not unusual.

Death: A Family Decision

Abe Tomoko, a pediatrician employed for many years in a hospital that specializes in neurological disorders, has been part of the grass-roots movement in Japan against the legalization of brain death as the end of life. She is also a member of the original Tokyo University Patients' Rights Group. In discussing her objections to recognition of brain death, Abe emphasized that the concept was created primarily to facilitate organ transplants. She is emphatic that when a dying person is understood

---

1. Aside from living related donations, until the law was amended in 1997, the only legal source of kidneys for transplant was cadaver donors.

as the focus of both a concerned family and a caring medical team, then it is difficult to interpret brain death as the demise of an individual.

Her opinion is derived, Abe states, from reflection on her own feelings:

> The point is not whether the patient is conscious or unconscious, but whether one *intuitively* understands that the patient is dead. Someone whose color is good, who is still warm, bleeds when cut, and urinates and defecates, is not dead as far as I am concerned. Of course I know that cardiac arrest will follow some hours later—but I think even more significant is the transformation of the warm body into something that is cold and hard—only then do the Japanese really accept death.

When asked the reasons for her views, Abe replies: "It's something to do with Buddhism, I suppose. I'm not really a Buddhist, but it's part of our tradition."[2] Abe is categorically opposed to organ transplants that make use of brain-dead donors and also has strong reservations about transplants from living donors.

I interviewed nineteen emergency medicine physicians in Japan in 1996, 1997, and 1999 (the medical specialty of intensivist does not exist there). The majority of these were neurosurgeons. None of them took as extreme a position as Abe. However, her sentiments, which are shared by many other Japanese, including other clinicians, are well known among the Japanese public from television appearances and publications: for example, Abe played an animated part in the panel discussion during Tachibana's 1990 program.

All the emergency medicine clinicians with whom I talked believe that brain death is an irreversible condition, provided that no errors have been made in diagnosis. Their reasoning is essentially the same as that of physicians in North America. However, the Japanese physicians are in close agreement (with two dissenters) that although biological death is inevitable, a brain-death diagnosis should not necessarily be equated with human death. Even so, most of these doctors are not opposed to organ transplants. Although none of them has ever participated in procurement of organs from a brain-dead donor, several have made cadavers available to transplant teams.

I conducted most of these interviews in the year before the Organ Transplant Law was passed. Interviews from 1999, just after the first

---

2. In Buddhist tradition, signs of warmth and of reflexes are recognized as indicative of life (Becker 1993:131).

donation from a brain-dead donor had taken place, suggest that clinical practice has changed very little as a result of the new law.[3] The physicians are unanimous that, even though they are not in principle opposed to organ donation, to declare brain death and promptly ask a family about organ donation is inappropriate.

If the family indicates that the patient signed an official organ donor card, then a transplant coordinator may be called in, but this happens only if the patient is in one of the university, national, or major regional hospitals designated to deal with organ procurement.[4] Since the passing of the Transplant Law, all such hospitals have ethics committees specifically set up to review procurement from brain-dead donors. About two hundred hospitals fulfill these requirements. Many people consider that government control over these hospitals is appropriate and their number sufficient. However, transplant surgeons are in woefully short supply: as of 2000, there were only nine teams for liver and three for heart procurements in the whole country. Should the number of donations increase, these surgeons would soon be physically exhausted. Procurement from cadaver donors is not regulated nearly so stringently.

If a patient becomes brain-dead in a hospital other than a designated transplant center, the body is not transported to a recognized center. The president of the Emergency Medicine Association announced that his specialty opposes the relocation of brain-dead bodies, and the Ministry of Health and Welfare made a similar statement. Several neurosurgeons told me that with the media watching every move physicians make in connection with brain death, any transfer of patients to another hospital to procure organs would certainly receive negative media coverage. Thus, even if Japanese should prove willing to donate more organs, the prior wishes of many brain-dead patients will never be met because of bureaucratic restrictions.

The physicians I talked to agreed that if the family does not raise the question of donation, as they rarely do (although this has begun to change since the passing of the new law), then it is unlikely to be discussed. Everyone agreed that extreme caution is needed for several more

3. Informants have been given pseudonyms. I was told repeatedly that emergency medicine facilities in Japan are not as up-to-date, as extensive, or as efficient as those in America. Very few hospitals have trauma units; accident victims are taken to tertiary emergency medicine departments and centers, but the triage system often does not work well, and patients may end up in hospitals without specialists available (Ikegami, personal communication, 2000).

4. Any hospital may do kidney transplants; restrictions apply to heart, liver, and lung transplants.

years and that doctors must do everything they can to avoid appearing aggressive. Two doctors stated, however, that they plan to start taking a firmer position now that the first legal donation from a brain-dead donor has taken place.

Most physicians emphasized that families need time to come to terms with sudden, "unnatural" deaths, and that no pressure should be placed on them. It is not uncommon for families, especially families of dying children, to take up to two weeks before they ask for the ventilator to be turned off. Physicians with experience in Europe or North America agree that in Japan there is a much greater willingness to keep patients on ventilators, even when treatment is deemed futile. It is as though families are permitted to hope for a miracle. There is a growing movement for "death with dignity," but, thus far, concerns about premature death far exceed fears about the prolongation of unnecessary treatment. Several Japanese doctors who have worked in chronic care units in North America have been surprised at how many DNR (do not resuscitate) orders are written into charts at the patients' wishes. No DNR policy exists in Japan, and one study reached the conclusion that "futile" CPR is often performed, even when death from cancer is imminent (Fukaura et al. 1995).

Hospitals in Japan are reimbursed for beds occupied, but the amount of government repayment for an ICU stay is reduced dramatically every two weeks. Even so, one never gets the impression in a Japanese ICU, as is so often the case in North America and in England, that doctors are under pressure to free up beds. Because in many Japanese hospitals organ donation is not a consideration, there is neither a sense of urgency nor a need for an accurate diagnosis of brain death. Several physicians stressed that "Japanese people like a 'natural death'" and so, once physicians are satisfied that the patient is brain-dead, gradual withdrawal of treatment is common. Matsumoto Harumi, an emergency medicine specialist, commented: "Perhaps this is unique to Japan, but we believe that it is best to tell the family that we are continuing to do our best for their relative even though brain death is 'approaching,' rather than to say, as they do in America, 'The patient is brain-dead, here are the test results, we are going to terminate all care.'"[5] He added that, once convinced of brain death, he "gradually reduces the treatment." Medications are no longer administered, and the amount of oxygen delivered from the ventilator is reduced ("weaning" is the technical term for this

5. Of course, in practice things are not handled so abruptly in the United States.

process). In Matsumoto's mind nothing more can be done for the patient, but he continues catering to what he believes are the family's desires.

Physicians interviewed all agreed that they "more or less" follow the Takeuchi criteria, that is, the standards set out by the Ministry of Health and Welfare in 1985 for determining brain death, in which the apnea test is required. However, several of the doctors interviewed prior to the passing of the Organ Transplant Law indicated that the apnea test could actually hasten death, and so they would very rarely resort to this procedure. Several added comments to the effect that "we do not always rigorously establish the diagnosis, even when we suspect brain death. We often guess, which is much easier for the patient and the family."

What is meant here, I believe, is that, especially in severe trauma cases, the attending neurosurgeon will carry out the required clinical tests for determining brain death, including pupillary response and reflex reactions. If the diagnosis is confirmed, the doctor informs the family that their relative is *hobo nōshi no jotai* (almost brain-dead), that the situation looks *zetsubōteki* (hopeless), or that it is simply a "matter of time." Some doctors use the concept of *ishiki shōgai*—"damage to the consciousness"—but this expression is most often used in connection with PVS patients. It was intimated to me that terms such as "brain death" (*nōshi*) are too technical to use with patients' families, and that it is much more appropriate to stress simply that the condition is irreversible or hopeless. Alternatively, some doctors choose to emphasize that the patient can no longer breathe for herself, or that she cannot think or feel any more. No one describes the condition as death unless they feel certain that the family has fully come to terms with the situation.

A neurosurgeon, Suzuki Makoto, described his feelings of ambivalence:

> Brain death is a kind of "end stage"; in other words, there is nothing more that we can do for the patient, but we are ambivalent because brain death is not human death. There was a case I had a while ago where a child stayed alive for six or seven days, even when the ventilator had been turned down. If the family had said early on that they wanted to donate the kidneys, I would have stopped the ventilator at once,[6] and called the transplant team,

6. I talked with this doctor before the new law was passed. At that time, kidneys intended for transplant would be removed right after the ventilator was stopped, as happened in the Yanagida case. This doctor, in contrast to the one attending the Yanagidas,

but there was no suggestion of this. As far as they were concerned, I would have been killing their child if I had turned off the ventilator—and in a way they are right. After all, we don't sign the death certificate until the heart stops beating.

Another neurosurgeon, with more than fifteen years of clinical experience, states that he would never approach a family about donation, nor does he turn off the ventilator until the family requests it. In his experience the family usually waits three or four days; then the ventilator is turned off at their request, "and the patient dies."

Like his colleagues, this physician, Fujita Kenji, reduces the oxygen supplied by the ventilator once he is convinced that the patient is brain-dead: "We do the basics and leave the rest to nature, but we always leave room for a miracle, just in case someone comes back." Fujita notes that he has recently been getting firmer with families who refuse to accept that the situation is hopeless. If he has time, he will do an EEG and show the family the flat line it produces as evidence of the finality of the situation. Several physicians with experience of turning off the ventilator and then watching over the patient until the heart stops beating expressed discomfort at this process. They stated that this interval had on more than one occasion taken over an hour, and one of these doctors described the patient as *kawaisō*, "piteous."

Among the four Japanese nurses whom I interviewed, none of them evinced any difficulty with turning down a ventilator once it was clear to the medical staff that brain death was close. Like several of the doctors, these nurses insisted that "life" and "death" are not fully medical matters, and so the feelings of families must be considered. Families, in their estimation, do not think of relatives as dead when diagnosed as brain-dead. Moral and ethical issues in connection with the brain-dead are not the same as for the living, but, the nurses argued, brain-dead patients are in a "micro world" of their own where "something continues to exist" that demands "moral sensitivity."

When told about this gradual withdrawal of care in Japan, North American intensivists often feel uncomfortable. One said spontaneously, "That's unethical." Others believe that their own approach is better: once it has been established that the patient can no longer breathe without assistance and is brain-dead, then the appropriate procedure is to

suggests that he himself would have determined when the ventilator should be stopped, independently of the family.

disconnect the ventilator immediately, unless organ procurement is to follow. Continuing mechanical support after a declaration of death intrudes into "death with dignity."

For the time being, the national health insurance plan in Japan continues to pay for care of brain-dead patients, and so there is no incentive to change these practices. Since only about three hundred centers can legally procure organs, precise determination of brain death continues to be of relatively little importance in the majority of Japanese hospitals. By contrast, in facilities that perform organ procurements, physicians responsible for clinical and legal diagnoses of brain death will no doubt take extra precautions, and scrupulously follow the rules and regulations, after the faux pas associated with the first legal case of procurement in March 1999.

Consciousness, Brains, and Persons in Japan

In complete contrast to the practice in North America, no one in ICUs in Japan talks with patients' families about the shell of a body remaining after the departure of the "person" or the "soul." Physicians are acutely aware of the ambiguous nature of a living cadaver and refrain from pushing families towards recognition of death. One reason is that medical practitioners do not believe it is appropriate to persuade families that their relative is no longer alive, not least because doing so might, even today, expose the physicians to media criticism.

Second, many physicians do not believe that families are prepared to accept this assessment. A neurosurgeon, Nogami Akira, told me that for him "80 to 90 percent of the 'person' is located in the brain—perhaps 100 percent," he added, after pausing for thought. But he added that most families of brain-dead patients would not agree with him. Emergency medicine specialists in effect try to infer and then defer to the family's understanding of the situation.

A third important reason comes into play: even in medical settings, death is above all a family matter. Doctors in tertiary care hospitals are *soto* (outsiders) to the family, and therefore they leave control over the process of dying to the family. This deference contrasts with the attitudes of Japanese medical practitioners in general, which lead so often to accusations of paternalism.

Several respected scientists have argued in widely circulated magazines that an individual—a person—is more than a collection of body parts, no doubt reinforcing the intuitive opposition to the brain-death concept held by so many people. Kawakita Yoshio, a recently deceased biologist who was also a Christian, stated, for example, that he could not accept brain death as the end of life, and was explicitly opposed to organ transplants. He argued that it is "superficial" to suggest that one person can live on in another as the result of a transplant, even though it is claimed that this is a "humanistic" move. On the contrary, Kawakita said, it is simply a rationalization for technological intervention into the process of dying (Kawakita and Sasaki 1992).

Such opinions are supplemented by those of eminent physicians. Watanabe Yoshio, writing in the *Japanese Heart Journal,* summarizes his opposition as follows:

> If the entire brain including the brain stem has indeed sustained irreversible damage, cardiorespiratory arrest would inevitably ensue, bringing about the person's death. However, the duration of this stage may well last for several days to several weeks when a respirator is used, and hence, this stage at best only predicts that death of the individual is imminent, not that it is confirmed. The fact that some brain-dead pregnant women have given birth to babies can be taken as strong evidence that the person is still alive, and the use of terms such as biomort or heart-beating cadaver is nothing but a sophism to conceal the contradictions in transplant protagonists' logic. . . .
>
> There is a crucial difference between brain death and death judged by the classical criteria. Cessation of blood circulation due to cardiac arrest would promptly result in the lowering of body temperature and discoloration of the skin that are evident even to lay people. . . . Death of a human being should be announced when everyone can indeed sense the occurrence of such irreversible processes and accept the sad fact. . . . To regard a human being only as an assembly of mechanical parts and utilize its organs and tissues as materials for recycling would completely negate the dignity of humans.
>
> (Watanabe 1994)

Watanabe goes on to assert that severe side effects are experienced by up to 76 percent of heart transplant recipients because of the constant use of immunosuppressants, and that a rapid progression of coronary atherosclerosis takes place in 90 percent of patients within five years of receiving a new heart. He likens transplant recipients to AIDS patients in that they are constantly "under the threat of severe infectious disease," and he argues that maintaining the balance between infection and rejection is like walking on a tightrope.

Watanabe further argues that he opposes the transplant enterprise primarily because it produces inequities among individuals. Because of the shortage of donors, recipients compete with one another. Watanabe demands ironically: "Is it my mistaken impression that transplant protagonists would like to see an increase in car accidents?" (705). Watanabe concludes that prevention and treatment of heart disease should take priority over the heroics of heart transplants.

Among Japanese physicians opposed to the recognition of brain death, a permanent loss of consciousness or of cognition in patients is not a deciding factor. They instead emphasize the liveliness of brain-dead bodies, together with a concern that death is being proclaimed too early along the continuum of dying. Like Watanabe, many physicians (and commentators from all walks of life) also worry about social injustice and inequity in connection with transplants. When talking to me, individuals spontaneously burst out again and again with assertions that the transplant enterprise is unfair. The cost of procurement, transportation, and transplantation of organs was frequently criticized after the first legal transplants. In contrast, living related transplants—donations from relatives—are not usually opposed by the general public, but a good number of surgeons, including Watanabe Yoshio, are adamantly opposed to deliberately causing harm to a healthy person.

In this climate, emergency medicine doctors are unlikely to impose their opinions on families of dying patients. However, I did find several intensive care physicians who were fully supportive of organ procurement and who, now that they no longer risk murder charges, plan to do everything possible to increase donations. These physicians agreed that many of their colleagues were much more reticent, no doubt fearing media exposure and even lawsuits.

One major difficulty is a long-standing lack of cooperation across medical departments. Several emergency medicine doctors told me that they have no time to look after brain-dead donors, which can take up many hours before procurement, and do not believe that this taxing work should be expected of them or of their staff.

At a national meeting of Emergency Medicine doctors in 1998, the final session was devoted to brain death. Usually people start to leave such meetings before the last panels, but this particular session was packed. Toward the end the audience was asked how many people had signed their donor cards. Approximately one-third of the doctors raised their hands, a much higher proportion than among the Japanese public at large, and higher than among intensivists in North America (if it is fair to generalize from the small sample who talked to me). This response suggests that if some of the pressure in their working environment were removed, a good number of emergency medicine doctors might well cooperate with procurements.

Many Japanese remain concerned that dying patients will be "sacrificed" so that their organs can be procured. Ohara Shin, a professor at a leading Japanese university, claims that "now that brain death is accepted legally, an increasing number of doctors may be eager to hasten death to obtain fresh organs, rather than doing everything possible to keep a dying person alive, as in the past" (1997:4). Yet my interviews and the experience of the Yanagida family suggest that physicians are exceedingly cautious about imposing brain-death diagnoses on the families of patients, with the result that families are very often left to make their own decisions as to when the ventilator will be disconnected. Many families, perhaps most of them, apparently keep hoping for a miracle.[7] Even when relatives suspect the worst, they are not encouraged to think of this condition as human death.

By contrast, doctors in North America are very much in control of decisions about when ventilators will be turned off, and they usually succeed in bringing reluctant families gently but firmly around to the view that a brain-dead patient should be freed from life-support machinery and allowed to rest in peace (unless organ procurement is planned). We trust doctors and believe them justified in ruling out all hope of miracles. In Japan the public has been incited by the media to worry about hasty decisions and possible error. This atmosphere is somewhat reminiscent of nineteenth-century concerns about premature burial in an era when techniques for "reanimation" were hitting the news. However, fears about misdiagnosis are not the driving force in the brain-death debate. Much more pertinent, in my opinion, is that the ambiguity heightens reflection about the worth of the newly dead to individuals, families, and society. Attempts to resolve this ambiguity have gone in different directions, as clinical practices clearly reveal.

Working to Arrest Brain Death

In 1997, before the Transplant Law was passed in Japan, another program dealing with brain death was shown on prime-time television. Yanagida Kunio was the guest commentator for this program, most of which was filmed in the unit of Hayashi Nariyuki, an emergency doctor specializing in brain injury. Yanagida briefly reviews his experience with his son's death. The program then presents the case of a woman who

7. Susan Long has come to similar conclusions on the basis of her work on terminal care in Japan (2000).

suddenly lost consciousness and showed no reaction of any kind for six hours, but eventually recovered in Hayashi's unit with the use of "cerebral hypothermia treatment." Yanagida says that this case was a "shock" for him. He had hoped for a miracle when his son died, but in this woman's case "it really happened." What disturbed Yanagida most was that the two CT (computerized tomography) brain scans of his son and the woman, shown side by side on the screen for the benefit of viewers, looked very similar.[8]

Although hypothermia treatment—cooling tissue to prevent swelling and permanent damage—is not new, it has not been used extensively because it has proved difficult to control. Hayashi's innovative technique uses detailed computer-assisted measurements of the patient's condition to monitor the cooling efficiently. Among other things, Hayashi demonstrated successfully that if the abnormally high temperature in a traumatized brain can be reduced to normal, or even decreased to $33°$ C, then the rate at which brain cells die is radically reduced.

The program showed several patients, including one whose entire frontal brain was severely traumatized in a motorcycle accident, who recovered at least sufficiently to resume life outside the hospital. Hayashi estimates that in the past year he saved the lives of fifty-six out of seventy-five patients who would ordinarily have become brain-dead. To highlight the point, the program shows a patient in San Francisco who was brought to an emergency department with severe brain trauma. This patient was declared brain-dead the next day, and with the family's consent organs were removed for donation.

In contrast, viewers are shown a patient undergoing intensive treatment in Hayashi's care. This patient has a brain hemorrhage and is reported to be in a very similar condition to the San Francisco man. Because it can disrupt body functions, the cooling therapy must be minutely monitored and adjusted. Eleven days later, once the brain appears to be reasonably stabilized, the patient's body is very slowly rewarmed.[9] Now the concern is about infection. The audience sees the patient's wife coming to visit him on the twenty-second day, when he opens his eyes in response to her voice. Yanagida is overwhelmed. The final scenes show the patient going home, nearly seven months after first being hospitalized, and being greeted tearfully by his grandchildren. He

8. Yanagida recently published a new book that elaborates on the television program. To date, 40,000 copies have sold.

9. It is claimed that this therapy is continued for much longer in Hayashi's unit than elsewhere in the world.

is by no means fully recovered, but he can talk to some extent, and he responds with a full range of emotions to events around him.

The Hayashi hypothermia technique was reported in Japanese newspapers prior to the television program, followed a few months later by a front-page report about new drugs added to the treatment regimen to improve survival rates (*Asahi Shinbun* 1997a). Thanks to the media, the Japanese public was once again involved in debate about the management of severe head trauma. Hayashi Nariyuki is a genial, dedicated surgeon who, when I interviewed him, showed me numerous modifications he had personally designed and installed to make his hospital unit more functional. He makes no claims to saving brain-dead patients but rather seeks to prevent deterioration to brain death. He has been quoted as saying that if transplant medicine is always given priority, then progress in emergency medicine may be slowed because patients are given up on too easily. Hayashi argues that "functional" death means that there is a "suspension of the cells' activity, but that this does not mean that the cells are necessarily dead." Hayashi is nevertheless satisfied with the Takeuchi criteria because once a patient has reached what is currently conceptualized as brain death, the condition is, at present, irreversible. Hayashi insists that in the future, with advances in technology, we will be better able to prevent brain cells dying after major trauma (*Asahi Shinbun* 1997a).

Hayashi's articles are read worldwide, and he has given numerous talks in Europe and North America. While showing me around his unit, Hayashi expressed his unhappiness that he receives little financial support from the Japanese government, in large part because his research continues to be classed as experimental. Because other units in Japan have not yet been able to reproduce Hayashi's results, mainstream recognition is slow in coming. Yet when the first procurement of organs was made from a brain-dead donor in March 1999, several critics, apparently believing that hypothermia treatment should be used routinely on all patients approaching brain death, asked rather aggressively why Hayashi's treatment had not been used with the donor.

Reflections on Brain Death: Japanese Health Care Professionals

In the mid 1990s I conducted interviews with twenty-three Japanese physicians from various medical specialties other than emergency medicine, ranging from obstetrics and gynecology to internal medicine and psychiatry. I also interviewed eight nurses and a social worker. All worked in hospitals in the cities of Tokyo and Osaka or in Nara and Shiga prefectures. My questions in these open-ended interviews were designed primarily to find out what these particular health care professionals think about *nōshi mondai* (the brain-death problem).

Among the thirty-two respondents, twenty-two reported little or no difficulty in accepting a diagnosis of brain death as an irreversible condition, and, with some provisos about regulations and cautionary measures, they think of it as physical death. But beyond this broad agreement lies a considerable range of responses, revealing just how inadequate are public opinion surveys with their simple, dichotomous choices. Of the remaining respondents, four said that they really had not thought about the matter very much, and six were opposed to the recognition of brain death as human death, again for a range of reasons.

Among the twenty-two who think of brain death as biological death, fifteen gave unqualified answers and went on to state that organ transplants would be acceptable to them. Others gave less straightforward answers. A head nurse said, for example, that she would donate her organs when brain-dead, but she would never want to have a transplant. If her child needed a transplant, she would hope that she or her husband or other relatives would be compatible and able to make a "living" donation; otherwise she would not want the procedure to take place. This nurse believes that nothing remains of an individual after death except others' memories of the deceased.

A male nurse, Hara Keigo, stated that he accepts brain death with his rational mind, but when directly involved with cases, he finds it emotionally difficult to accept that brain death is the end: "I keep wishing for a miracle to happen." Hara remains "a little insecure" about the accuracy of a brain-death diagnosis because he believes that inexperienced practitioners are sometimes involved. Nevertheless, he wants transplant technology to be supported and would himself donate organs. Yamada Kazuo, a psychiatrist who also has training as a Buddhist priest, regards brain death as human death, but he argues that organ transplants should not be routine until the lack of cooperation among the various specialties in the Japanese medical world has been remedied: otherwise too many mistakes will be made, and organs will go to waste.

Amano Keiko, a nurse, does not recognize brain death as human death and is opposed to transplants from brain-dead bodies. She states, "Death is the end, nothing remains once you are dead, but I have seen death a lot, both at work and in my family, and I can't think of the person as dead until the heart has stopped beating. So I'm uncomfortable with brain death . . . I'm hesitant. I can understand the difference between brain death and heart death in theory, but emotionally I'm still uncomfortable."

Kobayashi Yoshiko, a social worker, argues that without technology, brain death would not exist, and that the brain-death argument is always tied to the question of organ transplants, making her ill at ease:

> You might think I'm just being emotional, but I want to believe that something inside me is still alive, even if I become brain-dead. Anyway, an individual's life is integral to the family in Japan, and so it's difficult to think of giving "life" (*inochi*) to others. But that's just my opinion, I don't want to say what others should think. I personally don't really trust doctors. Patient's bodies are just "things" (*mono*) for doctors, so I'm uncomfortable with the whole idea of transplants.

Among the physicians, Noda Junko, a psychiatrist, is solidly opposed to the recognition of brain death as human death. She says:

> Even when the body is dead, the soul (*tamashii*) remains in each organ of the body for quite a while, so in brain death, when the body is still warm, I don't find it possible to think about taking organs out. Anyway, I don't think we really understand what is going on in the brain at death, and a death that can only be understood by a doctor isn't death as far as I'm concerned. The distance between doctors and patients is growing greater because of technology, and I think this causes a lot of distrust.

She adds, "I think many people in Japan find it really hard to objectify the body completely—these ideas don't come from any specific religious belief, but they are 'Japanese characteristics.' I definitely believe in fate and that one's time of death is determined at birth. It just doesn't seem right to try to prolong life through such invasive technologies like organ transplants."

A retired physician and historian of medicine, Sonoda Hirokazu, focuses on the way in which the technological determination of brain death excludes families and precludes a subjective, human determination of death through "feelings." Recalling several of the legal cases where murder charges had been brought against doctors, Sonoda lamented the lack of trust that doctors inspire in people in Japan. He criticized the usual Japanese decision-making system, which demands consensus before any action can be taken:

> In Japan, if you have 30 percent opposition to something, you can't do it. So in order to bring about change, you have to go around to people individually and in effect bribe them. You ask them to agree with you, and offer

them something in return . . . this is what's called *nemawashi* [prior preparation: literally, to dig around the roots of a tree]. That's how you get things done in Japan, and it means that no one feels really responsible about decisions because we all did it together.

Sonoda is himself opposed to organ transplants until the medical profession is "made to be more responsible," but he believes another issue is at work when people say they are against recognition of brain death:

> I don't think the problem is to do with Buddhism, absolutely not, we've never really believed in Buddhism in Japan, we just follow a few rituals. Nor is it to do with ghosts or ancestors or anything like that. If anything, Buddhism encourages organ donation because people are supposed to help others. No, among ordinary people the problem is to do with *uchi* [insiders] and *soto* [outsiders]. We are raised to stick with *uchi*, that is, to support our family and other people we have obligations to; so it's fine for a mother to give a kidney to her child, but she doesn't have to worry about her next-door neighbor when he is dying. You know, people in Japan still don't leave their bodies to medicine or permit autopsies very often. I think the big problem is that we don't like to give anything to people if we don't have a familial or an established working relation with them.

Numerous people made similar comments to me and have also noted that the Christian tradition specifically encourages giving to strangers in a way unheard-of in Japan. With modernity, altruism blossomed in the West; Japan, unhappily in most people's estimation, lags behind in this respect.

When Persons Linger On

Several surveys of clinical practice in Japan have shown that in comparison with physicians in the United Kingdom and the United States, Japanese doctors are reluctant about withdrawing nutrition and hydration from patients who have been in a persistent vegetative state (PVS) for months or even years and are unconscious but breathing independently (Asai et al. 1999; Fukuda 1975). Half the physicians surveyed in the United States on the subject thought that patients in a permanent vegetative state (lasting more than a year) should be considered dead and treatment withdrawn, and two studies showed that only about 10 percent of these physicians would want to be left to live under these circumstances (Fox and Stocking 1993; Payne et al. 1996). Japanese responses were quite different. About 4 percent of physicians would withdraw treatment from patients (rising to 30 percent if the patient acquired an infectious disease), and 60 percent of these physicians would want treatment continued if they themselves were in PVS (Asai et al. 1999).

The authors who compiled these findings, themselves Japanese physicians, believe that religious attitudes toward death, notably those of Shinto, which associate death with pollution, are a major contributory factor. I tend to disagree with this conclusion but concur with the others: "Regardless of [an irreversible loss of] consciousness, PVS patients still remain the same persons who had lived meaningful lives with their families," and so PVS patients engender sympathy from family members (Asai et al. 1999:306). They remain not only biologically alive but also social agents who elicit emotional responses from those around them. Susan Long, in her research on dying patients in Japan, concluded that families are in effect "expected" to maintain hope. This is part of their "job" as family (Long and Long 1982; Long 2000). Furthermore, the expression of hope is intended to help the patient toward some sort of recovery. Along these lines, Asai et al. argue that a widespread belief exists that miracle recoveries (many of which have been portrayed on television) are always possible (1999:306).

These authors also observe that doctors worry about lawsuits arising from the withdrawal of care. The concept of futility is not recognized in Japan, even among medical professionals. Patient autonomy has only recently been recognized as a credible issue, and so support for recognition of medical futility would inevitably be seen as a regressive move by doctors reverting to autocratic behaviors common until recently.

In Tokyo I visited a children's hospital that cared for a number of PVS children. I had seen such patients in London and Montreal, and as usual I was deeply moved by their profound helplessness and by the care they received from their nurses. Parents visit in all the units I have observed, wherever their location, and it is common to see them talking with, stroking, and kissing their unconscious children. But in Japan families seem able to sustain hope for a longer time and are very reluctant to entertain the possibility of allowing a patient to die. The guilt associated with such thoughts, it seems, would be insurmountable.

The most shocking sight in the Tokyo children's hospital was of a child born with deformities so massive that she did not look like a child at all. She had been unable to breathe independently from birth, but instead of letting this infant expire, someone had placed her on a ventilator and started artificial feeding. Three years old when I saw her, she was totally blind, deaf, apparently fully unconscious, stunted, and hideously contorted. She had survived several major infections with the help

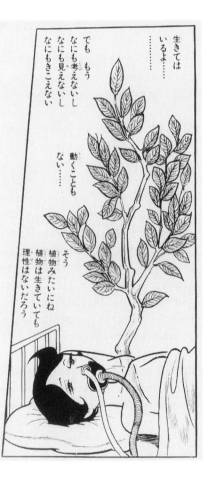

Shokubutsu ningen (a plant person), a translation of persistent vegetative state. The text says, "She *is* living . . . even though she no longer has any thought, sight, hearing, nor the ability to work. So, it's like being a plant; even though plants are living, I don't suppose they can reason." Reproduced by permission of Tezuka Production, Tokyo.

of medication. Student nurses came to visit this child as I observed her, and, barely casting a glance at the patient, they were shown how to check the ventilator and the feeding tubes. I was told that the child's mother visits every week and that while there, she performs all the care of her child.

When I asked tentatively why this situation continued, I was told that obviously no firm decisions had been made during the first few days of life, and that the parents, in shock, had probably indicated that everything possible should be done for the newborn. Several Japanese physicians told me this was clearly a case where someone had failed to take control in the first few moments after birth to put an end to the tragedy.

Others speculated that the mother gains some inner peace from caring for her child.

Citizen Reflections about Brain Death

In 1997 I interviewed three groups of people in and around Tokyo about brain death and organ transplants. The groups were composed of seven to ten members, comprising twenty-seven in all, and everyone within each group knew the other participants well. One group was composed of individuals who work together in a volunteer women's health organization; another was composed of men and women who work together on various community projects; and the third was composed of psychologists, social workers, and administrators who work in a clinic that is part of a community mental health program. I am well acquainted with one or more persons in each of these groups, and these people organized the discussions on my behalf.

Despite the public furor and hundreds of publications on the subject, many of which explain brain-death diagnosis in considerable detail, few individuals professed to having a reasonably clear idea about what exactly is signified by brain death. Only three had read anything other than newspaper articles on brain death prior to our discussion (although four had rushed out and bought books especially to prepare for the group session). However, more than twenty people had seen television programs on the subject, and nearly everyone had seen the 1990 program produced by Tachibana. Many shared the view that brain death was invented by doctors to facilitate organ transplants.

Several people commented that Japanese families keep hoping for a miracle even if their relative is unconscious, and that they cannot possibly allow treatment to be stopped while there is any possibility, however remote, of recovery. About half the informants said they had heard of cases in which people recovered from brain death, although others were emphatic that recovery was impossible. In other words, these informants did not necessarily take medical judgments on death as authoritative or trustworthy. More than half insisted that a warm body cannot be dead and that families want to be able to judge death for themselves. Several people asserted that they had read stories about or heard directly of doctors who pressure families into making decisions about disconnecting the ventilator in order either to save money or to obtain organs for donation. Most of these stories, it turns out, were those widely reported in the media.

Complaints about a gap in communication between doctors and patients were frequent; twenty people stated that it is very hard to get information out of doctors. One woman said, "When a patient wants more information, a doctor is likely to get angry. Patients are in a really weak position in Japan." Another woman noted that "it is hard to tell if a doctor is giving you facts or if he is just speaking in his own interest." In other words, doctors may be prescribing drugs because they will profit from it, and similarly they may diagnose brain death so that organs can be procured. Yet another woman insisted that "doctors don't explain things well. We have to infer what they mean because they never set things out clearly," and another said, "Why do they have to call it brain death if it's really death? Why can't they just say death?"

Eight of the twenty-seven people claim that they would sign donor cards once things were legalized in Japan and that they have no difficulty thinking of brain death as the end of life. Several of these individuals thought the idea of being kept on a machine once permanently unconscious and brain-dead was offensive. Others equivocated in one way or another against donation. One woman said, for example, that families as a unit must decide about brain death and organ donation. Several people noted that the opinion polls apparently show that people would like to receive organs but not to give them, and that such an attitude does not seem fair or just. Two people recalled that the history of surgery in Japan had been curtailed by prohibitions against cutting into corpses. One man said that he had heard that in the past dead bodies had been dug up so that medical students could practice dissections, and this surely would account for why people are cautious about organ donation. (It is possible that this man has read about body snatching in nineteenth-century England. I have come across no such accounts in Japan.)

Several people spontaneously observed that should they agree to the donation of organs from a relative, they would want to know who received them. More than ten people stated that organ donation would be a positive way of contributing to society (see also Hosaka 1992), although several of them nevertheless expressed considerable reservations at the idea of actually doing so. Only two individuals had made their willingness to donate clear to their nearest relatives. (These interviews were conducted while it was still illegal to procure organs from a brain-dead body.)

Ten group members believed that something resembling a *reikon* (soul or spirit) survives after physical death. The feelings of the others are expressed by a middle-aged woman: "I suppose I'm not very sensitive about these things, I don't have any sensation of a spirit or something like that." Another woman stated that she has never "seen" a spirit, but believes that something must continue: "If my husband should die, then I will have my memories of him, and this will be like his spirit." One man stated that his parents believed in the spirits of the dead, but that he himself most certainly does not: "Once you're dead, that's it." Half of his group agreed. Clearly it is not possible to extrapolate from such a small sample, but this limited foray into beliefs about *reikon* shows how varied they are.

Two people thought that some kind of animated entity, more than just biological life, continues to exist in individual organs after transplant, and that transplants inevitably transfer some of the special characteristics of the donor. Some people characterized this entity as *tai-shitsu*, meaning individual bodily constitution or predisposition, but they were clear that they did not mean simply biology. Four informants commented that organ transplants are "unnatural," in particular because of the need to take immunosuppressant drugs. Others said that if their child needed an organ, they would consider going to India to buy one, although they probably would not go on their own behalf. Once again, the responses were very varied, and clearly the media barrage on brain death has not succeeded in turning people completely against it. Two of the three groups spontaneously returned toward the end of our discussion to the question of doctor-patient relationships and lamented that they are so poor in Japan. At the practical level, this is what seems to trouble people the most. But in the clinical setting, the inability of family members to make decisions seems to be the major stumbling block.

One person had watched her father being kept on a ventilator for two weeks after doctors had intimated that he was brain-dead.

> We didn't want to think he was dead, but I think we really knew, because the pupils of his eyes were dilated all the time. We could have asked for the ventilator to be turned off, but we were all quite young, and none of us wanted to take the initiative. I think we all understood rationally that he was dead, but we hoped for a miracle, and none of us wanted to be thought of as selfish by being the first to say that we should resign ourselves to his death. I think that looking for a national consensus is stupid. No one knows how they will respond until they have been through something like this. Individuals should make up their own minds without being subjected to all this self-reflection that goes on the media. It's up to each of us to deal with our own emotions as we think fit.

Another woman responded to this statement by saying, "Technology is supposed to save people from dying, but another way of looking at it is that it's linked to our ideas about human happiness. We have to ask for what purpose we are all born. Are we just machines, just part of the work force? We're all so overworked, no wonder people need organs sometimes." All three of these sessions were interspersed with questions to me about the situation in North America and in other countries; most people were very surprised to find out that Japan was one of the few "developed" countries not to recognize brain death and that there had been so little public opposition to the concept in other countries.

When I interviewed the president of the Japanese Transplant Recipients' Organization, Ohkubo Michikata, himself the recipient of a kidney from his sister, he insisted that "there is nothing especially stingy about Japanese compared to other ethnic groups when it comes to donating organs." The real trouble lies, in his opinion, with the poor organization of organ procurement and distribution in Japan. He said, "Unless a doctor is himself interested in transplants, even if he has a brain-dead patient under his care, he's not going to bother informing others." Ohkubo is careful to add that the position of individuals opposed to organ donation must be scrupulously honored.

Okhubo is certain that the public outcry by groups opposed to the recognition of brain death has created anxiety in those who might have become donors, and he devotes a large amount of his time in trying to change this situation. He produces a newsletter and gives numerous public talks. Even though he is himself a recipient of a living donation, Ohkubo believes that organs should be taken primarily from brain-dead bodies, and not from people who are alive.

These interviews reveal the heterogeneity of thinking among Japanese on the subjects of brain death and organ transplants. Despite a public debate lasting thirty years, and massive media coverage of the subject, no dominant line of reasoning has emerged. It is questionable whether, despite this exposure, Japanese are any more knowledgeable on the subject of brain death than are North Americans. But it is clear that public discussion of the brain-death problem and numerous polls have fostered doubts and outright opposition.

These interviews also suggest, however, that if organ transplants from brain-dead donors become routine, then a good number of people will be willing to participate. For others, the body at death is not understood as a "mere thing" but continues to represent the "personality" of the individual (Watanabe 1988), and such people are unlikely ever to come to terms with commodification of a body that is legally dead but biologically alive.

Continuing medical scandals will not help the Japanese to gain trust in their doctors. Recently the president of a medical clinic and six of his employees were arrested for illegally treating cancer patients with lymphocytes that had not been properly prepared. The clinic president does not have a medical license but was nevertheless directly responsible for treatment of patients, and the lymphocyte blood product he used was also sold to other medical institutions at enormous profit (Watts 1998c: 1368).

The situation in Japan is unlikely to change radically for some time. If ICU doctors remain uncomfortable with asking families about organ donation and shy away from facilitating procurements, few donations will take place except at the donor family's insistence. (There are some exceptions to doctors' reticence: see Kawashima et al. 1994.) No doubt hospitals designated as transplant centers will show more initiative in bringing about changes, but other difficulties remain. For one thing, many more transplant coordinators will have to be trained; but, above all, Japanese families will have to be prepared to relinquish their brain-dead relatives to the medical establishment quite early, often a few hours after brain death is declared—something that most families at present appear unwilling to do.

Four months after his birth, Kodama Yasutoshi was diagnosed with Werdnig-Hoffmann's disease, an untreatable and progressive congenital disorder in which the spinal muscles atrophy. At four months he was put on a ventilator, and before he was a year and a half old he had a tracheostomy. At three years of age he had lost all voluntary movement in his fingers. It was not known how long Yasutoshi would live, even on life support, and his parents, who had been married for eight years before Yasutoshi was born, coped from day to day and then from year to year.

Yasutoshi is now nineteen years old. He can move his eyes, hear, and shed tears, but he is able to do virtually nothing else. He has been hospitalized all his life and has spent most of his time watching television and listening to music. When I met Yasutoshi at age fifteen, his hospital room was filled with toys, pictures, and other eye-catching memorabilia.

The Kodamas' family life was, of course, entirely transformed in order to care for their son. While his father remained at home, several hours' journey away, Yasutoshi's mother virtually lived in the Tokyo hospital, where she looked after her son together with competent and caring nurses and doctors.

Yasutoshi seemed to enjoy listening to music and, when he was twelve years old, Ishimoto Takumi, a teacher of children with disabilities, started coming to the hospital to see if he could help Yasutoshi express himself through music. During the first year, teacher and pupil listened together to many different genres of music. In the second year Ishimoto played scales and simple tunes on a keyboard at Yasutoshi's bedside until it was clear that Yasutoshi understood that he too could make melodies if he could convey what combination of sounds he wanted to put together. A computer that detects eye movements and converts them into yes or no signals was rigged up. With this Yasutoshi could select TV channels, learn Japanese ideograms, play video games, and make music. Gradually teacher and pupil began to compose bars of music and then eventually whole tunes. Yasutoshi's father says it was "like water flowing from a dam." When Yasutohshi was fifteen, after hours and hours of work, a carefully orchestrated CD comprising eleven of his tunes was released and sold by the thousands in Japan. He has recently put out a second CD.

In the booklet that came with the first CD, his father writes that Yasutoshi is no longer a child: "We have to accept him as a person who has the personality of an ordinary junior high school student. I want to encourage him to continue making music because it is the only way of expressing himself. In a way, I envy Yasutoshi. He has done something my wife and I cannot do, and has left a CD in this world."

Sakakihara Yoichi, the head of the hospital department where Yasutoshi lives, has tracked what happens to children on long-term life support in Japan. He notes that the incidence of Werdnig-Hoffmann's disease is one in 25,000 and that the average life span is about fifteen months. Each year about fifty cases are diagnosed in Japan, of which about 20 percent are placed on ventilators. The data from other countries suggest that very few such children are placed on ventilation, and even in Japan pediatricians disagree as to whether these children should be given life support, particularly because no government funding is available to support families in looking after the children at home (Sakakihara et al. 1996). The estimated expense to the health care system for hospital care of the children is just over $6,000 a month, but because they are few, their care has little effect on the overall budget.

The Nobel Prize winner for literature, Oe Kenzaburo, and his wife Yukari have a disabled son who is also a musician and whose compositions are no doubt better known in Japan and elsewhere than Yasutoshi's. In reflecting frankly on life with his son, in his book *A Healing Family,* Oe writes that Hikari appears mostly completely at "home" when he is composing music: the music Hikari creates "is itself the expression of that feeling." Oe goes on: "I wonder if I haven't been writing novels all these years as an expression of this same most basic feeling: that I, too, am at home in this world. Moreover, though I dream of finding a way in my writing to express something that transcends this world, it is in Hikari's music that I most often get a premonition of a world beyond our own" (1995:127).

TWELVE

The Body Transcendent

Then shall be brought to pass the saying that is written,
Death is swallowed up in victory. O death, where is thy sting?
O grave, where is thy victory?

1 Corinthians 15.54–55

Brain death, a concept that permits the commodification of body parts for transplant, is an invention of the West. I turn here to a consideration of the uses to which bodies have been put in Europe, for this is a singular history to which both Christianity and medieval medicine made major contributions. Biomedicine, with its anatomical foundation in which dissection of human organs is indispensable, is based on a long tradition of body commodification, a tradition that has been virtually absent in Japan.

Relics and Regeneration

No argument can be made for simple historical continuities, but certain concepts and practices may have been at work in medieval times that are not totally unrelated to the apparent ease with which the idea of brain death and organ transplants have been accepted in the majority of European countries and in North America. The purpose of the following exploration is to be provocative, perhaps iconoclastic.

The culture of medieval European death is deeply entangled with Christian values. Writing about medieval representations of death, the art historian Paul Binski starts out with the raising of Lazarus. He reminds us that, when hearing of Lazarus's sickness, Jesus makes it clear that illness furnishes an opportunity for the glorification of God. Lazarus had been dead for four days when Jesus arrived in Bethany, whereupon, troubled in spirit, he went to the cave where the body was laid out, and asked for the stone to be rolled away. Lazarus emerged, shrouded, prefiguring the resurrection of Christ himself. Binski describes this remarkable rebirth as one of "absolute normality" for the medieval Christian, a scene made vivid fact through its portrayal by artists such as Giotto. From the vantage point of earlier traditions, however, it was a moment of complete transgression. In Judaism, the freshly dead corpse was a site of impurity, and in pagan Rome the dead body was abhorred by the gods (Binski 1996:10).[1]

The raising of Lazarus is the first great event in the Christian triumph over death. The cross from which Christ redeemed the world is, in Binski's words, "an implement of lethal torture" transformed into a symbol of eternal life (9). Early Christianity retained beliefs and practices about life and death characteristic of the Greco-Roman world and earlier periods, but this transgressive move, the gradual systematization and defeat of physical death, was to become one of the forces peculiar to the new religion. The souls of the Roman dead lingered by the body for three days, a liminal, dangerous time. For Binski, the resurrection of Lazarus after four days, and of Jesus after three, is a triumph imbuing the physical body with special meaning. The physical body itself, and not simply the memory of persons, lineages, and communities, is valued as something that will be resurrected.

The Romans, troubled by the preaching and practices of the early Christians, burned and scattered the charred remains of Christian martyrs in an effort to diffuse the power associated by believers with their bodies. Binski suggests that this response reveals how, from its inception, Christianity was a religion of the body as much as one of the soul. Moreover, "From the time of St. Paul onwards, the great transgression implicit in the Christian attitude to the dead threatened both to reorder the old worlds of nature and divinity and, more importantly, to adjust, or renegotiate, the sensitive boundaries between the dead and the living" (11). One of the first moves by Christians as they amassed confidence and power was to bring sainted bodies into the church and bury them near the altar (Brown 1981). Although some believers were troubled by this practice, one that Ariès claims came from North Africa (1974:15), it became widespread. Christians wanted proximity to these holy bodies for protection and for the transmission of miraculous healing powers.

---

1. Although certain Rabbinical texts debate the possibility of resurrection, many scholars believe that this idea was not present in Judaism before the birth of Christ.

Bodies retained power whether intact or dismembered. Human relics were bought and sold, stolen and divided, given and bartered, much like any other commodity between the eighth and twelfth centuries. Fakes circulated along with authentic items, and if they were associated with miraculous cures, their worth multiplied accordingly. Like slaves who were at once persons and things, relics held an ambiguous status, both living and dead (Geary 1994).[2]

Contact with body parts enabled the spread of positive "spiritual contagion" (Binski 1996:16) and the remains of powerful people accumulated particular worth. Royalty willed parts of their bodies to their subjects as a sign of largesse and as a means of accruing symbolic capital. The heart was highly valued, and so were the bones, the durable, pure essence of the individual. Burial in churchyards ensured that the living always had close contact with the remains of the dead, perhaps reducing fears commonly associated by ordinary people with dead bodies and body parts.

In classical Greece and Rome, individuals were recognized in society on the basis of their position in a line of ancestors and descendants and the accomplishment of certain deeds; a life history was understood as a small part of the continuum of society. Personal biography ended at death, but human happiness was ideally achieved with a good reputation that transcended death (Binski 1996:22). Evidence of these beliefs can be detected in early Christianity, in which the dead, the ancestors, were understood as an "age group"—a cohort that continued to act on society after death. As part of an ongoing system of exchange between the dead and the living, the deceased could warn, admonish, or chastise their living descendants through dreams and omens, as they still do among the Greeks living in Inner Mani. Parents gave life, property, and identity to their children. After death such gifts had to be reciprocated through memorials and in the form of material wealth (Geary 1994:78).

These practices were gradually replaced with ideas of individual salvation. Like Christ, individuals "under[went] a series of transformative crises—conversion, baptism, and death," to emerge ready for instant assessment "whose qualities are inscribed in the Book of Life to be judged" (Binski 1996:22). An individual life course was reconceptualized as a linear progression, a personal journey. This change is in turn

2. Other major religions, such as Buddhism and Islam, value relics taken from the human body, but these are for the most part limited to the hair, teeth, and other body parts whose detachment does not desecrate the body.

linked to new ideas about time and history as a teleology, a movement toward a clearly demarcated end. Time was now governed by an awareness of individual destiny orchestrated by God, so that by the twelfth century, for many Christians, the meaning of life became the seeking out of personal fulfillment. Happiness lies not in reputation, as it did for the Romans, but in personal transcendence (Binski 1996:23).

Medieval Christian scholars were acutely aware of the body and its parts as more than "mere things" (Rabinow 1996:149), and survival beyond death was envisioned literally as a form of material continuity: as a resurrection (Bynum 1991:247). Caroline Bynum quotes Peter the Venerable in this connection: "I have confidence more certainly than in any human thing that you ought not to feel contempt for the bones of the present martyrs as if they were dry bones but should honor them now full of life as if they were in their future incorruption. . . . Fresh flowers from dryness and youth is remade from old age" (264). Dead bodies, as is commonly believed throughout the world, were considered fertile. Bynum also points out that many medieval stories imply that the body is in some sense alive after death; claims of miraculous resuscitations were made repeatedly. She notes that medical writers "spoke of cadavers that continued to move or grow while on the embalming table or in their tomb" (266), and that some worried about premature burial.

The Art of Dying

As theology became increasingly complex, so did the art of dying. The *Ars morendi,* a layperson's version of rituals developed in the medieval Church, comprises eleven woodcuts depicting a series of deathbed temptations. Binski describes these woodcuts as a form of bedside drama in which the central character controls his own death and thus his own destiny. Death is clearly a process: a "good" death, prepared ahead of time by the dying person, is a "tamed death" culminating in a ceremony in which sin is absolved.

Joachim Whaley (1981) argues that the *Ars morendi* is modeled after the Egyptian *Book of Coffins,* but in the Christian version a preoccupation with the solitary character of death is evident from as early as the eleventh and twelfth centuries. In the literary genre arising from the *Ars morendi,* commencing in approximately the late fourteenth century, the death of Christ, alone and suffering on the cross, is clearly the model for individual death. It is the dying man, Moriens, who is judged in these

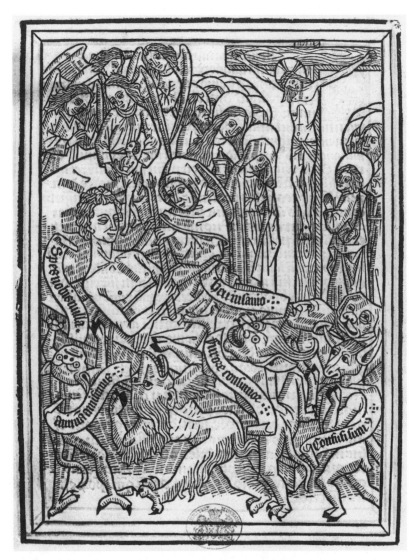

The good death as depicted in a late-fifteenth-century *Ars morendi* (The art of dying). Reproduced by permission of The British Library (no. IB 23).

scenes, rather than society or humankind as a whole (Binski 1996:42).
Moriens controls the character of his own death and therefore his destiny. Individuals who give in to the temptations of devils succumb to a
bad death; but there are other forms of bad death, those that are out of
place, unprepared for, untimely, or violent. The socially dead—the un-
baptized, heretics, lepers, Jews, suicides, and excommunicates—were
all, by definition, denied a good death, destined to remain forever in
Limbo or Purgatory rather than enter Heaven. Lepers and heretics in
particular were treated as dangerous objects of spiritual contagion
whose liminal status could be transferred to others. But anyone could
succumb to a bad death if caught unprepared.

The medieval Japanese, like the early Christians, formalized death
rituals. A tenth-century Buddhist priest, Genshin of Hieizan, wrote
down "Rules for Dying" (*Rinjū no gyōgi*). Genshin's rules were designed
to teach people how to achieve an ideal death, culminating with entry
into paradise. Buddhist texts and practices such as those espoused by
Genshin were first brought to Japan in the sixth century from China
and Korea. They mingled with indigenous Shinto concepts that hold
death as polluting. Matsumoto argues that the fear of death in classical
Japan lessened once Buddhist dogma and practices became widely disseminated (1993).

A series of fourteenth-century pictures, the *Kyusōshi emaki,* shows
nine stages of dying, in the last two of which maggots eat the body,
leaving only the bare bones. Many Japanese, as Abe Tomoko suggests,
still think of exposed, clean bones as the sign of physical death. The
close attention to the process of decay during dying and death in medieval Japan recalls similar European practices of the same period, and
Yōrō Takeshi argues that this preoccupation suggests that physical death
was understood, as in medieval Europe, as a process and not an event
(1992).

Piero Camporesi argues that for men of God in Renaissance Italy
there was little difference between the flesh (*caro*) and decay (*putrado),*
and life was understood as "camouflaged death." Putrefaction was not
"a *post mortem* process but one that ran concurrently with life, was
inherent to life, inside life itself, for life was but corruption and stench"
(1988:78). Nature was conceptualized as "a swarming cosmos full of
myriads of ephemeral metamorphoses," and the corpse was understood
as in some sense still alive and capable of feeling, even as the fine machinery of the body dissolved into horror, stench, and worms—a process
particularly repugnant in women. The possibility for transcendence was

everywhere, for all God's creatures were born from decay—humans from fetid sperm and stale blood—but individual transcendence could be brought about only if one overcame a fear of the flesh.[3] The idea of physical death as process and as incipient regeneration was repeatedly expressed through the use of powerful, earthy metaphors. Certainly there were differences among occupational groups and classes in mortuary practices and in attitudes toward the corpse, but regeneration was undoubtedly a powerful image.

Ariès argues that by the seventeenth century indisputable evidence of a new preoccupation exists, a concern not only about physical mortality but with the "death of self." These ideas gradually weaken the power of religious and communal belief with its dogma of rebirth (1974; see also Cohen 1973). Nevertheless, a "deep-rooted refusal to link the end of physical being with physical decay" persists (Ariès 1974:33), as do perennial concerns about the power and even the life that inheres in the body itself and in body parts after physical death. Bynum argues that concerns about regeneration can easily be detected in the transplant world, and human organs are frequently anthropomorphized and attributed with something more than biological worth when transferred from donor to recipient (1991). Thoughts of personal regeneration die hard.

Both Buddhism and Christianity promulgate a doctrine of salvation, but medieval Christianity, with its focus on the physical body, differs significantly from Buddhism. In Buddhist doctrine, the soul does not depart until the body is cold. Following decay of the body, what is left, in the words of the philosopher Kaji Nobuyuki, is simply a thing—*tannaru mono*—with little or no value (1990). In most Buddhist sects, one seeks to escape entirely from earthly travail and the relentless cycles of rebirth. However, Robert Smith and others argue that Buddhist ideas about reincarnation never really took root in Japan, and that one must look to the treatment of ancestors to understand Japanese ideas about death and continuity (1974).

Even though, in the new Buddhist sects in Japan, much is made of wandering, neglected spirits who hold grudges, Kaji insists, in support of Smith and others, that this is not authentic Buddhist teaching (1990: 12). Kaji is explicit that because living related organ donation supports

3. Buddhism too advocates overcoming an abhorrence of the flesh by meditation on and contemplation of dead bodies, as is particularly evident in the *Tibetan Book of the Dead* (Evans-Wenz 1981), but the emphasis is on a marked transcendence of worldly flesh, a complete liberation from the karmic cycles that confine one to this world.

and revitalizes the family, it is rarely resisted in Japan; in contrast, cadaver and brain-dead donation contravene Confucian edicts because they require defilement of the body.

Ancestors with agency seem decidedly odd to most people today, wherever they live, but the ancestors' power, weakened though it is, remains evident in Japan and influences the brain-death debate. Ideas about personal salvation and resurrection on earth appear equally odd to many of us. However, as Bynum suggests, medieval Christian beliefs, notably about the life and power inherent in dead bodies and body parts, may have contributed to the promiscuous commodification of the human body in the service of European medicine.

Dissection and Transcendence

Vivisection and dissection were practiced before the time of Christ; but a close association exists between the medieval Church, especially in southern Europe, and practices of medical dissection. This fascination with dissection led directly to the flowering of anatomy in European medicine, enabling unparalleled developments in surgery.

When Jean Baudrillard states baldly that "for medicine, the body of reference is the corpse" (1993:114), he has in mind so-called Western medicine.[4] In no other literate medical tradition—such as East Asian medicine, Ayurvedic medicine of South Asia, or the Unani tradition of the Islamic world—has anatomy been held as the key source of knowledge about the body. In early Greek medicine, after the time of Hippocrates, an interest in anatomy is well-documented. Anatomical thinking may have crystallized as a result of the practices of Aristotle, who performed both anatomization and vivisection of animals, but it was Herophilus, with his vivisection of humans (criminals and outcasts) in Alexandria in the fourth century B.C., who was recognized as the "father of scientific anatomy" (Potter 1976).

This early interest in anatomy fell into decline, perhaps because of opposition from state officials (Von Staden 1989), but in Italy the dissection of corpses, initially for autopsy, was taken up again in 1286, and by the fourteenth century autopsies to ascertain causes of death had become quite common (Park 1994). Many of these autopsies took place in private houses, usually to determine if the deceased had been poi-

---

4. In training for biomedicine today, although gross anatomy remains important, actual dissection of a body is sometimes dispensed with.

soned. Such dissections did not greatly disfigure the body. Dissection of a different sort, practiced in universities for educational purposes, commenced during the fourteenth century. In these, the body was systematically and entirely exposed. The idea that the truth about life and death can be found in the interior of the body is of long standing, at least in southern Europe. In Italy, attendance at one or more dissections was required to obtain the degree of doctor of medicine, although only one or two public dissections took place each year.

Katherine Park challenges the current assumption that a taboo on autopsies and dissection existed prior to Vesalius in the sixteenth century. She insists that only in the mid-sixteenth century is there clear evidence in Italy of opposition to tampering with the human body, when it was rumored that several anatomists practiced human vivisection. Vesalius is reported to have taken a beating heart out of an individual involved in an accident, and by his own admission he and his students desecrated graves, forged keys, stole corpses, and ransacked ossuaria to obtain human material; they were particularly keen to get their hands on the bodies of women (Harcourt 1987; Park 1994). Many commentators on anatomical practices in Europe, influenced by Foucault, refer to the violence, punishment, and transgression associated with dissection (see, for example, Harcourt 1987). Outdoor dissections of the bodies of criminals are described as "punitive spectacles" that violate the sanctity of the human body. Francis Barker argues, for example, that the spectacles of public dissections were remarkably similar to corporal punishment, still prevalent until the early seventeenth century, and to the familiar sight of the body on the gibbet. When dissected, the body is transformed, in the name of science, into a "gruesome spectacle," one exhibited in an anatomy "theatre" (1984:74). Although Park acknowledges that a raucous crowd often attended public dissections, she insists that in Italy it was family honor and the correct performance of funeral rituals that stopped people cooperating with autopsies and dissection, rather than any aversion to cutting into the body itself (1995).

Before anatomical theaters were built, dissections were sometimes performed inside churches. Anatomical treatises published before Vesalius's *De humani corporis fabrica* depicted *écorchés*—flayed bodies—that closely resembled saints holding their own instruments of martyrdom. The figures, beautiful despite their flaying, are set in pastoral landscapes. They give every appearance of willingly participating in their own death and dissection; the body often resembles the crucified Christ.

The criminal and the saintly body are closely associated in Renaissance Italy. These bodies are exemplary, sites of special power (Park 1994), and this association persisted after secular anatomy theaters were built and dissection became medicalized. When criminals were executed, they believed that their sins would be forgiven after dissection, and that their bodies would be identified with those of Christ and the saints (Park 1994). The brutality of the criminal act and that of the dissection could both be transcended.

Whether for this reason or others less exalted, dissections became popular spectacles. Park writes about Jacopo Berengario da Carpi, who claimed to have demonstrated the placenta of a hanged woman to "almost five hundred students at the University of Bologna, together with many citizens" (1994:15). Once this kind of public performance became common, pressure was exerted for more public dissection theaters to be built. By way of compensation, after the dissections were complete, medical students were required to pay for transportation of the corpses to the church and for the appropriate rituals to be carried out (1994:13). Evidently, as Park suggests, mutilation of a dead body was not totally abhorrent in southern Europe, nor did it violate Church teachings; nevertheless, participation must surely have incited prurient fascination and horror, especially when women's bodies were the object of the exercise.

Holland and Italy were closely associated in the sixteenth century, and Holland too became an important site for anatomical practice. A dissection theater built in Leiden was modeled on the one in Padua, but larger, with plenty of space for public viewing. Paying spectators enjoyed music and refreshment. Rembrandt's *Anatomy Lesson of Dr. Nicolaas Tulp* is among the most memorable representations of anatomical practices at this time. This painting shows the dissection of a petty thief from Leiden, thirty-six hours after his death by hanging. (It was perhaps an exercise of artistic license to depict the anatomist working on the thieving hand and forearm while leaving untouched the internal organs, which must be dealt with quickly because they are the first to putrefy.) *The Anatomy Lesson* has been interpreted repeatedly as a demonstration of medical mastery over death and of death made into a source of knowledge. Meike Bal even claims that Rembrandt deliberately creates ambiguity by permitting this corpse, and other corpses in earlier paintings, to exhibit signs of life (1991). This device incites a fascination in the viewer and suggests that the artist, along with early Christians and many people of his own time, saw life and death as not easily distinguishable. This ambiguity also indicates, to Bal's mind at least, that the surgeon has the potential power to bring the corpse back to life and has become, in effect, the "Divine Maker" (1991:394).

The Emergent Corpse

With the recognition of anatomy as the key to medical knowledge, the corpse became commodified as a unique, irreplaceable object for the advancement of medicine. Whereas in early Christian society esteem was reserved for the relics of saints, for modern medicine all corpses, whatever their source, have social worth. The importance of the work of anatomists is evident from statements by individuals such as Ercole Lelli, who performed public dissections in Bologna in the early eighteenth century. He was convinced that dissection would reveal the "grammar" by which the "language" of the body could finally be understood (Barsotti and Ruggeri 1997). Dissection also permits students of medicine to acquire, in the words of the eighteenth-century anatomist William Hunter, the "Necessary Inhumanity"—a clinical sense of detachment from the human body.

Equally important was the preservation of dissected body parts. Portions of the body were made into anatomical preparations through drying, bottling, salting, or pickling (Richardson 1996:68–69). The knowledge of members of religious orders about preserving holy relics would have been valuable in this work.

Although the majority of bodies dissected in medical schools today are donated, this has not always been the case. Concern about a shortage of human material for dissection is not new (Richardson 1989). For example, in England there was no legal supply of bodies for medical purposes until 1540, when the king bestowed an annual gift of four executed prisoners on the Companies of Barbers and Surgeons. These proved insufficient, however: the physiologist William Harvey, urgently desiring research material, dissected the corpses of his own father and sister.

Ruth Richardson argues that demand intensified because bodies were in short supply, and this shortage in turn encouraged illicit procurement. She speculates that between 1675 and 1725 human corpses, and not simply human relics, were bought and sold in Europe like any other commodity, and that grave-robbing became fashionable around the same time. In northern Europe, dissection was disowned entirely by the Church and recognized, in law and among the public, as a mutilation—an extension of the prisoner's punishment post mortem, as *The Anatomy*

Lesson suggests. Dissection represented, in Richardson's words, a "terrible aggravation of the death penalty" (1996:70).

Despite an increment to the original royal gift, the supply of gallows corpses continued to fall short of the medical profession's needs, particularly because the number of teaching hospitals was increasing. Peter Linebaugh argues that an increase in the private trade in corpses in the early eighteenth century reveals a significant change in attitude toward the dead body: "The corpse becomes a commodity with all the attributes of a property. It could be owned privately. It could be bought and sold. A value not measured by the grace of heaven nor the fires of hell but quantifiably expressed in the magic of the price list that was placed upon the corpse" (Linebaugh 1975:72). He documents in gruesome detail the "hanging matches" that took place in England, notably at the gallows in Tyburn, outside London. Surgeons and kin of the hanged person would fight over the body, tear it down—perhaps only half dead—from the gallows, the family hoping to give the body a decent burial, and the anatomists wanting a body to dissect. The "Tyburn crowd," often in their hundreds, became restless with the passing years, and riots were staged against the anatomists, to which the military had to be called to restore order (Linebaugh 1975). Incomplete hangings were common, and "resurrection" sometimes happened, in which case the victim was usually released—unless the doctors got hold of him first.

Popular opposition to dissection was so vocal that members of the medical profession turned increasingly to "body snatchers" for assistance. The poor rapidly became more valuable dead than alive, and several notorious murderers and traders in corpses were eventually brought to justice in England. The most famous of these, Burke and Hare, plied their victims with whisky before smothering them. The bodies were then sold to reputable London hospitals with no questions asked (Richardson 1996).

English common law has long stated that there can be no ownership of dead human bodies, but over the years a concept of "legal possession" of the body evolved. Those who own the property where the person dies have "possession" until someone with a greater claim arrives to take possession of the corpse for burial (Lawrence 1998). The result is that the corpse and its parts have no standing under the law for damage, theft, exchange, or inheritance. The Anatomy Act, signed in 1831, was designed to prohibit the sale of dead bodies. It was later adopted, with some minor modifications, by the Commonwealth nations and the existing American states, and it remains the foundation for modern laws

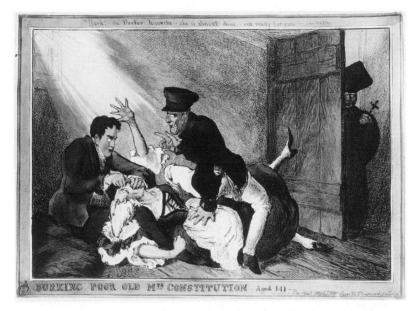

Body snatching: Burke and Hare's suffocating of Mrs. Docherty for sale to Dr. Robert Knox. Colored etching after William Heath ("Paul Pry"), 1829. Reproduced by permission of the Wellcome Library, London.

on these matters. Prior to the passing of this act one could not be prosecuted for "stealing" a dead body. Even after the act, workhouses and other institutions that housed the poor, including hospitals, were defined as "lawfully in possession of the dead."

As a result of the quasi-property status of the corpse, these institutions were able to confiscate the bodies of those who died when no claimant came forward or when no money was available for a funeral, and make use of them as they wished (Richardson 1996:73). Richardson remarks that to die without provision for burial was a sign of social failure, and the Victorian poor did everything they could to avoid such a fate. Friends and neighbors would take up collections to pay for funerals; corpses were hidden at home; or more than one body was placed in a single coffin (1989).[5]

In the interests of medicine, the poor were effectively defined as socially dead, their bodies not entitled to the respect given the rest of so-

5. The anthropologist Patricia Pierce Erikson, when she asked her mother about death rituals, was startled to be told that the wake was held in order that the body would not be stolen. Her family was originally from Ireland (personal communication, 2000).

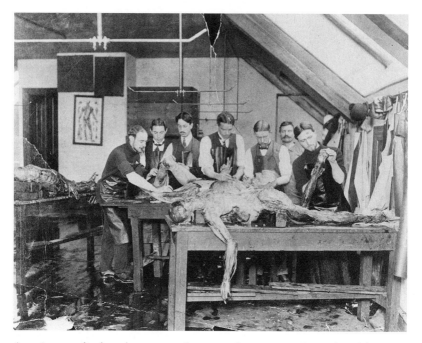

American medical students at work on a cadaver, 1890. Reproduced by
permission of the Minnesota Historical Society.

ciety (although, after eight weeks, anatomists were required by law to
provide a "decent" burial for the remains; see Lawrence 1998). This
situation still prevails today: if someone dies in hospital and the body
goes unclaimed, it can be used by the hospital for educational purposes.

There is evidence that, despite the Anatomy Act, in certain hospitals
dissections were done hastily, in the face of blatant opposition by family
members. Richardson cites Sir Robert Christison, a doctor who wrote
about his early career in a London teaching hospital in the 1820s. There
was, he said, "usually a race between the relatives and the students—
the former to carry off the body intact, the latter to dissect it. Thus,
dissection was apt to be performed with indecent and sometimes dangerous haste. It was not an uncommon occurrence that, when the op-
erator proceeded with his work, the body was sensibly warm, the limbs
not yet rigid, the blood in the great vessels fluid and coaguable" (Richardson 1996:97).

The utilitarian philosopher Jeremy Bentham took decisive steps to
counter the horror generated by such practices. When he died in 1832,

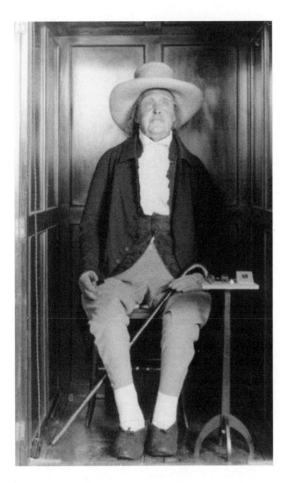

Jeremy Bentham. "Auto-icon" on display at University College, London. Bentham directed that his head be dried and preserved and his skeleton reassembled, clothed, and exhibited in a glass case. His head did not survive and was replaced by a plaster model. Reproduced by permission of University College London Library.

Bentham bequeathed his body for anatomical dissection, to be carried out by his anatomist friend Thomas Southwood Smith. The public dissection took place in a tiered amphitheater filled with spectators, many of whom, including John Stuart Mill, had helped Bentham to chivvy the Anatomy Act through Parliament. The spectacle was designed to encourage the donation of bodies to medicine.

In a speech before the dissection, Southwood Smith acknowledged the relatives' "natural" emotional attachment to the dead body. He insisted that although such sentiments have their foundation in the human heart, they belong to that class of feelings "which require control, and sometimes even sacrifice" (Richardson and Hurwitz 1987). When heart transplants were made into public spectacles for a brief time in the late

1960s, notably due to the activities of Christiaan Barnard, the idea that, through these spectacles, the public could be educated into donating the bodies of their relatives was clearly at work. A backlash soon set in when fears arose that if these procedures were thought of primarily as spectacles rather than as sound medical practice, a public revulsion to the whole transplant endeavor could easily result.

Despite Bentham's magnanimous gesture, public suspicion of medical imperialism prevailed for many years and fears about premature burial and living corpses were common. Richardson documents a similar course of events in North America. There, however, it was not only the bodies of the poor but also a disproportionate number of Native American and African American bodies that ended up in medical institutions (1996).

No sustained public outcry against these unscrupulous practices was heard before the end of the nineteenth century, but by this time people in some regions flatly refused to send their unburied dead to medical schools for dissection. The rate of voluntary donation, already very low, became negligible during the first part of the twentieth century. After World War II, a major shift in public attitude toward the medical profession and medical research contributed to a large rise in the number of bodies donated to medical schools.

The Physiological Body

Differing attitudes toward dissection at different times and places in Europe hint at contested meanings attributed to the dead body; moreover, Europe was unique in its early institutionalization of autopsies and dissection.[6] In Japan, as in most other regions, even those with well-established medical institutions, autopsies were not routinely practiced until the latter half of the nineteenth century. Bodies of beheaded criminals were occasionally dissected, but the dissections were performed either by members of the former outcaste group known as *burakumin* or by convicted criminals. Doctors, having paid the dissectors, usually watched the spectacle from a discreet distance (Low 1996).

The first dissection in Japan to be carried out by a physician, Tōyō

---

6. E. E. Evans-Pritchard documented the use of dissection among the Azande, who required an autopsy to see if witchcraft was a cause of death (1937). Similar practices have been documented in other nonliterate traditions, but among the literate medical traditions outside the European sphere of influence, anatomy was only rudimentarily developed.

Yamawaki, took place in a Kyoto jail in 1754 (Sakai 1982), followed in 1759 by the dissection of a female corpse by of one of Tōyō's students. Compared to Europe in the eighteenth and nineteenth centuries, dissections and autopsies were few and were performed exclusively on the bodies of criminals or purported criminals (Low 1996). The idea of practicing dissection in a religious precinct, as in the churches of southern Europe, would have been unthinkable.

Restrictions on dissection are usually attributed to powerful Confucian edicts against tampering with the dead. However, Nathan Sivin documents regular autopsies in China (1988). A much more compelling explanation is that prior to contact with European medicine, East Asian doctors had little interest in anatomy. East Asian medicine is based predominantly on physiological conceptions of the body, and emphasis is given to the relationships among corporeal systems. Curiosity about the anatomical structure of the body was never apparent in Japanese medicine (Kuriyama 1992), and those doctors who participated in dissections were trying to gain an understanding of European medical practices, which were becoming known in Japan from the beginning of the seventeenth century.

Probably because of this lack of medical interest in dissection, grave robbery does not appear to have been a cause for public anxiety. Moreover, particularly in the crowded cities, bodies were cremated rather than buried. The result, reinforced no doubt by Confucian edicts, was that commodification of human bodies for medical purposes, other than those bodies designated as beyond the pale of society, was uncommon in Japan until well into the twentieth century. The policy in Japanese hospitals today is similar to that in North America: bodies that go unclaimed may be used for educational purposes prior to cremation.

Human Experimentation

During the twentieth century Japan participated in various activities that reinforced public reluctance to cooperate with medical science. The biological warfare programs carried out by Japanese scientists in Manchuria between 1932 and 1945, and particularly the exploits of the infamous Unit 731, received considerable media coverage in Japan and abroad throughout the 1970s and 80s. These involved the use of many hundreds, perhaps thousands, of subjects, most of them Chinese. Scientists initiated this program under the auspices of the army and with the full knowledge of the Japanese government.

The extent of the atrocities is still not known because a good quantity of archival materials remains sealed. Manchuria was, in Sheldon Harris's words, turned into "one gigantic biological and chemical warfare laboratory" for well over a decade. But this knowledge was deliberately suppressed for years, not just by the Japanese themselves but as a result of an extensive cover-up by the United States government. Knowledge obtained from the experiments was deemed too valuable to the military to be exposed to public scrutiny (Harris 1994). The United States, the former Soviet Union, South Africa, and no doubt many other countries were all deeply implicated in developing programs for biological warfare; the Japanese were by no means alone in this aberration.

Since the war, the media have exposed experiments on prisoners, babies, and patients in psychiatric hospitals that took place in Japan without consent until the mid 1950s. Among more recent incidents to come to light was the involuntary subjection of members of the Japanese Self-Defense Force to experiments involving the bacterium shigella. In May 1985, two hundred hospitalized children were made into experimental subjects for an unapproved encephalitis vaccine without the consent of their parents. From 1987 to 1989, a genetically modified influenza vaccine was tested on about forty hospitalized children, again without their parents' permission. These activities took place despite Japanese endorsement of international treaties against involuntary human experimentation (Harris 1994).[7]

In Japan, the media and various activists now work to make sure that citizens are alerted to such events. Media coverage of the Manchurian wartime atrocities, of doctors procuring organs from patients when consent has not been given, and of experiments on human subjects carried out without consent contribute enormously to the widespread distrust of the medical profession and unwillingness to cooperate with organ donation.

In both Germany and Japan there has been extensive public opposition to recognition of brain death as the end of human life. In Germany, concern is almost certainly motivated by the racial hygiene programs in the early part of the twentieth century that culminated in systematized eugenics and the Holocaust (Hogle 1999). In Japan, resistance arising from the horror of the atrocities in Manchuria is compounded by memories of Hiroshima and Nagasaki. Victims of the bombs were made into

---

7. Similar incidents happen in virtually all countries with competitive scientific programs (British Medical Association 1992).

unwitting research subjects by both American and Japanese doctors, and they were often refused medical care by the same researchers (Todeschini 1999). There seems little doubt that public antipathy to anything that smacks of human experimentation in Japan is fueled by memories of the recent past.[8]

When the profound distrust on the part of many Japanese about the motives of medical science and the practices of certain doctors is coupled with the short history of body commodification in that country, it is not surprising that the public resists the idea of organ donation. Added to these concerns are worries about respect for the recently deceased and improper tampering with their bodies, serious doubts that brain death represents human death, and the fact that many people do not locate "person" in the brain. In light of these diverse influences, the brain-death problem begins to appear inevitable. It is, moreover, evident that the metaphor of the "gift of life" is not appropriate in Japan. Not only has a resistance to the concept of brain death inhibited organ procurement, but many Japanese are also reluctant to make "gifts" of the organs of their deceased relatives to unknown others.

8. Germany has exhibited much more public opposition to genetic engineering and to the genetic screening and testing of human populations than has Japan. This type of technology appears less tainted to many Japanese, it seems, and the possibility of manipulating reproduction and producing "perfect" babies through biomedical technologies is welcomed in some quarters (Lock 1998a).

A COURT ORDER

K'aila was born in June 1989 near the Slave River in northern Alberta, in tranquil surroundings with neither telephones nor piped water. During most of his eleven-month life he was the unknowing center of a disturbing controversy. His mother, Lesley Paulette, a midwife, has written about his story and recounted it in public. Her hope is that we may learn from it.

K'aila, whose name means "willow tip" in the Chipewayan language, gave every sign of good health at his birth, although his mother noticed early on that he frequently showed spontaneous bruising. She wondered at the time if this could be a premonition of the future. Their local doctor, after checking the baby, insisted that there was nothing particularly unusual about K'aila's health, even though the baby was somewhat jaundiced. Nevertheless, two months after K'aila's birth, with the doctor's support, his parents took him to a hospital in Edmonton, where his liver function was checked. Following some inconclusive test results, K'aila was admitted to hospital and submitted to a further battery of blood tests. The final report stated that although the liver was slightly enlarged, no identifiable liver disease could be found.

In mid-September, when K'aila was three months old, his father François, a former Dene chief, received an unexpected phone call in his office from a doctor in Edmonton. He informed François that K'aila's medical records indicated that K'aila had one of two very serious liver diseases—either biliary atresia or giant cell hepatitis—and that he would in all likelihood require a liver transplant if he was to live for more than one

or two years. The family were, of course, appalled; Lesley was reminded
of her premonition. The doctor asked them to bring K'aila back to Edmonton at once. Later that day, without discussing anything directly
with K'aila's parents, he called their local physician (who was out at the
time and whose wife took the call) and prescribed phenobarbital, with
instructions to administer it right away.

When Lesley met the Edmonton doctor, Adrian Jones, for the first
time, he explained to her the effects of the two deadly diseases. He was
certain K'aila had one, but was not sure which. He made it clear that
there was no cure for either. Lesley returned home to discuss the situation with her husband and then informed the doctor that she and her
husband were doubtful that a transplant was the right choice. Adrian
Jones responded by telling them about one of his patients whose mother
was a Jehovah's Witness. Jones had the child made a ward of the court
to ensure permission for treatment. He intimated that the courts would
in all likelihood perceive K'aila's case as similar.

Adrian Jones informed the Paulettes that the survival rates from liver
transplants for end-stage liver disease approached 80 to 85 percent. He
pointed out that it would be difficult, however, to procure the small liver
needed for a baby and added that he would wait until K'aila was very
ill before doing the surgery, because there was always some chance of
losing the infant as a result of the operation.

By the end of January, K'aila was beginning to show signs of distress
and becoming anemic. His parents took him back to the University Hospital in Edmonton. K'aila's father asked Jones how long he estimated
the baby would live; the doctor responded, "About three months." He
suggested that they prepare right away to travel across the country to
London, Ontario, where K'aila would be assessed for a transplant and
undergo the operation as soon as an organ became available.

Lesley, writing about the family ordeal a year or two later, does not
doubt that Adrian Jones acted in what he believed was K'aila's best
interests, but she and her husband, while they agonized over what to
do, arrived at a very different perspective. They had an overwhelming
sense that a transplant would be "unnatural." They believed that they
would be playing God if they went ahead with the operation, and that
they "would run the risk of violating K'aila's spiritual as well as physical
identity" (1993:14). Lesley thinks that Adrian Jones never understood
these feelings, even though she tried to explain them, and she and her
husband both grew to fear Jones as their difference of opinion became
evident.

As the months went by, Lesley's spiritual convictions were supplemented by her increasing knowledge about transplant medicine. The family consulted with two other families whose children had received liver transplants. One of these children had an ear infection that had been out of control for over a year, destroying the eardrum. Everyone concerned agreed that the child's medications were in some way implicated.

Lesley's mind was made up by an almost casual comment by a nurse's aide about the side effects of long-term use of immunosuppressant drugs, especially in babies. Only then did Lesley understand what she had never been told by the doctor: that organ rejection has to be averted through the use of powerful immunosuppressants, taken not just for a few months after surgery but for life. Immunosuppressants leave the body vulnerable to infections, bacterial and viral. Chicken pox can be fatal. In addition, these drugs can cause progressive damage to the kidneys, elevated blood cholesterol, increased hairiness (creating enormous psychological and social problems for children), and many other side effects. The risk of cancer is increased tenfold in young children taking immunosuppressants. When pressed, Adrian Jones explained most of these side effects, although not the increased cancer risk. He also acknowledged that death from the disease that K'aila had is relatively painless.

Lesley also found out that official reports on transplant survival rates do not agree. Some sources estimate survival at 70 to 75 percent and often even lower for infants; Adrian Jones had given her the best possible estimates. Then Lesley learned that these percentages are for one year only.[1] Five years after surgery, the survival rate is 60 to 65 percent. The survival rates for infants beyond that time are not well-documented, but they decline significantly.

Even after clarification of these discrepancies and gaps in information, Adrian Jones insisted that he would have to act in what he perceived to be the child's best interests; if Lesley and François did not consent to the transplant, he would allege neglect on their part to Social Services. However, Lesley and François concluded that they "would be doing violence" to K'aila if they went ahead with the surgery: "He would have to live in a state of coercion for the rest of his life, his little body a veritable battleground for antigens, antibodies, immunosuppressants, viral and bacterial agents, antibiotics, cancers, assorted chemo-

---

1. Survival rates have improved over the past decade, but complications remain common in infants.

therapies and other unforeseeable yet continual problems" (Paulette 1993:16). In the end, the Paulettes refused to have their son considered for a transplant. Lesley recalls that in reaching their decision they looked at K'aila and wondered what he would want for himself. She and François were concerned above all that they should not go ahead with the operation simply for their own sakes—because they could not bear to lose K'aila. They were overwhelmed by sadness at the thought of letting him go, but they came to believe that K'aila supported their decision, that it was what he would have chosen.

The Paulettes believed that Adrian Jones saw their refusal as a challenge to his professional integrity. He informed them that if K'aila had been a "white" child, he would have had him taken into custodial care right away, but he admitted that he was "leery" about a court battle because he could be seen as trying to "impose his standards on Indian people." Nevertheless, Jones eventually reported the Paulettes to the Department of Social Services of the province of Alberta. As François said on the television program *Man Alive,* "We knew then that Social Services and the police could come at any time to take our baby away." The only way to avoid this catastrophe was to leave the province. Through Lesley's father, a retired academic in Montreal, the Paulettes found a pediatric gastroenterologist in Saskatchewan, Garth Bruce, who agreed to care for K'aila even though they had declined to go ahead with a transplant. They supplemented his services with indigenous medical care to keep their baby as comfortable as possible.

Social Services in Alberta contacted the agency in Saskatchewan, alleging that K'aila was being denied essential care and asking that the child be apprehended immediately. A social worker arrived on the Poundmaker Reservation where the Paulettes were staying. She warned them that it was within her power to take K'aila away, but that she did not plan to do so as yet. The court hearing, at which both Lesley and François testified, took place in mid-April. Ultimately, the court upheld the position of the parents, and the Crown did not appeal. In the case summary, the judge stated: "There is considerable uncertainty as to the future quality of life for a 'successful' recipient. There is no real way to look into the future to determine what may be visited upon this child. The 'successful' candidate may be committed to a life of prolonged suffering." Testimony was given by Richard Hamilton, a senior physician who had formerly been the teacher of both Adrian Jones and Garth Bruce. Hamilton indicated that a transplant recipient cannot expect to live a "full, normal, active life" and added that in his opinion the parents' views warranted respect, particularly because "a transplant is a major operative procedure with very significant, intense post-operative care required, and a significant mortality." He said that he himself would not be critical of any parents who made a caring and informed decision to withhold consent for a transplant. Garth Bruce gave very similar testimony and added an account of his experience with another infant. The child was seven months old at the time of the liver transplant, had been in a coma ever since, was being kept alive by tube feeding, and had multiple seizures every day because of severe brain damage he suffered prior to the surgery. The statement of a third doctor in support of Hamilton and Bruce added further doubts as to whether liver transplants are necessarily in infants' best interests (*Saskatchewan v. Paulette*, F.).

The judge concluded that although things may change in the future, given the degree of uncertainty at the time, it would be inappropriate for the state to compel the child to undergo a transplant. In other words, the parents were not neglectful of their child in any way—quite the contrary—and a decision to participate in or refuse transplant surgery cannot be based solely on medical grounds. Social Services Saskatchewan decided not to appeal the provincial court decision.

Lesley writes of what happened later:

> In the weeks that followed, K'aila's body grew weaker and more frail, yet his spirit seemed to grow immense. He had a powerful way about him that touched everyone who met him. Sick as he was, he loved to eat, to dance and to spend time in the company of good friends. He taught us by example to enjoy each day as it came, and when we became downhearted he uplifted us with his courage and quiet will. In his own way he reassured us and let us know that everything would be alright.
>
> On the evening of May 27, 1990, after a thanksgiving feast, K'aila died suddenly and quietly at home at the age of 11 months. As he was taken gently from us, we held him in our arms and talked and sang to him. . . . In the moment that he left, my heart broke wide open and I experienced a love and sense of inner peace that I had never known before.
>
> (Paulette 1993:17)

The Paulettes still had to face one more round of heartless indifference to their plight. A doctor who lived near the Poundmaker Reservation, where K'aila died, refused to sign the death certificate because he was aware that the case was controversial. Lesley was obliged to drive the body of her baby hundreds of miles to Saskatoon to procure a death certificate from a colleague of Garth Bruce.

A year or two later, when I asked K'aila's mother and grandfather if I might recount this story, they simply said, "K'aila continues his work."

The Social Life
of Human Organs

In his celebrated book *Essai sur le Don* (The gift), Marcel Mauss argues
that gifts, like commodities, must be understood as part of an economy
of social exchange. In premodern society, Mauss concluded, all gifts
carry reciprocal expectations, and gift exchange is a means of establishing lifelong commitments that create the structure of social institutions
and their hierarchies (1990). Mauss argued that individuals in effect give
away a modicum of themselves with a gift, an animated "essence" that
should, therefore, be returned in kind (1990:10).

The idea of a gift economy has been all but lost in contemporary
society; the word *gift* is used today fairly interchangeably with *present*,
to which we attach no weighty meanings. But organs, donated as "gifts,"
cannot be divested of their social meanings as easily as the transplant
world would have us believe.

With Mary Douglas (1990), Annette Weiner (1992), and others in
different contexts, I believe no clear demarcation can be made between
altruism, gift giving, and commodification. Whether body tissues and
organs can be counted as alienable in the first place, and under what
circumstances they may enter into systems of exchange, must be examined in context. "Donation" of human body parts is not necessarily
altruistic (and in any case the very concept of altruism and what it means
merit scrutiny). Moreover, donations are rarely made without expectations of a return (Lock 2000). In Japan, where people are finely tuned
to the reciprocal obligations of gift giving, a deeply entrenched moral

economy of exchange has acted as yet one more deterrent to the donation of organs. This deterrent strengthens skepticism about the concept
of brain death and the reasons for its invention and also creates discomfort about the possible transfer of an animated essence with body parts.
In North America, too, even in the absence of such an economy of formalized reciprocal exchange, organs represent much more than spare
parts.

An Economy of Gifts

Since the mid-1950s the metaphor of the "gift of life" has been used
with considerable success to promote organ donation in both Europe
and North America (Fox and Swazey 1992). But what kind of a "gift"
are human tissue and organs? Richard Titmuss, writing about blood
donation when transplant technology was still at the experimental stage,
posed a fundamental question: "Why give to strangers?" Categorically
opposed to the sale of blood, Titmuss argues that contemporary society
is strengthened when individuals exercise the moral choice to give to
strangers in nonmonetary form; he believes policies on blood donation
should encourage this form of social solidarity (1971).

When considering donation of blood and organs, numerous commentators, Titmuss included, return to the work of Mauss, who believed
that his theory of the gift has relevance for contemporary society (Mauss
1990:68). Mauss, Bronislaw Malinowski (1922), Titmuss, and numerous other thinkers who have written about systems of exchange believe
that an unbridgeable gulf exists between reciprocal gift exchange and
exchange in the modern market. Mauss, for one, exhibits nostalgia for
premodern solidarity. One assumption built into this dichotomy is that,
unlike premodern societies, the contemporary economic system is a rational endeavor, free of cultural constraints. However, research into
economies of exchange has shown that the imposition of a capitalist
economy does not replace a preexisting system of reciprocal exchange;
rather, pluralism results (Thomas 1991; Weiss 1996). Nicholas Thomas
argues for a "promiscuity" of objects, meaning that they may be assigned more than one value and have several meanings associated with
them, depending on the specific circumstances and the vantage of participants. In the hands of some people, certain objects are simply disposable things-in-themselves; but the same objects in the hands of others
may be imbued with social meaning. Something of this sort clearly happens in organ donation.

Donation of human organs is not, of course, of the same order as giving twenty dollars to UNICEF. It must first be determined whether human organs are alienable, either as gifts or for the market. The argument of the anthropologist Igor Kopytoff, that objects can be thought of as having "social lives," is useful here (1986). If less attention is paid to the objects themselves, and more to the systems and sequences of exchange—thus inserting a time dimension into the analysis—the shifting value of objects becomes evident as they change through time and space. At one moment objects may be understood as inalienable, even as sacred, but later they may gain commodity status and then occasionally return to their former status, or become only partially alienable under specific circumstances.

In Kopytoff's phrase, then, objects have a "life history": one that reflects local desire, demands, and specific social situations (including whether technologies exist to transform human materials into living substitutes). These life histories are intimately related to relationships of power (blood and kidneys are sold almost exclusively by those economically compelled to do so). Furthermore, symbolic meanings are crucial to the way in which objects are valued: in North America, for example, sperm donors are routinely paid, but advertisements by women selling their eggs have caused public offense. The commodity status of things is contestable and subject to revision.

Human body parts have been commodified for hundreds of years as religious relics, talismans, medication, and so on, but only in the last fifty years have they gained value as living substitutes. Today, the commodification of body parts is a vast global enterprise; human tissues and organs are scarce, and enormous pressures are exerted to persuade the public to allow their body parts to be put to use, either for the benefit of sick individuals or indirectly, in the name of scientific advancement (Lock 1999; Machado 1998).

The "gift" of organ donation can perhaps be understood as an act of charity—a benevolent act to assist people urgently in need. Charity is, of course, a fundamental Christian virtue, a moral position associated with selflessness, fellowship, and a concern for others. In practice, however, it has very often taken the form of benevolent donations from the wealthy to the poor. In eighteenth- and nineteenth-century Europe, the free distribution of goods from the rich to the needy, often their employees, became routine and disposed of almost all sentiment of communal fellowship associated with charitable giving. Today it is the plight of individuals in the Third World and heroic airdrops of food and medicine that make news. But the "needy" often resent being turned into recipients of charity (Douglas 1990:vii), for they find it both condescending and humiliating. In any case, many are well aware that their marginalized position is the direct result of exploitation by institutions and individuals related to those that are praised for their life-saving donations.

Organ donation is not, in my estimation, associated with this calculated charity of modernity but rather with the biblical sense of charity. Moreover, the charitable act is carried out by the family rather than the donor. People waiting for organs are described as being "in need," and many of them will die without a transplant. However, individuals who sign donor cards may place little value on their own dead bodies; and so their act costs them little. Nor is it especially selfless, given that they will be irreversibly unconscious at the time of the procurement. Families, on the other hand, are thrown into confusion by a traumatic death; they must face up to the ambiguities of the brain-dead body, and in this state of shock they must make a decision they will live with for the rest of their lives. These decisions do not emerge from everyday experience (Kaufman 2000:79). Surely it is these acts that are charitable, selfless, and filled with generosity for unknown others?

It was assumed from the outset in North America that gifts of organs would be "free" gifts, that is charitable donations grounded in altruism. Altruism, so often claimed to be the reason for organ donation, is, in effect, charity made modern. Auguste Comte created the concept at the end of the last century in opposition to egoism, a condition that he feared would destroy the tattered remnants of solidarity in urbanized, modernizing society. Altruism, deliberately stripped of any religious connotation, is a thoroughly secularized form of charity that expects no direct return; however, the knowledge that society, and the unknown individuals who constitute it, will benefit, may substitute for any material reciprocity.

Use of the "gift" metaphor has had the effect of representing the act as a personal choice—one that "fits" with a dominant ideology in North America of having the right to dispose of one's property as one wishes. Some potential donors assumed that they would be able to name, if not an individual, then at least the ethnic group to which the organ should go. But altruism, in contrast to gifts, is not directed toward individuals. Altruism is a modern form of fellowship building.

Confusion multiplies because, where bodies do not "belong" to individuals, as is the case in Japan, individuals do not necessarily have the "right" to choose to donate their bodies. This is why families are still able to veto donation in Japan.

Organs as Things

Mixed metaphors associated with human organs encourage confusion about their worth. On the one hand, the language of medicine insists that human body parts are material entities, devoid of identity whether located in donors or recipients. However, in the rhetoric promoting donation, organs are animated with a life force, and donor families are not discouraged from thinking of their relatives as "living on" in the bodies of recipients. Organ donation is very often understood as creating meaning out of a senseless, accidental, horrifying death—a technological path to transcendence. All that donor families can hope for in the way of a return gift for this selfless act, however, is a letter of heartfelt thanks, often belated, written anonymously, and delivered through the local transplant coordination service with all identifying features deleted. Any thought of creating tangible human ties through this act is nipped in the bud. Reciprocity is reduced to an act of the imagination, and donors must be content with the thought that should they or their families ever need an organ, then perhaps another family will be willing to donate to them.

Similarly, many recipients experience a frustrated sense of obligation toward the family of the donor for the extraordinary act of benevolence that has brought them back from the brink of death (Fox and Swazey 1978, 1992; Simmons et al. 1987; Sharp 1995). The "tyranny of the gift" has been well documented in the transplant world (Fox 1978: 1168), but recipients' curiosity about the donor stems not merely from a desire to settle accounts. Donated organs represent much more than mere biological organs; the life with which they are animated is experienced by recipients as personified, and this agency manifests itself in some surprising ways.

Lingering Animism

I recently spoke with a heart transplant surgeon about a debate taking place in several American states as to whether prisoners on death row should be able to offer their organs for transplant. The idea is that condemned prisoners should be allowed to make a "gift" to society. Perhaps prisoners with religious beliefs may even go straight to heaven.

This surgeon was uncomfortable about the idea of organ donations from death-row prisoners not so much because of the highly question-able ethics (can one make an "informed choice" in such circumstances?) as at the idea of receiving the heart of a murderer. He said to me, with some embarrassment, "I wouldn't like to have a murderer's heart put into my body," then added hastily, glancing at my tape recorder and trying to make a joke out of the situation, "I might find myself starting to change."

Many organ recipients worry about the gender, ethnicity, skin color, personality, and social status of their donors, and many believe that their mode of being-in-the-world is radically changed after they receive a do-nated organ. That some surgeons also think this way suggests that fetish-ism is doubly at work, even in the materially oriented world of biomed-icine. Marx argued that the fetishism of commodified objects—their objectification as things-in-themselves—disguises the relations among individuals involved in the production and consumption of those com-modities. In theory, this is the way human organs are understood in the transplant world, and anonymous donation is designed to create objec-tivity. But fetishism in its original sense, the animation of objects with magical or religious power—closer to what Mauss suggests happens with gift exchange—is clearly at work as well. Body parts remain infused with life and even personality. Contradictions are rife. Once an organ is procured and transplanted, the recipient is severely reprimanded, even thought of as exhibiting pathology, if he attributes this life-saving organ with animistic qualities (Sharp 1995).

Among thirty organ recipients I interviewed in Montreal in 1996, just under half are very matter-of-fact about the organs they have received. These people insist that after a few months they ceased to be concerned about the source of the new organ and resumed their lives as best they could, although their routines were disrupted by a massive regimen of daily medications. However, the other recipients produced emotionally charged accounts of their donors (about whom they actually knew very little), the particular organ they had received, and often about their own transformed identities.

Yasmin Rizk is a first-generation immigrant from Europe who had a major heart problem that had been misdiagnosed over many months.[1]

---

1. The names I give for all those interviewed are pseudonyms. Of the four women I interviewed who had received heart transplants, three reported that they had been mis-diagnosed for several months or more before the severity of the problem was recognized.

(At one of her trips to the hospital, she recalls, "The doctor threw the curtain back and said in an aside to the nurse, 'Goddamn women in their forties, it's menopause, menopause, menopause.'") She told me, "Three different doctors, including my own family physician, and heart problems run in my family, and they still took months to recognize that I had a serious problem. . . . I had to have a heart attack right in the doctor's office before something was done." Once the severity of her condition was recognized, Yasmin received a heart transplant without enduring a long wait. She has appeared on Oprah Winfrey's television show to talk about the experience, and she claims, one year later, that she feels "fantastic." When asked how she felt about the donor, she replied, "I thought about who the heart had come from just for a little while, but I don't any more. I'm getting more out of life than I ever did, and I'm not going to die at a young age, I know I'm not." She considered writing a letter of thanks to the donor family, but decided in the end that they would probably want to forget about their sad experience and that a letter would do nothing to help them.

Forty-one-year-old Stefan Rivet, doing well five years after a kidney transplant, says:

I heard about the donor, even though I wasn't supposed to. It was a woman between twenty and twenty-five. She was in a car accident. You know, don't you, that you can't meet the family because the doctors think it would be too emotional? But I wrote a letter to them, it must have been a terrible time for them, and I wanted to thank them.

Did you find it hard to write that letter?

No, no, it wasn't hard for me. Like saying "thank you" to someone if they do something for you, that's just the way it was.

Did you feel at all strange because it was a woman's kidney?

No. At first you wonder how could a female kidney work in a man. You think about it. But once the doctor tells you that it works exactly the same in men and women, you don't question things any more. It doesn't bug me. I have my kidney, and I can live, that's all you really worry about.

When I first woke up in hospital, I was worried. Of course, I didn't know whose kidney it was then, all you know is that there's a strange organ in there and you hope that it works; you don't want anything to go wrong. After a while though, you adapt and you stop thinking about it, except that it's really important to take the pills. I just say now that it's my second life.

.   .   .

Lithuanian by birth, Juo Dilys has lived most of his sixty-seven years in Montreal. He says that he knows nothing about the donor of his new heart, sewn into place five years before the interview. He wrote a thank-you letter to the donor family, and his wife also wrote one and delivered both letters personally to the transplant coordinating office. Apparently the Dilyses expected a reply from the donor family, even though it is not customarily permitted. "We didn't hear anything at all, and now we don't know if they've accepted the letters with a good understanding or not. Perhaps they're still grieving, we don't know. Maybe they just want to forget." Then, after a small pause, Juo Dilys adds:

Anyway, I don't want to develop a relationship with them, I would feel uncomfortable about that. I don't think of it as a donated heart any more now—it's *my* heart. This is the way I look at it. When you stop to think about it, it's sad to say that I'm alive because of another person's death, but that person was dead before they took the heart out. I don't know what caused that death—a traffic accident, a gunshot wound, some sort of disease. But I was lucky.

Did it feel strange at first, having someone else's heart inside you?
No, not for me. The heart is just a pump.

.   .   .

Ellen Biron is a Christian who grew up in Lebanon and then immigrated to Montreal with her husband ten years ago. She had a heart transplant when she was thirty years old, exactly five years before I interviewed her. She was hesitant about having the operation, hoping that her heart might somehow recover, but once her mind was made up she did not have to wait long for a suitable donor, and she has never regretted going ahead with the surgery. She describes the operation as easy, with a hospital stay of only ten days and not much pain afterward.

I know that the donor was a girl, she was seventeen years old, a young girl.

Did you send a letter to the family?
No. Like some people warned me, it can be hard to do that. I felt sometimes I wanted to write a letter, and then other times I thought,

no, just leave it alone, you have your own family, you have to take care of them, focus on that. It's done. Accept it. I feel really good now—that's it.

. . .

In contrast to these recipients, many others undergo a dramatic transformative experience (see also Sharp 1995). One such was Katherine White, who received a kidney transplant in 1982, and then in 1994, after that kidney failed and her liver was also in jeopardy, a double transplant of a liver and a kidney. Six months after surgery, she said:

I have no idea who the donor was, all I know is that both the kidney and liver came from one person because you can't survive if they put organs from two different people into you at once—your body would never be able to deal with it. I wrote a thank-you note right away that I gave to the nurse. But they don't like you to know who it is, sometimes people feel that their child has been reborn in you and they want to make close contact. That could lead to problems. I still think of it as a different person inside me—yes I do, still. It's not all of me, and it's not all this other person either. Actually, I might like some contact with the donor family . . .

You know, I never liked cheese and stuff like that, and some people think I'm joking, but all of a sudden I couldn't stop eating Kraft slices—that was after the first kidney. This time around, the first thing I did was to eat chocolate. I have a craving for chocolate, and now I eat some every day. It's driving me crazy because I'm not a chocolate fanatic. So maybe this person who gave me the liver was a chocaholic?! It's funny like that, and some of the doctors say it's the drugs that do things to you. I'm certainly moody these days. You do change whether you like it or not. I can't say that I'm the same person I was, but in a way I think that I'm a better person.

You know, sometimes I feel as if I'm pregnant, as if I'm giving birth to somebody. I don't know what it is really, but there's another life inside of me, and I'm actually storing this life, and it makes me feel fantastic. It's weird, I constantly think of that other person, the donor . . . but I know a lot of people who receive organs don't think about the donors at all.

A while ago I saw a TV program about Russia, and it seemed as though they were actually killing children in orphanages to take out their eyes and other organs. This disturbed me no end. I hope to God it's not really like that. My parents and my uncles all thought I shouldn't have a transplant, they said you can't be sure that the patient is really dead. Brain-dead is not dead, they said. But I know that's not right. I had a friend a few years back who had a bad fall off a bicycle and her husband donated her organs. Once you're brain-dead, that's it.

What do you think happens when people die?

I hope I go to heaven! I don't believe in resurrection, but I do believe in a heaven and hell and an in-between, you know? I think there's a person up there who knows that I'm carrying a part of her around with me. I always think there's somebody watching me . . . but you know, I don't *really* believe in religion . . . I really don't. In a way I wish I could have a pig's liver or kidney—it would be much simpler then.

.   .   .

Now in his fifties, George Papadopoulos, an immigrant from Greece, had a kidney transplant twenty-three years ago, and has had no serious health trouble since. He says that he changed a great deal after the transplant, and that never a day goes by but that he thinks briefly about the woman who was the donor: "I never had any idea who she was. I wanted so much to help her family, but no way, they wouldn't let me do anything. But I changed after the transplant. I care about people more, and I care more about myself and my wife too."

A nurse, Elizabeth McLean, originally from Guyana, received a kidney two years prior to the interview. She says that she badly wanted to know who her donor was but that no one would tell her anything.

At first I was a bit happy and a bit sad. I was happy because I felt much better, but on the other hand I kept wondering if it was a child had died. It took me a long time to get used to the idea of having someone else's kidney inside me, even though I am a nurse. Now I'm just thankful, but it still comes back in flashes, like a daydream sometimes, wondering, wondering who it was.

Do you feel now that the kidney is completely part of your body?

Oh yes, it's part of me—it's me, it's me. I even call it my baby! I take so much care, I feel protective, it's a really special part of me. You know, at first, when I went through periods of rejection, I would pray about it. I knew it was in the Father's hands, but I felt I must be responsible for this other person's kidney.

.   .   .

Forty-four-year-old Marie Laplante, who had a heart transplant two years before I interviewed her, took some time to make up her mind before putting herself on the waiting list. She says:

I had spiritually based objections. I thought, "You come into this world whole, I think you should leave with all the same parts." I kept thinking, "Does God really approve of this?" Is it the right thing to do, it is morally right to mutilate another's body?

Are you a practicing Christian?
Yes. I go to church. I did a lot of soul searching. I went to talk to a couple of priests, and one of them was very understanding about my dilemma, but he told me about a friend of his who had had a transplant and how that had worked out fine.

So you decided to go through with it?
Yes. I found out in the end that it was a woman donor from Quebec City in her early thirties. She'd had a brain hemorrhage—a blood vessel had burst in her brain—that was a bit of a shock when I heard that. I have children; chances are she has too. What's going to happen to them? You do feel a sense of guilt, you can't help that. You know, some people when they're waiting for an organ to turn up for them, they keep their eye on the newspapers every day to follow up on car accidents, and they read the obituary columns—it's bad.

Did you write a letter to the family?
I wrote the letter and I never sent it. I could never seem to get it right. I wrote reams, and then I thought, "Are these people going to want to hear this from me?" The transplant people said I shouldn't worry about writing it right away, but I kept trying and trying. I kept a bit of a journal too. I just couldn't decide if I would be opening up new wounds for those people or not. I didn't know what was for the best. You feel like you're inflicting pain again on people who already have pain. You can never get away from this—that's for sure. If it's any other kind of surgery, it heals and it's finished. But this is never finished.

You know, I can understand those people in Japan that you told me about, I'm sure my feelings are pretty close to theirs. I had a kind of a resistance all right, a need to keep the body whole. I saw a psychiatrist afterwards once or twice. He said I was mourning for the loss of my old heart and that I hadn't learnt to accept the new one because I kept calling it "It"!

I never said then that it was my heart, and I won't say it even now, because it doesn't feel like it totally belongs to me. It's on loan. I know how those Japanese feel, but it's terrible that they miss out on having transplants. That shouldn't happen because when a person's brain dead, they're dead . . . but I still have trouble with this, and I do think spiritually that we are more whole than we allow ourselves to think we are. We're not just bits and pieces. So there's really no heart transplants at all in Japan? Do you think the next generation might overcome that?

Maybe. I think a good number will, and they'll start donating when it's made legal in a year or two.[2] So far, the only Japanese who've had heart transplants have had to go overseas to get it.

That must be incredibly expensive. If I'd had to pay, then we'd have had to sell our house and our car and everything. My sister-in-law was Japanese, so I was a bit aware of these things already, but they're divorced now.

Life on a Roller Coaster

One day I received a call from a psychiatrist who works at a local hospital and does liaison work with a transplant unit. Having heard that I was interviewing transplant patients, he suggested that we get together and talk, and perhaps even design a research project. A few days later I took my lunch to the psychiatrist's office. During our conversation, Robert Wilson proved to be a thoughtful man:

I'm very influenced by Friedrich Schiller's ideas about body image. I think it's very relevant to what transplant patients go through. The mind and body are always interrelated in ways that we don't understand, and so the transplant becomes, in effect, a subset of other major concerns that have been going on with the patient, sometimes over their whole life. Patients in the initial phase after a transplant have a mixture of emotions, but often for a while euphoria and high expectations dominate. Not long after that, they get depressed, and they sort of come back down to earth. And then they realize, "OK, I'm reborn, but unfortunately I'm reborn back on earth!"

And so it's back to everyday life with all its troubles?

Exactly. It's, sure, I have my body back, but now I have back all the problems that I had all the time anyway. . . . For a long time, sometimes

2. This interview took place before the Organ Transplant Law was passed in Japan.

up to six months or a year, people can have big swings between euphoria and depression. They're on a roller coaster. Along the way they tend to go over things in their own minds, quite consciously, about the new organ. They're self-conscious about telling me this sort of this thing. Some of them are really embarrassed, but once they feel it's safe to talk then they say: "Oh yes, I talk to it every morning. I get up and I say, 'Oh, hi.'" And then I ask, "What do you call it?" And they're always surprised when I ask that, because they didn't think anyone else had given their organ a name! They've given it a persona, a story, and they have a whole relationship with it. And I think this repeats what we do as kids when we first understand that we have and are a body. What we do is we anthropomorphize different parts of ourselves, we get to know ourselves, but eventually we don't think about it any more—we are at peace with ourselves, more or less. This is what transplant patients do. They talk with their new organ, they try to get in touch with it, they think about it, they tell little stories about it, and exchange dialogues with it, they strike deals with it, and then after a while they don't give a damn about it! They just make their peace, and they carry on their lives with that all in the background. When that works well you see a comfortable patient. When it doesn't work, then you see a lot of depression.

Because patients don't know their donors, doesn't this leave a lot of room for the imagination to go a little wild? Doesn't this make it harder to become a "comfortable" patient?

Yes, but I don't know if that's good or bad. Remember, what these patients are thinking is *all* in the imagination, no matter where the organ came from.

But you just told me about the Anglo Protestant adolescent who had a kidney from an Italian, and what happened to him.

Yes, he did feel more laissez-faire, and he thought he liked garlic for the first time. And men who get kidneys from women often feel feminized—although I haven't noticed a problem the other way around. But the point is that it doesn't matter how closely the image corresponds to reality—it's the image that counts. Like this particular eighteen-year-old who felt he was Italian, he thought he was making his body into a good home for an Italian. He wanted the kidney to be happy, so he struck a deal with it, mostly unconsciously. That's good. If you can't strike a deal, then I think you're at much higher risk for immunological rejection. Often after a transplant there's a series of mild rejections. I bet this reflects closely what's going on in the patient's mind. It's a leap—not very scientific yet—but it's a wonderfully enticing idea.

Do you think some patients might be ambivalent about the "gift" they have received? Some patients might be wondering about whether brain death is death or something like that, and that might influence episodes of rejection?

You know, it's difficult to be ambivalent about a gift when that gift is connected to your survival. If you don't want the gift, then you have to accept that you're dying. Maybe they do worry about where the organ comes from sometimes, but they don't talk about that to me; maybe they just can't say it. But it's clear that patients do try to become what they think the donor was like. This has been observed by everyone. There is no doubt that there's a shift in the sense of self.

Ties That Bind: Gift Giving and Reciprocity

Gift giving remains central to social solidarity in Japan, and perhaps these activities can be thought of as part of the collage of postmodernity in that country. The very word for gift giving, *zōtō,* connotes a formal reciprocity. Ideally, when a family moves to a new location, small presents are distributed to the nearby neighbors to set social relations on the right footing. Groups of neighbors participate together in wakes and funerals and make appropriate monetary donations for funeral expenses, as well as prepare and serve food at the reception after a funeral service. Social activities such as these foster relationships known as *tsukiai*—ties that are cultivated out of obligation, but with an awareness that reciprocity will be forthcoming when needed.

Both at New Year and in the middle of the year, gifts are sent to individuals, families, professionals, companies, and organizations to whom one is indebted. These gifts, often lavish these days, are usually household items such as oil, tea, meat, fruit, cakes, and sake, all elaborately and appropriately wrapped. In addition, gifts may be given for particular services rendered during the year, including medical treatment. This complex system of gift exchange requires an acute sensitivity to the obligations and the reciprocal worth embodied in a gift, and Japanese believe that foreigners simply do not understand how to engage appropriately in this economy of exchange. Today people also give presents for occasions such as birthdays, anniversaries, and Valentine's Day.

Not surprisingly, the metaphor of the "gift of life" has simply not taken root in Japan. One or two books published in Japanese make use of the awkward, deliberately created term *seimei no okurimono*—literally "the gift of life"—but this sounds artificial and simply cannot carry the metaphorical load associated with it in English. Advertising designed to increase organ donation makes use of the idioms of "life's relay" or "the present of love." Perhaps such idioms are in part designed to remove donations from the arena of reciprocal obligations. Following Buddhist teaching, advertising often emphasizes the relief of the suffering of others rather than the continuity of life transmitted directly from one person to another. An emergency medicine doctor told me that families considering whether to donate may briefly believe that their relative will actually "live on" in another body, but he thinks that once the immediate shock is over, no one mistakes this metaphor for reality. He feels that the "gift of life" and similar idioms suggesting a living continuity are likely to be much more effective in North America than in Japan. Like many of his medical colleagues and other Japanese commentators, this doctor believes that organ donation "fits" much better with the ethos of "Christian" cultures rather than with Japan's eclectic mix of Buddhism, Confucianism, and Shinto.

The concept of charity fares no better. The Japanese term for charity, *jizen,* created in the nineteenth century, connotes pity, and it is seen by many as a foreign concept, one associated with inequalities, cold relations, and anonymity. Although charitable giving is considered a decent, good thing to do, it is not associated with the warmth and sincerity that should infuse gift relationships. To try and rid the concept of its negative connotations, the English word *charity* has been incorporated into the charitable campaigns of community organizations.

Although the Buddhist understanding of life and death may complicate the recognition of brain death, Buddhist teaching does not oppose organ donation. Buddhism strongly supports the idea of spontaneous gift giving. A "true offering" is one that is given with pleasure, an offering from a compassionate heart "with no thought of return" (Bukkyō Dendō Kyōkai 1975). Those who work to encourage the donation of organs often use Buddhist doctrine to support their arguments (Iwasaki et al. 1990), and some point out that in Buddhist Thailand there has apparently been no resistance either to the recognition of brain death or to the donation of human organs (Ohkubo 1995).

The president of the Japan Transplant Recipients' Organization, Ohkubo Michikata, argues in an article in *Transplant Proceedings* that "in a truly mature democratic and cultured nation, the individual members should help each other in order to allow the citizens a decent life, and there should be a system in which citizens in crisis are supported by the society as a whole" (Ohkubo 1995:1452). He laments that, although Japan is a leading economic power, it has apparently not reached "social maturity" with respect to organ donation. He notes that the "spirit of mutual aid" has in the past been contained within the family and is, in his estimation, qualitatively different from the "spirit of Christian love" common to North America and Europe. However, Ohkubo believes that a willingness to help unknown others can be fostered with the dissemination of knowledge about the benefits of organ transplants.

Despite the efforts of individuals such as Ohkubo, spontaneous giving is rare when it comes to organ donation. Whether described as altruism or as a Buddhist-inspired act, donation is curbed by the measured reciprocity that is part of an economy of gift giving. Even though the new transplant law has passed, many potential donors and their families continue to feel uncomfortable about anonymous donation. Nearly half of the individuals I interviewed in Tokyo stated spontaneously that they would consider donation seriously only if it were customary to identify the recipients and a relationship could be established between the donor and recipient families. Lawyers in Japan, on the other hand, have repeatedly expressed concerns about just this eventuality, for they envision disputes over inheritance settlements.

This view affects the transplant enterprise in less direct ways as well. Doctors, themselves suspicious of the motives of many of their colleagues, have tended to reinforce the importance of personal relationships in medical care. Those relationships, part of the system of formalized exchange from which they can expect some sort of direct return, are put above the impersonal relationships required for cooperation across large segments of the medical profession and medical specialties. This makes for poor cooperation among transplant centers and contributes to the difficulty of procuring and distributing organs.

Since 1991, for example, a kidney transplant coordination center has operated in Japan, but it is well-known that those few kidneys that were procured from cadaver donors, and the even fewer obtained (illegally) from brain-dead donors, were rarely funneled through this center but rather were distributed through personal, informal networks, often inside the hospital where the organs had been procured (*Asahi Shinbun* 1991c).

The Tyranny of the Gift

Given the obligations involved with gift exchange in Japan, it would seem reasonable to surmise that potential recipients would not want to receive organs from named donors, for they would forever be indebted to the donor's family and might worry, as do some Japanese lawyers, about financial expectations of one sort or another. There can be no repayment to anonymous donors, but this situation in turn might result in guilt that could be overwhelming.

Interviews I carried out with twenty-one organ recipients in a Tokyo tertiary care hospital in 1996 suggest that, in fact, Japanese recipients do not always suffer from frustration over an inability to reciprocate.[3] All were adults who had undergone a kidney transplant. Seventeen of the procedures were living related donations: that is, a close blood relative had donated a kidney. The other recipients had received organs from brain-dead donors, all of whom were American. In three cases the patients had gone to the United States for the surgery, and in the fourth case the kidney, deemed unusable in the States because it had been procured from a seventy-year-old donor, had been imported into Japan.

Nearly a third of these recipients had been on dialysis for ten or more years—a long time by North American standards. Not surprisingly, several of them had serious, chronic health problems. All but one had entered their names on one or more hospital waiting lists in Japan, some of them years before, in the hope of receiving a kidney transplant from either a cadaver or brain-dead body, but had heard nothing at all.[4] Clearly these individuals had accepted the idea of receiving a kidney from an anonymous donor but were thwarted because so few donations are made in Japan. For most patients, even after the passing of the Organ Transplant Law, a living related donation is the only way to get off dialysis.

Only one recipient admits to having raised the question of living related donation with his family. Another young woman said that she wanted to ask her younger brother but did not dare do so. In the end, her brother took the initiative and arranged to become the donor—after establishing that he could take a month off work without any penalty other than loss of pay. In all the other cases, a relative decided to donate

3. I thank Dr. Ota Kazuo for facilitating these interviews.
4. Prior to the passing of the Organ Transplant Law, there was no central registry for patients waiting for organs in Japan.

without consulting the potential recipient; in ten out of these seventeen cases it was the recipient's mother.[5] The majority of these donors were over sixty years of age and therefore considered rather old for donation by North American standards. Three donations came from fathers, three from a younger brother, one from an elder sister, and one from an elder brother. In each of these eight cases, the mother of the patient was deceased or for some reason ineligible or unsuitable as a donor. In several instances it was clear that the father or a sibling had volunteered to be the donor and perhaps would have done so regardless of the mother's condition.

Only one respondent gave me a narrative that clearly "fitted" with my expectations about guilt in connection with anonymously donated organs procured from cadavers. This fifty-five-year-old man had been on dialysis for two years when his younger brother, who lives in Brazil, had written to say that he wanted to give him a kidney. The recipient's father was dead and his mother in her eighties, and so his brother was the only remaining possibility. The recipient told me that in Brazil people are "more open to donating organs; it's a daily event, but in Japan it's still a big deal." When asked if the relationship between the brothers had changed after the surgery, the recipient said, "Yes, I appreciate him more. I feel I have to treasure the kidney because I was the reason why my healthy brother was cut open."

Later in the interview, I asked this recipient if he had registered in Japan for a cadaver transplant. Alone among the interviewed recipients, he replied that he had not. His wife, sitting listening as we talked, interjected that her husband was resistant to receiving an organ from a stranger. I asked why this was so, and her husband replied: "I don't want another person's blood or body parts. I don't feel right about hurting another person." To which I responded, "But that person would be dead, surely," provoking the retort: "I feel he should be left alone to return to the other world—I don't want to receive something from a dead person in order to live. His organs are his, so he should go to the other world complete. I don't want to prolong my life by getting something from the dead." I then asked this man if he would himself become a donor, and he said he would have no hesitation at all. "It's only when I'm on the receiving end that I feel ill at ease (*ki ga hikeru*)."

5. Some organ recipients have received kidneys from both their parents or from a parent and a sibling. After the first kidney failed, the patient received another one from a second relative (Ohkubo 1995).

Three of the four individuals who had received kidneys from American brain-dead donors, in contrast, stated that they were opposed in principle to living related donation, even when family members had volunteered. They gave various reasons, among them that it is "too big a sacrifice to expect of family," that it is inappropriate to incur such an obligation of debt, or that to carry out surgery on a healthy body is "wrong." Two recipients said that their siblings had their own families to think of. Only one man went abroad *because* he had no relative who would make a suitable donor; the others apparently had a choice between living related and an anonymous donation from a foreigner. None of these four recipients admitted to any strange feelings about incorporating a kidney from someone who was not Japanese into their bodies, but all expressed enormous gratitude. When asked what feelings he has about having a kidney from a foreign donor, one man, who had the surgery in Boston, said "I'm just appreciative." This man did not write a letter for the donor family. He says that no one suggested that he might do so. He asked nothing about the donor, believing it better not to know anything at all.

A thirty-four-year-old woman who had received a kidney from her mother told me that she must "treasure" her mother more than ever now. She insists that she had never once thought about asking for a kidney, but her fifty-four-year-old mother had spontaneously offered to be the donor. This recipient is determined to follow all the advice given her by her doctors because things "*must* turn out well now that my healthy mother has been cut open for my sake." When asked if she had thought about going abroad for a transplant, she replied, "I *thought* about doing anything and everything, no matter where I would have to go. When you need to receive something as precious as life you're driven to extremes. Even so, if I hadn't had a kidney from my mother, I'd have hesitated to receive an organ from a stranger, but I suppose I would have done it if I'd had to." Further questioning revealed that this woman had in mind the purchasing of a kidney in the Philippines, India, or China. I then asked, "What about receiving an organ from a dead person or a brain-dead person?" She responded: "I'd be much less resistant if the organ was from a dead person. I'd be happy to receive from a person who had expressed a clear will before she died that she wants to donate. Then, I can't be held responsible for that person's condition after donation."

Further discussion revealed a great ambivalence on the part of this woman, an ambivalence that I also detected in other respondents. Living related donation encourages what in Japanese can be expressed as the "natural feelings of warmth among blood relatives," but it also brings with it an onerous responsibility. This responsibility is just bearable if the donor is one's mother—she, after all, is supposed to nurture her children without reservation—but it is usually much more difficult to bear if a father or a sibling is involved. If the donor falls ill, or if the transplant is rejected, even years later, then recipients experience overwhelming remorse and a sense of failure. Their bodies become tangible evidence of outright rejection of someone they love, who has made an unrepayable sacrifice on their behalf.

Receiving an organ from an anonymous, unrelated dead donor who had clearly stated prior willingness to donate would circumvent the burden of obligation incurred with living-related donations. That every informant but one had registered themselves to receive a cadaver organ suggests that they would have preferred not to involve a living relative. Any concerns about cutting into unknown dead bodies or incorporating a foreign organ are secondary to the worry about being directly responsible for the removal of an organ from a healthy relative, or for that matter any living donor.

When asked to reflect about organ transplants in the abstract, many Japanese visibly recoil at the idea of incorporating an organ from a stranger into their bodies. Most people simply dismiss the entire enterprise of organ transplants as "creepy" and "unnatural," but, not surprisingly, people personally confronted with death often overcome these feelings of revulsion.

Although Japanese often express a strong resistance, even an abhorrence, to the idea of receiving organs anonymously, outside the economy of gift exchange, I suspect that this reservation will be overcome as cadaver organs and organs from brain-dead bodies become more readily available. Unknown strangers, especially "outsiders" or foreigners, exist by definition beyond the world of formalized exchange, beyond the bounds of reciprocity and obligation. When it comes to survival, most individuals will no doubt accept the charity of strangers rather than endure a lifelong dread of either rejecting an organ donated by a living relative or of being the cause of suffering or impaired health in that relative. Over the years, public criticism has been aired about the violence inevitably involved with living related donation, making recipients of such organs feel ever more compromised.

Yet when one lives in a society bonded through networks of reciprocity and exchange, not only within families but in almost all forms

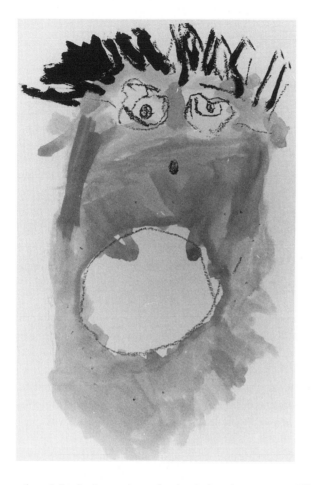

Daddy. Watercolor by Ogata Ami, done at the age of three after she received part of her father's liver as a transplant in 1992. Reproduced by permission of Japan Transplant Recipients Organization.

of social relations, then charity is hard to accept. The burden of being on the receiving end of a living related transaction is enormous; but a burden of reciprocity is potentially implicated in all organ donations.

Where anonymity is required, guilt can accrue about the debt, guilt that is by no means assuaged through public activities to raise consciousness about organ donation or by making sure that family members sign donor cards. Some people, such as the man who went to Boston for a transplant, are able to objectify the donated organ, to "strike a deal with it," as the Montreal psychiatrist put it: to turn the organ into a thing-in-itself and dissociate it from the donor. The gratitude that such recipients feel, whether they be Japanese or North American, are not then directed toward any specific individual or family. Nevertheless, this view does not preclude self-conscious reflection about debt. In part as a result of such reflections, Ohkubo Michikata has poured his energies into the creation of a fair and effective organ transplant system in Japan.

Kidney Trouble

Patients from many locations—North America, Europe, the Middle East, and Asia—have gone abroad for organ transplants over the years, presumably because they believed it was their only hope. The sole alternative, and only then for those with kidney failure, was to endure dialysis several times a week for the foreseeable future. The figures for Japan are not reliable, but it is estimated that about 200 individuals have gone overseas for liver transplants; many of these are children. Since 1984, 44 Japanese have received heart transplants and 6 have received lungs in the United States, Great Britain, or Germany (*Japan Times* 1999b). Among those who have received kidneys abroad, many have paid for an organ from a living donor, usually in the Philippines, India, China, or Taiwan. These transactions take place with the assistance of brokers, even though the buying of organs has been banned not only in Japan but in other countries.[6] Doctors find it hard to refuse care to these organ recipients on their return to Japan (Nishimura, personal communication), and they are eligible to buy immunosuppressants at minimal cost under the Japanese health care plan. Several patients who bought kidneys overseas have died from infections most probably contracted at the time of the transplant surgery (Aikawa and Kawai, personal communications).

Kidneys have also been shipped into Japan from the United States. During the first half of the 1980s, despite criticism in the Japanese media, about 100 kidneys were flown to Japan with the approval of UNOS (the United Network for Organ Sharing). These were kidneys that would have gone to waste or else had been rejected by UNOS because they were taken from elderly or diseased patients and deemed unsuitable for use in America. The resulting media coverage helped to stimulate, to a small extent, living related and cadaver organ donation within Japan itself because people felt embarrassed about this practice.

In the later 1980s exporting kidneys to Japan tailed off, in part because of improved immunosuppressants, and new techniques, fewer kidneys were deemed unusable in the United States. In 1991 a liver was

---

6. With the passing of the Organ Transplant Law in Japan, organ brokerage has been made a criminal offense.

imported into Japan from Belgium under the auspices of Euro-Transplant. Livers are much more fragile than kidneys, and even under the best conditions specialists calculate that they do not survive for more than fifteen or twenty hours outside the body. This endeavor was thus doomed from the outset; the Japanese surgeon involved had asserted that donated livers can survive for thirty hours, and also that the family was eager for the transplant. The recipient died twenty-four hours after surgery (*Asahi Shinbun* 1991c).

From 1992 until mid-1995, shipments of kidneys to Tokyo from the United States were resumed, and out of a total of eighteen kidneys (some reports say twenty-one), fourteen were transplanted into Japanese patients. It has been shown that, with careful preparation, kidneys can survive outside the human body for up to forty-eight hours, but the journey from America to Japan was slowed down by numerous bureaucratic obstacles, making the practice questionable.

By spring 1995 a National Kidney Transplant Network had been set up by the Ministry of Health and Welfare, with the express purpose of ensuring the fair distribution of organs. However, Ohkubo told me when I interviewed him in 1997 that because the network deliberately excluded transplant doctors from their organizational meetings, animosity existed between the surgeons and the network. Although the *Lancet* reported that the first transplants under the auspices of the network had taken place in early April 1995, Ohkubo states that the system was not really functioning until June.

Accounts of events at that time are conflicted. Ota Kazuo, an experienced transplant surgeon at a major Tokyo teaching hospital, was then head of the Japan Society for Transplantation and the Japan Dialysis Society. Of all Japanese doctors, he has developed the best connections with UNOS and with American transplant surgeons. In July 1995 Ota was informed about the arrival of four kidneys at Narita Airport. He insists that he immediately reported this to the Kidney Transplant Network, who responded that they were not yet in a position to deal with the organs. Under time pressure, Ota went ahead himself and transplanted the kidneys into waiting patients—his own patients, whom he judged medically as the most suitable recipients.

This event was rapidly pronounced a scandal by the media, but more was to come. One of the kidneys was known to be positive for the hepatitis C virus; and another came from a seventy-year-old donor and was therefore deemed unfit for transplant in America. It was also reported that at least seventy-two hours elapsed before this kidney was finally sewn into the recipient. Ohkubo defends Ota by stating that "no matter what other people say, people who are really sick would rather have a kidney, even if it will only last a few years, than not have one at all. I do not see a problem with what Dr. Ota did—kidneys should never go to waste." The media, however, did not concur, and their treatment of Ota was largely responsible for his resignation as president of the Japan Dialysis Society. The Japan Society for Transplantation decided in the end not to take the matter further, and Ota remained as its head.

Kidneys infected with hepatitis C have been used in North America for patients already suffering from that disease, provided that the recipient is aware of the situation. The Japanese media failed to note this in their critical articles about Ota. Yet many of Ota's colleagues defend him fiercely, and some throw a further complication into the story by claiming that Ota was set up as a target for the media, probably by a colleague jealous of his success.

International Bridge Building

Naka Yoshitomo, a retired school principal, was sixty-three years old when he received a kidney from a seventy-year-old American donor. The operation took place sixty to seventy hours after the kidney was first procured, having traveled halfway across the world and then languished in a cooler while people disputed its final destination. Exactly one year later, when I interviewed him, Naka was experiencing mild rejection and was having his medication adjusted, but since that time, by all reports, he has done exceptionally well:

I've become ten years younger since I had the transplant. I was on dialysis for thirteen years, every Tuesday, Thursday, and Saturday, afternoons and evenings. It was impossible for me to have a transplant from one of my relatives, so I registered ten years ago to receive a kidney from a cadaver, but nothing came along.

How did you feel about having a kidney from such an old donor?
My wife was opposed, partly because of the cost. But my son agreed as soon as he understood that I was keen. I felt really lucky to be right at the top of the list of waiting people just because I happened to be the best match. I didn't want to lose this chance—really this seemed to be a "gift of love and health" (*ai to kenkō no okurimono*), finally, after all the waiting.

. . .

In his book, written after the transplant surgery, Naka Yoshitomo notes that he was told in detail before making his decision that the kidney was from an elderly man but was functioning quite well (Naka 1996). He was warned that after its long journey the kidney might take a few weeks to recover and begin producing urine. He was also informed about the long-term side effects of the medications he would have to take. In the event, after the operation, the kidney started functioning after only five days. Naka describes his happiness, but goes on to recount the outcry over his case and the reasons why his family had denied him television in his hospital room and made sure he did not see any newspapers right after the transplant.

One morning, shortly after the operation, Naka heard the sounds of one of the noisy loudspeaker vehicles used by the extreme right wing in Japan to stir up nationalistic sentiment. As it crawled back and forth outside the hospital, he gradually became aware of the strident and abusive message from the loudspeakers: "Bad doctors have taken part in a cover-up. Importation of defective kidneys." Naka was attacked by serious doubts. He began to feel that in his haste to get a transplant he had done something wrong. He had been told that the chances of success for the transplant were about 80 percent, but now he wondered whom he should believe.

One year later, Naka lives daily with thoughts about his donor:

Hopefully I will understand how he felt one day. We must change our ideas in Japan, and that is why I wrote the book.

Did you write a letter to the donor's family?

Oh yes! I was happy to send that letter. I told them that the donor is living with me now. He is smiling and walking with me wherever I go. I sent a copy of my book to UNOS as well.[7] Now I'm working hard on cultural exchange between my hometown and our sister town in America. I go to America all the time arranging visits and events. I can't think of a better way to thank that family for what they did for me.

. . .

Clearly the altruism of unknown strangers has inspired Ohkubo and Naka to find ways to reciprocate to society at large. Surely their activities exemplify modern charity at its best? But what of those families of po-

7. The book is in Japanese. I hope someone in UNOS will translate at least parts of it.

tential donors who hesitate unless they can be assured of someday meeting the recipient? And what of those recipients who hope eventually to meet the family who facilitated the donation? Is the price we pay for anonymity too high? Is the shortage of organs perhaps exacerbated by an insistence on anonymity? Could anonymity be a matter of choice, carefully mediated by coordinators, but left up to donors and recipients rather than an imposition? These questions take us beyond the scope of this book; but, given the ambiguities inherent in the "gift of life" as it is presently managed, the time is ripe for a reconsideration of human organs as mere material entities.

One more facet of this complex story remains to be told: efforts to alleviate the shortage of organs for transplant that encourage new definitions of being as-good-as-dead.

A RELIABLE MAN

I was born with a bladder infection and a problem that needed surgery. That's twenty-five years ago now. They did the surgery when I was six months old, but the doctor was an alcoholic and he botched things up, and it caused permanent kidney damage. I had about six more surgeries to try to correct things, and my kidneys were fine for about thirteen years, and then they gradually started to give up.

Did you go on dialysis?

Just for a little while. I knew that I wanted to be a candidate for a transplant right away. They put me on the list but warned me that it might take a long time in Quebec. I was told it was because I'm Jewish and there'd be a problem with tissue typing. There's so much inbreeding with the Jewish religion, you know, and not much intermarriage, so they said I might have to wait three or four years.

My parents decided to try to put me on a list in the States because I'd had some of my surgeries there, in Pittsburgh. But they wanted a quarter of a million dollars—I was like, "What, it's not a gold kidney!" They said they'd push me right up the list. It was around the time the Governor of Pennsylvania received a heart really quickly when he needed one. We asked around in New York and the New England states, too, but they all wanted at least $150,000.

My family and I are extremely involved in the Jewish community here, and a lot of people had approached us asking if they could help.

They really wanted to give us the money, but I didn't want anything to do with it. They said, "Listen, you've invested your life in our community, so for us it's an investment." Anyway, in the end it was done behind my back, they raised $150,000, but I didn't need it because I got my kidney in Quebec, so the money is in an endowment fund for people who need transplants but can't get them in Quebec. It's wonderful how this community works—it's so nice. They put me and my family in an awkward position, but the money will be put to good use.

Do you know anything about the donor of your kidney?

No, we're not allowed to know anything in Quebec. There's a part of me would really like to know. I've named it—he's a friend.

Was it from a man, then?

I've no idea. But I'm convinced it is, and I say to my friends, "Most reliable man I've ever dated." He's with me in the morning, and in the afternoon and at night, we're perfect together! I've done a lot of publicity to encourage donation, and I told the last journalist I talked to that I've named him Fred. They said in the article that "he follows me everywhere I go," and made me sound like a real idiot!

You know, the doctors don't deal with this—this is my biggest complaint about the transplant world; they just don't understand the emotional aspects of being a recipient. There's so much to deal with emotionally. I feel now, I'm really driven about this, that I'm not just living my life for me, but for whoever this person was who wasn't able to continue their life. It's a big deal.

So, have you taken on their life as well in some way?

Yes, in some respects, and I don't know if that's really fair for me. I've been brought up in a family with tremendous Jewish guilt, everything is like . . . I don't look at it as a burden, but it's an extra responsibility, and what if I can't live up to that?

I was so happy when I got my transplant. I remember that I got the phone call just two days before my twenty-fifth birthday. Lorraine, the transplant coordinator, called and she said, "Your kidney's here, Esther!" And a month before it had been, "Don't expect it for a long time." My parents were out of town at the time, and my sister ended up being home, and she's never home. She goes: "It's the weirdest thing. My car broke down; I was just going out, and I couldn't start the car, and now you get this call." So she came with me, and I was very happy. I knew it had to go well. Of course I got Dr. L., who everyone knows emphasizes all the negative stuff. But I take him with a grain of salt. I love that man. He comes in and he goes, "Esther, you know you're taking a risk here." And I said, "OK, can't you sound a little more optimistic?" But that's him. I had two really good friends in med school at the time who came down to surgery with me, just until I went to sleep. I was nervous, but when I woke up, I was fine. And then a few days later I was able to urinate, and that was fantastic.

There's no other surgery like a transplant. I can't compare it to anything. It's the only surgery where you *gain* a body part. I'll tell you something, it's completely psychological. I hated mustard, I swear. I never touched it. It was never in the house. Now I put it on everything. My mother looks at it: "What are you doing? Are you pregnant or something?" I go, "Seems like it." It's very funny. I wonder if they've done any research on this? Because I think it's very necessary.

I think there's been very little research of that kind, and it's not the kind of thing the medical profession encourages.
Well, I'm in social work now, and I'd like to do research like that.

By the way, are you religious?
I don't think of myself that way really. I'm a traditional Jew. I'm kosher in terms of I don't eat meat or chicken or shellfish outside of the house. So I have a very strong belief, yet when I was sick I asked myself, why did I do all these things? I was such a good Jew, dedicating my life to community and to family and to the religion. Well, not really religion, but to tradition. But then I went through a whole Jewish identity crisis. Very severe. And my sister is religious, and she looked at me and said, "I don't know where you're coming from now, you had enough belief for both of us."

There was an article about me in the *Canadian Jewish News,* and I got a lot of calls about it, asking me, "Is this true?" And what happened was I had people come up to me and ask if my kidney was Jewish or not—about ten or fifteen people or more. One man had the audacity to say, "If that wasn't a Jewish kidney, why couldn't you have waited?" And I looked at this man and I said, "I don't want to wish harm on you, but I'd like you to feel what it's like to be on dialysis, even for one day." And I started to think about the stupidity of some religious people. I go to an orthodox synagogue, and after this fifteenth person asked me if it was Jewish, I said, "No, not only is it not Jewish, but it's gay and it's black," and I turned around and walked away. Afterwards my mother said, "I can't believe you said that, you should have seen that man's face!" It's so stupid. Who cares? So my whole identity was a bit messed up for a while. But now I do all I can to encourage donation by giving talks and organizing meetings and so on.

AN UNSATISFACTORY INTELLIGENCE

The case of seventeen-year-old Terry Urquhart, which made front-page news in Canadian newspapers in 1995, encapsulates many of the contradictions rife in the transplant world. Terry, now deceased, had Down syndrome and impaired lungs and was given at most another five years of life. His parents applied to an Alberta hospital to have their son placed on the waiting list for a lung transplant, not in the expectation that it would "save" his life, but, in the words of a newspaper reporter, because "the medical miracle of a new lung means simply the chance to live out his last few years without gasping for air." It was reported that Terry did not meet the written criteria of the transplant program for "satis-factory intelligence," and his application was therefore turned down. His parents went public with their story, with the result that the hospital hastily rewrote its policy and then placed Terry on the waiting list (Mitchell 1995). A representative of the transplant program told me in 1999 that the newspaper report had been inaccurate: in fact, the selec-tion committee had been slow to meet, causing Terry's parents to assume wrongly that he had been turned down.

As a result of the newspaper article, phone calls flooded the hospital, accusing it of "wasting" organs, and hundreds of callers threatened to tear up their donor cards if mentally impaired individuals were routinely to receive transplants. A smaller number of callers agreed with Terry's parents that to be denied a transplant on intellectual criteria amounted to discrimination.

Approximately twenty-five single-lung transplants are done in Canada each year; this number has not changed dramatically in recent years. About 12 percent of patients die within thirty days, and only about half the survivors remain alive three years later. Terry underwent assessment and was placed on the waiting list with the likelihood of waiting for up to two years for a suitable donor. He died a few weeks later, but had a donor been located and the operation performed, he would have faced between one and three months in hospital. For the remainder of his short life he would have taken powerful immunosuppressants daily, together with other types of medication producing unpleasant and possibly life-threatening reactions. The hospital's transplant program, which must demonstrate "success" in order to remain competitive, would have intervened aggressively so that Terry's statistic did not adversely affect its "survival curve." Meanwhile, someone else would have died waiting for a lung.

Revisiting Vivisection in a World Short of Organs

I think, therefore I am is the statement of an intellectual who
under-rates toothaches. *I feel, therefore I am* is a truth
much more universally valid, and it applies to everything that
is alive. . . . The basis of the self is not thought but
suffering, which is the most fundamental of all feelings.

Milan Kundera, Immortality

In North America the public today is repeatedly told of a shortage of
organs for transplant. Forums and symposiums are held and committees
are convened to investigate why so few people donate their organs and
how more could be procured. We read regularly about the agony of
waiting and the sorrow of losing a loved one for want of a suitable organ
(see, for example, *Globe and Mail* 1999b). Many argue that unless we
master the technology of cloning, there never will be enough organs to
meet the demand. We need more and more because patients who formerly were considered too sick, too old, or too young to be recipients
are now placed on waiting lists. The cutting edge of transplant technology is concerned with "cluster" transplants (transplanting multiple organs into one recipient), brain tissue implants, the paring down of large
organs to fit children, and other innovative measures. Repeat transplants
are commonplace; some patients undergo four or five. At the same time,
there are fewer organs to procure because we have reduced the number
of fatal traffic accidents.

Arguments about "maximizing" the availability of organs are
grounded in the utilitarian assumption that organs must be made available for the greatest good of all. These discussions address xenotransplants,[1] permitting the sale of organs, and whether the category of pa-

---

1. The transplantation of organs from animals into humans.

tients counted as good-as-dead can be expanded, in order that we may harvest their organs. In contrast to the situation in Japan, this debate is taking place long after the routinization of organ transplants from brain-dead donors.

Perhaps it is expedient to think animistically of donors "living on" in other people, and of transplants unequivocally as life-saving procedures. One transplant surgeon talks of the "alarming number of patients who die waiting" (Peters 1991:1302), and another commentator describes this situation as a "public health crisis" (Randall 1991:1223). But by no means everyone understands this crisis in the same way. The physician and ethicist Leon Kass, for example, observes: "Now, embarked on the journey, we cannot go back. Yet we are increasingly troubled by the growing awareness that there is neither a natural nor a rational place to stop. Precedent justifies extension, so does rational calculation: we are in a warm bath that warms up so imperceptibly that we don't know when to scream" (Kass 1992:84).

Virtually the same justifications used by the Harvard Committee in 1968 for creating a new death are today made by medical professionals and bioethicists who seek to designate another class of patients as potential donors. Most of these are in a persistent vegetative state (PVS) (Jennett 1992). As trauma medicine has developed, an increasingly large number of patients are now placed on ventilators. Improvements in resuscitative and supportive measures mean that more patients survive, but recovery is often minimal, creating numerous patients in persistent or permanent vegetative states. As the Harvard Committee noted more than thirty years ago, caring for such patients places a considerable burden on their families, on hospitals, and on those in need of hospital beds. The Harvard Committee also argued that "obsolete criteria for the definition of death can lead to controversy in obtaining organs for transplantation" (Ad Hoc Committee 1968:85).

In the intervening years, one more concept has been added to the armament of medical rationalizations for terminating patient treatment, that of futility. In cases such as those of anencephalic infants or patients in PVS, the concept of medical futility is often deployed as an ethical trump card that overrules patient autonomy and can be used to justify denial of treatment. Thus far, very few doctors have ended up in court when they have withdrawn treatment on this basis, and it is very rare indeed for them to be found guilty of negligence.

Forcible arguments of futility circumvent disagreeable discussion about medical costs. Pope Pius XII sanctioned the idea of medical futility in 1958, but it is nevertheless a concept that has run into trouble. Trauma specialists and intensivists argue about the accuracy of prognoses, and some suggest that the answers about futility all depend on who is asked (Poses et al. 1989). Other critics within medicine point out that the concept is often used simply to impose unilaterally the values of attending physicians on patients and their families (Weijer and Elliott 1995; Carnevale 1998).

Sentience Does Not Make a Person

Proponents of "higher brain" or "neocortical" death have argued all along that, inasmuch as individuals diagnosed as in PVS are irreversibly unconscious and have lost all capacity for cognitive functioning, treatment is futile because they are no longer persons. Moreover, the majority of neurologists argue that such patients have no capacity to experience pain and do not suffer (Cranford 1996; Multi-Society Task Force on PVS 1994a). This argument against personhood is made even though PVS patients usually breathe without assistance, have sleep-wake cycles and reflexes, and can swallow and yawn. A few patients can, with great patience on the part of their attendants, feed themselves when food is placed in their mouths.

Opponents of the higher-brain formulation insist that neurological experts cannot be certain that loss of higher brain function ensures no consciousness or awareness. Current theory holds that consciousness is activated by the lower brain, which in PVS patients continues to function at least partially. The issue is made more difficult because the sentience— the aliveness— of PVS patients is beyond dispute. Neocortical death, as even its most dedicated proponents acknowledge, is not biological death; neocortical death must, therefore, be interpreted as death of the person, or the "unmaking" of the person.

At the request of involved families, the courts have permitted life support to be removed from patients in PVS, with the result that upper brain death has, on occasion, been legally recognized (Hoffenberg et al. 1997). No request has yet been made to procure organs from such patients, but as early as 1988 it was argued that medical recognition of neocortical death would increase the number of organs procured:

> A neocortical death standard could significantly increase availability and access to transplants because patients . . . declared dead under a neocortical definition could be biologically maintained for years as opposed to a few hours or days, as in the case of whole brain death. Under the present Uniform

Anatomical Gift Act, this raises the possibility that neocortically dead bodies or parts could be donated and maintained for long-term research, as organ banks, or for other purposes such as drug testing or manufacturing biological compounds.

(Smith 1988:129)

One of the difficulties about assessing PVS is that it is a "syndrome of behavioral features and not a single entity of pathology, site, or even volume of brain damage" (Andrews 1993a:109). Shortly after discussion about neocortical death began in the literature, David Lamb asked, "How much neocortical damage would be necessary for a patient to be considered dead?" (1985:43). He pointed out that there is no "clinical homogeneity" in patients in PVS, since there are no firm criteria for defining the condition. Efforts have been made to rectify this situation (Bernat 1992; Grubb et al. 1997; Multi-Society Task Force on PVS 1994a,b; Ramsay 1996), but diagnosis remains difficult, particularly in children (Mejia and Pollack 1995; Shewmon 1988). A permanent loss of consciousness and self-awareness is difficult to establish definitively, and cases of significant and occasionally complete recovery have been repeatedly reported (Andrews 1993a,b; Dougherty et al. 1981:997; Falk 1999; Rosenberg et al. 1977:167–68). One particularly worrying issue is that the vast majority of patients in PVS (approximately twenty thousand adults and up to ten thousand children in the U.S. alone) receive only maintenance care. However, in those few facilities dedicated to intensive therapy, some patients recover. We simply do not try as hard as we might with the majority of cases. Keith Andrews, a gerontologist who dedicates his life to working with PVS patients in England, states that the irreversibility of the condition is a self-fulfilling prophecy because so little is done for patients (1993a:117). Similar assertions are made in Japan, where rehabilitation of PVS patients is taken much more seriously. The 1992 film *Lorenzo's Oil* is a moving portrayal of what can be done for at least some PVS patients who have dedicated and determined families.

In Andrews's unit, where intense efforts are made at rehabilitation, out of forty-three cases, eleven regained awareness at least four months after suffering brain damage. Of these eleven, six were able to use non-verbal means of communication, and four were able to speak; only one patient never recovered any ability to communicate. Two of these patients became totally independent in daily life (1993b). Andrews concludes that even patients with profound brain damage should be offered specialist rehabilitation, and he questions the received wisdom that no worthwhile recovery can be made by patients who remain unconscious three months after the initial injury.

Although Andrews admits his assessment is subjective, he asserts that the majority of patients are not depressed after a partial recovery and that they exhibit signs of pleasure more often than distress. He argues that many people with disabilities would heartily support his findings and suggests that physicians tend to project their own fears about disability onto patients, assuming that the patient would prefer to be dead than to live with a major impairment. Andrews also reminds his readers that very occasionally PVS patients make a significant recovery after a year or more of no improvement. One year is the cut-off point at which persistent vegetative state is usually rediagnosed as "permanent" and therefore hopeless.

Recently Andrews reported that among forty patients referred to his unit, seventeen had been misdiagnosed: although severely impaired, they were not in PVS (Andrews et al. 1996). When Andrews showed me round his bright, busy unit in the Royal Hospital for Neurodisability in west London (one of the very few charity hospitals left in England), he explained that one of the patients in his care at that time was "locked in": that is, fully conscious, aware, and able to feel pain but, due to irreversible damage to the brain stem, unable to speak or make any movements other than blinking. This patient had been treated as though in PVS for months at another institution, where physicians had assumed that he was fully unconscious and unable to experience pain.[2]

Andrews's work has provoked controversy among neurologists. Robert Cranford, a leading American neurologist, published a commentary in which he questions whether Andrews's patients are representative of PVS patients in general. Andrews himself considers this unlikely, because only patients with persevering families will be referred to his facility. Cranford goes on to express the dominant medical position on PVS:

> It is interesting to note that all 17 patients who were found to be conscious were severely disabled; all were severely paralysed and anarthric,[3] most were either blind or severely visually impaired, some were substantially cognitively impaired, and all were presumably dependent upon feeding tubes. Reasonable people may differ in their views of the quality of life of these conscious individuals, but I would speculate that most people would find this condition

2. Perhaps the most celebrated case of a locked-in patient is that of Jean-Dominique Bauby, who "dictated" the deeply disturbing book *The Diving-Bell and the Butterfly* (1998) with the only part of his body that remained mobile—one eyelid.

3. Anarthric means paralyzed.

far more horrifying than the vegetative state itself, and some might think it
an even stronger reason for stopping treatment than complete unconsciousness.

(Cranford 1996:6)

An editorial in the *Bulletin of Medical Ethics* reported Andrews's research incorrectly and argued that it was of "great propaganda value to
pro-life groups," but it concluded that his findings might encourage neurologists to define their terms more precisely in language intelligible to
most lay people. This would facilitate decisions about when medical
treatment is futile (1996).

A recent article in the *Lancet* called for renewed discussion about
ending the lives of certain patients in PVS. It noted that if such a decision
was made, then the possibility of organ procurement might be raised
with the family, but this step would be entirely independent of the decision to end the patient's life. This article insists that no discussion of
any kind about end-of-life decisions should take place until patients have
been in PVS for twelve months or more and have shown not the slightest
sign of recovery (Hoffenberg et al. 1997). Obviously doubts about diagnostic error would have to be completely ruled out. Medical practitioners other than the patient's attending physician would be called on
if organ donation were to be considered. If donation were agreed on,
then death would have to be "accelerated," for it would not be possible
to starve the patient to death, as is the current practice once treatment
for PVS is withdrawn. The deliberate administration of an injection to
bring about death is, of course, illegal (except in Holland).

This paper, to which I am a signatory after protracted discussion and
exchange with my coauthors, argues that since it is already legally acceptable to terminate treatment for certain PVS patients, hastening death
might well be better for all concerned. In Britain and in North America
it has been argued that any separation between active and passive euthanasia (that is, between "acts" and "omissions," as these practices are
sometimes called) is, in legal terms, "a distinction without a difference."
Organs are already procured from anencephalic infants, who are alive
by current legal definitions. If guidelines were developed to cover withdrawal of treatment and hastening of death, a conscience clause could
be inserted so that health care professionals could opt to remove themselves from involvement in these procedures.

A flurry of letters appeared in response to this article, all of which
categorically opposed organ donation from PVS patients. The letters
raised the specter of Nazi Germany in particular and of totalitarian re-

gimes in general, as well as the fear of destruction of trust in doctors (Engelhardt 1998). But euthanasia is already practiced frequently, although few people outside Holland dare to talk about it in public, so perhaps we are simply being duplicitous by not entertaining this possibility. It remains exceedingly difficult to separate the debate about death from that about organ donation, a shortcoming that tends to preclude any engagement with the matter. The article in the *Lancet* maintained a sharp distinction between the decision to end a life and considerations about organ procurement. And Keith Andrews, for all his extensive experience with PVS, is not adamantly opposed to ending the lives of patients who are permanently vegetative and for whom there is absolutely no hope, provided of course that this is what the family wants (Hoffenberg, personal communication, 1998). Under these circumstances some families might welcome an opportunity to donate organs.

Anencephalic Infants and the Organ Shortage

Anencephaly is a congenital defect in which infants are born without a scalp or cranium and the cerebral cortex is virtually absent, although a brain stem is present. Only 25 to 45 percent of such babies are born alive (about one thousand every year in the United States), and approximately 95 percent of them die within one week of birth. Even though anencephalic babies can breathe independently, their status after birth—alive or dead—is debatable. For physicians and philosophers who define life in terms of whole-brain activity, anencephalics are alive because the lower brain is functioning, although death is imminent. For those who ground their arguments in a concept of "meaningful life" and "personhood," anencephalics, lacking any potential to become persons, may be counted as dead. The majority who subscribe to this view have promoted the use of their organs for donation, even though the quality of organs taken from these infants is questionable (Shewmon et al. 1989).

These incompatible positions are made yet more complicated because it has been shown that the diagnosis of anencephaly is by no means infallible and in any case covers a continuum of conditions (Fost 1988:8; Meinke 1989). Infants who are not anencephalic have been referred for organ procurement in error (Council on Ethical and Judicial Affairs 1995:1616); and some survive longer than anyone had anticipated, independent of life support, prolonging the anguish of all concerned (Baird and Sadovnick 1987).

The first surgeons to procure organs from anencephalic infants justified their position in several ways. They frequently argued that they were persuaded into organ procurement by parents wishing to create a meaning for their infant's existence: "Much of the interest in organ donation stems from parents of anencephalic infants who desperately desire to see some good come from their personal tragedy" (Walters and Ashwal 1988:24). Involved physicians resorted in the late 1980s to "definitional gerrymandering," arguing for an amendment to the Uniform Declaration of Death Act so that anencephalic infants could be counted as dead on the grounds that they are anomalous and therefore constitute a special case. Others conceded that anencephalics are alive but sought nevertheless to remove organs on utilitarian grounds; or else they tried to create an entirely separate category for such infants, stating that they are in effect nonhuman.

In these arguments, the life of the infant is dismissed as without meaning because it has no capacity for consciousness or mental functioning and its prognosis is uniformly terminal (Caplan 1987). A 1969 article boasted of surgeons making use of an "anencephalic monster" as a donor (Martin et al. 1969). A surgeon at Loma Linda Hospital in southern California declared that an anencephalic infant is preferable as a donor to a baboon: "Not only does the [anencephalic] have human genes," he stated, "but it is a nonperson and sure to die; whereas the monkeys are living and, well, there's a down side to that" (Gianelli 1987). Terms that mark the anencephalic as human—*baby, infant, newborn*—are conspicuously absent from the literature in support of procurement of their organs. Interest has been expressed in harvesting organs from other types of "anomalous" infants, including those with hydranencephaly and microcephaly.

Various individuals and groups have contested this view. J. C. Willke and Dave Andrusko, one a physician and President of the National Right to Life Committee, and the other the editor of the *National Right to Life News,* respond that no one faults the desire of a parent to "redeem" the death of their baby, but they regard it as profoundly misguided to believe that the only way an anencephalic child's life can have significance is through organ donation. They argue that "the perspective underlying much of the public clamor is an application of raw utilitarianism, reducing a person to a function" (Willke and Andrusko 1988: 33).

Other criticism comes from medical professionals with no obvious axe to grind. The pediatrician Norman Fost comments on donation from anencephalics: "If our leading medical centers and practitioners tell us that it is responsible to 'act first, talk later,' that doctors are entitled to make profound policy, what message does this send to the hospital and surgeon inclined to cross yet newer boundaries . . . ? Just as war is too important to leave to the generals, transplantation policy is too important to leave to the physicians" (1988:9). One way of achieving social consensus, Fost observes—the usual American way, he suggests—is to act and then to invite society to accept or reject the action through legislation, litigation, prosecution, or public criticism. He cites one hospital ethics committee that has explicitly adopted a policy of acting first and talking later (10). An alternative method is to seek social approval and consensus prospectively, through professional and lay publications, the legislature, the courts, national commissions, hospital ethics committees, and the like. Fost believes that the latter method is more likely to include careful consideration of the relevant facts, interests, and arguments (1986), and is much closer to the course charted by the Japanese in connection with brain death—with a strikingly different outcome.

Heroics and Medical Moratoriums

A close association between medical heroics, nationalistic inclinations, and culturally constructed values is sometimes evident in North America as well as in Japan. For example, the author of a "family doctor" column in a Montreal newspaper, which is usually about relatively trivial matters such as warts, hernias, and lower back pain, writes about the Schoutens, a couple who carried their anencephalic baby to term expressly so that they could donate the organs:

> I have never met the Schoutens, but as a father, a physician, and a person proud that they are Canadian, I feel compelled to tell their story one more time.
>
> In an age of crooked politicians, unscrupulous business deals and newspapers filled with stories about prostitution, nuclear weaponry . . . and war criminals, we must continue to think about the Schoutens, not only to maintain our sanity, but as an inspiration for all Canadians.
>
> The world has an acute shortage of heroes, we cannot afford to let the memory of these people fade.
>
> (Seiden 1987)

To my knowledge, neither the media nor the family doctor reported that the infant born by caesarian section who received Gabriel's heart died shortly after the transplant surgery.

Not everyone is as laudatory as this family doctor; in particular many physicians and nurses directly involved with cases like that of the Schoutens have misgivings. As a result of both peer group and public concern, involved hospitals in Canada imposed a moratorium on the use of anencephalic infants as donors in early 1988 (Lipovenko 1988), followed later by most American hospitals, and finally the Californian hospital that had conducted the majority of such transplants. At the time, few of those involved believed that this was anything more than a temporary retreat. Sure enough, in 1995, after years of debate, the Council on Ethical and Judicial Affairs of the American Medical Association reversed the decision. This expert committee announced that it should be permissible to take organs from anencephalic infants "while they are living" because such babies "never have thoughts, feelings, sensations, desires, or emotions" (Council on Ethical and Judicial Affairs 1995: 1615). They referred to a survey showing that two-thirds of bioethicists and medical experts agreed with this decision (1614). Some of these ethicists had argued for years that a strong "ethical case can be made for the permissibility—even the obligation—to utilize anencephalic donors if certain basic precautions are taken" (Walters 1987).

In temporarily renouncing the procurement of organs from anencephalics, the AMA noted the discomfort of involved doctors, but it seems these sensitivities can be overcome when the "need" for organs is great and the parents of the baby are in strong support. However, both the American Academy of Pediatrics and the Canadian Pediatric Society take a conservative position, arguing strongly that the law should not be changed to count anencephalics as dead. Both these organizations have insisted since the early 1990s on extreme caution about organ procurement from anencephalics, although they do not state categorical opposition provided the procedure is classified as experimental (American Academy of Pediatrics 1992; Canadian Pediatric Society 1990).

Usually an anencephalic infant receives warmth and food but no medical interventions. If organs are to be procured, however, the situation is radically altered. One method entails placing the baby on a ventilator at birth for a predetermined time, between seven and fourteen days. If during this time all brain function is lost, then organs can be procured rapidly. In one study, only one of six infants became brain-dead. The majority of clinicians are extremely uncomfortable under these circumstances.

Non-Heart-Beating Cadaver Donors (NHBCDs)

Virtually unnoticed by the public, two more sources of organs are already being used, although to date they involve a very small number of donors. Prior to the recognition of brain death, organs were usually obtained from living related donors or, alternatively, from donors whose hearts had already stopped beating. The great disadvantage of this second type of procurement is that the organs are likely to be damaged by a lack of blood flow during their retrieval from the donor; and the heart is not usable.

However, if a patient is perfused with specially prepared cold fluids immediately prior to or after cardiac arrest, then the organs remain in reasonably good condition even after cardiopulmonary death and can be removed for transplant. The difficulty with this approach, known as "uncontrolled donation" because death is unexpected, is that it is usually not possible to obtain prior consent to remove organs, and hence body cooling usually takes place, on the assumption that donation will proceed, before the next of kin have been contacted. A second, equally troubling feature is the question of whether every effort is made to carry out resuscitation prior to declaring death.

The second form of NHBCD donation, known as "controlled donation," takes place when patients and their families opt to donate organs after the patient, who is terminally ill, has decided to forgo further treatment. Usually the patient, after saying goodbye to relatives, is taken to the operating room, where "treatment" is stopped. The surgical team waits (outside the operating room, one hopes) ready to remove organs immediately after death has been declared. It comes as no surprise that these practices were first implemented at Pittsburgh University Hospital, which, it is widely agreed, has the most aggressive transplant program in the United States. Alan Weisbard, a lawyer, in commenting critically on these practices (as others have done; see Arnold et al. 1995), insists:

> In its rawest form, the Pittsburgh protocol envisions wheeling a . . . still living prospective donor into the O.R., prepping the individual's body for subsequent removal of organs, presiding over a series of events . . . hopefully culminating in the individual's death (or, at least, the individual's being "declared" dead by a new and scientifically unvalidated set of criteria), and finally removing the individual's organs for transplant—all this unless something goes dreadfully wrong, and the patient survives. . . . Enormous pains are taken to characterize events as an allowing to die, rather than a killing, and as a series of stepwise "adjustments" of respiratory support and pain medication, each portrayed as "intended" to respond solely to the patient's

needs of the moment. The protocol has the secondary or "unintended" (if
foreseen) effect of bringing about the patient's (desired) death.

(Weisbard 1995:147)

Arnold and Youngner (1995) point out that society has assured itself
that potential donors will be protected from harm because of what is
known informally as the "dead donor" rule (Robertson 1988): that is,
all donors must be declared dead before organs can be removed. Clearly
we have already quietly subverted the intent of this rule and are now
embarked on the process of "allowing patients to die" and "accelerating
death" to retrieve their organs expediently. These protocols are apparently driven by feelings of urgency about alleviating the suffering of
potential organ recipients and the shortage of organs (Arnold et al.
1995).

The Slippery Slope of Truth

Despite the general consensus, in North America and Europe doubts
have persisted all along among certain professional commentators, as
they do in Japan, as to what actually constitutes human death (Arnold
and Youngner 1993; Veatch 1993). Robert Truog, a pediatric intensivist
and anesthesiologist, argues that "despite its familiarity and widespread
acceptance, the concept of 'brain death' remains incoherent in theory
and confused in practice. Moreover, the only purpose served by the
concept is to facilitate the procurement of transplantable organs" (1997:
29). Truog insists that we should maintain a "clear and simple distinction between the living and the dead" (1997:34), and therefore we
should return to the "traditional" cardiopulmonary standard for determining death. He argues that we should, nevertheless, permit retrieval
of organs from patients who have indicated their willingness in advance
directives or when permission has been given from a recognized surrogate. Included would be those individuals who are permanently and
irreversibly unconscious (but whose hearts still function either independently or through assistance from a respirator) and those who are im-
minently and irreversibly dying. Truog argues that we have had twenty
years of experience in making decisions about withdrawal of life support, which stands us in good stead in dealing with patients who are
"beyond harm" (1999).

Robert Taylor, a neurologist, comes to similar conclusions. He
stresses that "death is a biological phenomenon, not a social construct."
For Taylor, nature and culture are separate and must remain so. He

insists that "the proper biological definition of death is 'the event that separates the process of dying from the process of disintegration' and the *proper* criterion of death in human beings is the 'permanent cessation of the circulation of blood' " (1997; emphasis added). Taylor finds the concept of brain death unconvincing, but, with Truog, he does not wish to undermine the transplant enterprise. He suggests that, similarly to "legal blindness" (a social construct designed to provide assistance to those who are not completely blind), we could maintain brain death as a social construct, permitting individuals, although living, to become organ donors, provided that prior consent has been established.

Alan Shewmon, a pediatric neurologist from Los Angeles, circulated a letter to several of the participants following the Second International Conference on Brain Death in Havana in February 1996. In it, he summed up the most critical points of dispute at the conference. He asserted that the majority of individuals who presented papers lacked a "coherent and universally accepted conceptual basis for why brain death should be equated with death." Shewmon believes that by the end of the conference there was virtually unanimous agreement that loss of all brain function is not equivalent to loss of biological life, although obviously brain destruction is a fatal injury. The brain should be understood, argues Shewmon, as the organ critical to "consciousness and personhood." The question of its role in the "somatic integrative unity" of the body remains unsettled, but in any case this function should not be crucial to a diagnosis of brain death. By extension, argues Shewmon, "*If* the brain-dead patient is dead, then so too is the PVS patient," because the only *coherent* argument that brain death is death [an irreversible loss of consciousness] logically applies to PVS as well (emphasis in the original, unpublished letter).[4] Shewmon writes that society "tacitly adopted a new concept of human death, namely that human death is the permanent absence of consciousness" (personal communication, March 1996). However, loss of spontaneous breathing is also crucial to a diagnosis of brain death. Shewmon's conflation of the PVS condition with a brain-dead patient hooked up to a ventilator, and thereby breathing, is inappropriate in my opinion.

Truog, Taylor, and Shewmon, together with an increasing number of their colleagues in neurology and related specialties, suggest that we should abandon the dead donor rule. However, they agree that organ donation will be severely curtailed if we can no longer obtain organs

4. Presumably what Shewmon means is a "permanent," irreversible vegetative state.

from brain-dead donors. Hence these physicians argue that individuals, including those currently diagnosed as brain-dead, with their prior consent, should be permitted to become donors even though they remain alive, once it is clear that no chance exists for recovery of consciousness. Ironically, this position is not entirely at odds with what has become law in Japan, where brain-dead patients are counted as legally dead only if they have indicated that they want to become organ donors.

Increasing time of survival of patients after a diagnosis of brain death reinforces the doubts about the validity of considering this condition equivalent to death. Shewmon has documented the survival times of brain-dead patients kept on ventilators for more than a week after the diagnosis. Eighty cases survived for at least two weeks, forty-four for at least four weeks, twenty for at least two months, and seven for at least six months. Survival of more than four months has been seen only in children, three of whom survived for over two years. In some cases treatment was terminated by the medical staff.

Shewmon concludes:

> The phenomenon of chronic BD [brain death] implies that the body's integrative unity derives from mutual interaction among its parts, not from a top-down imposition of one "critical organ" upon an otherwise mere bag of organs and tissues. If BD is to be equated with human death, therefore, it must be on some basis more plausible than that the body is dead. Whether other rationales, such as loss of "personhood" from a biologically live body, might be conceptually more viable or desirable for societal endorsement is beyond the scope of this physiologic inquiry.
>
> (Shewmon 1998:1544)

Earlier, Christopher Pallis, in a study of over 1,300 patients diagnosed as brain-dead in whom life support treatment was discontinued, found that cardiopulmonary death followed rapidly within hours (1987). It is the extended use of the artificial ventilator and other life-support systems that permits this ambiguous entity to continue its existence. But even among these cases documented by Shewmon, in which "life" persists for weeks or months, no one ever regains consciousness, or the ability to breathe independently. This is what is significant.

Because of the 1981 legislation that a criterion for whole-brain death is the "irreversible cessation of all functions of the brain, including the brain stem," ambiguities are inevitable. Amir Halevy and Baruch Brody demonstrated in 1993 that standard clinical tests proposed by the advisers to the President's Commission do not ensure that the criteria have been met, and the various possible solutions to this discrepancy proposed over the years have proved unsatisfactory. These authors cite Morison's 1971 article in which he argued that a sharp dichotomy between life and death is biologically artificial because death is a process rather than an event. There *is* no detectable moment of death, and therefore the concept *must* be socially agreed upon. Brain-dead patients are on an irreversible course toward complete biological death, but organs must be taken before this point is reached. Shewmon's work makes it clear that for some patients on life support technology the liminal period of the process of biological demise is greatly extended, increasing the anxiety of all concerned as to what should count as the moment of death.

This dilemma cannot be resolved. Knowledge about the brain will expand, and ICU technology will become more effective, but these changes will not dispel the fundamental problem that the determination of biological death of an individual can never be definitively reduced to a point in time, no matter which criteria are applied.

Elusive Death

In North America, the trend is toward "coming clean" about the liveliness of the brain-dead patient. In a provocative 1999 article, the pediatrician Norman Fost asserts that it is not necessary to know whether or not brain-dead patients are "truly" dead; nor, he adds, "is it knowable" (1999:162). Similar statements have been made by the philosophers A. Halevy and B. Brody (1993), and the physicians Robert Arnold and Stuart Youngner (1993) and L. Emanuel (1995). Fost reminds us that death is not an entity, a substance, or the presence of something. On the contrary, "it is the absence of something—namely, life—whose definition is elusive" (1999:162). Moreover, death encompasses the loss of many functions, biological, personal, and social.

Fost, like Truog, believes that it was not necessary to redefine death at all, that doing so was simply a utilitarian exercise associated with the desire to procure organs. However, he observes that "the simple fact is that there never has been a single physician in the history of the United States found liable, in a criminal or civil proceeding, for withholding or withdrawing any kind of life-sustaining treatment from any patient for any reason" (1999:165). (The same can be said of Japan, although the suits filed in that country proved unpleasant and newsworthy.)

To support his point, Fost describes the situation in Wisconsin, the state that currently leads in organ procurement in the U.S. Because the state was late in enacting a brain-death statute, for ten years kidneys

were procured from brain-dead patients without legal protection and
with no difficulty. Even if it is agreed that statutory support is desirable
to promote organ retrieval (something that Fost finds doubtful), then it
is still not necessary to redefine death, he argues (1999:168). It would
be more candid, he suggests, to create a statute that permits organs to
be retrieved from brain-dead bodies without making the claim that they
are dead. Fost's position is that if no patient "interests" are violated by
organ removal, whether the patient be brain-dead or anencephalic, then,
with appropriate consent, there can be no ethical dispute.

Fost concludes that "over-treatment," the continuation of life-
sustaining treatment on patients who have no reasonable prospects for
meaningful survival and no clear interest in or desire for such treatment,
is more widespread today than it was in 1968 (1999:175). Redefining
death has not solved the problems first set out by the Harvard Committee, and the difficulty of not knowing what to do with patients on
life support who show no improvement is actually worse than formerly.
In closing, Fost puts his clinician's hat firmly in place:

> I do not address here the important role that declaring death plays in the
> ritual of saying good-bye and grieving for a loved one who is passing on. I
> believe it is helpful and desirable to select a point in time where it is appro-
> priate to say, "He is dead," not because it is true, or because we are expert
> on such questions, or because it facilitates organ retrieval, but because it is
> helpful.
>
> (Fost 1999:175)

In December 2000, a position statement appeared on the "Defining
Death" Internet site that was very different from that of Fost. It was
signed by more than 120 people from nineteen nations, including physicians and theologians, who are opposed to accepting brain-death criteria as indicative of death and believe that we are killing patients by
removing organs from them. This position statement makes clear that a
speech given in August 2000 by Pope John Paul II renewed interest in
the controversies surrounding brain death and organ transplants. The
hybrid of the brain-dead body remains suspended, between life and
death.

A DUBIOUS DEFINITION OF DEATH

From the *Ottawa Citizen:*

> Doctors are removing organs for transplant from "brain dead" patients who are actually still alive, a parliamentary committee was told yesterday.
>
> The controversial testimony came from a small group of doctors—including one who once had a clinical near-death experience herself—and sparked a sometimes gruesome debate on the ethics of organ transplant medicine.
>
> The Commons health committee is holding public hearings to examine ways to improve Canada's low rate of organ donation. So far, the committee has mostly heard from medical experts and patients who have told sad stories about how people have died while awaiting organ transplants.
>
> Yesterday, MPs were confronted with a different dilemma: from an ethical standpoint, are too many organs being transplanted?
>
> Critics of transplants complained the medical profession has made a fundamental moral mistake in allowing organs to be removed from patients who are still breathing but whose brains are declared to be clinically dead.
>
> "I'm testimony that people survive," said Ruth Oliver, a Vancouver psychiatrist who suffered internal bleeding of the brain after childbirth in 1977. For a time, she said, she was deemed clinically dead by doctors ... but emerged from her condition and was regarded as a "miracle patient."
>
> She told MPs her experience demonstrates that practitioners of transplant medicine should proceed with caution.
>
> "The value of each human soul created transcends what doctors can or cannot test of the functioning of the brain," she said.
>
> "Unconscious or dying people are not people of lesser value. More and

more ethicists, philosophers and churches are rejecting brain death specifically for that reason." . . .

Michael Brear, a Vancouver general practitioner, told MPs the criteria
used to diagnose brain death are seriously flawed.

"The so-called 'beating-heart cadavers' who are used as donors are, in
fact, living patients. They are sick, they are dying. They are living and not
dead."

But others disagreed. . . .

Rabbi Reuven Bulka, chairman of the organ-donation committee of the
Kidney Foundation of Canada, said major religious denominations have
closely examined the ethical questions surrounding the removal of organs
from brain dead patients and they have concluded there are no moral problems with such transplants.

"It's essentially the equivalent of decapitation," he said. "It's generally
agreed that if a person is decapitated they are dead."

John Dossetor, a leading medical bioethicist, said there's no doubt that a
brain dead patient is dead. He referred to a case documented in medical
journals that he said is "macabre" and "extreme" but that, nonetheless,
drove home his point. A pregnant woman suffered brain death, but her doctors kept her on life support for 10 weeks and delivered a live infant.

After the plug was pulled and an autopsy was performed, the woman's
skull was opened and there was nothing but water inside. The brain had
liquefied and the coroner could see right into the spinal column, Dossetor
said. . . .

John Yun, a Richmond, B.C. oncologist . . . testified against transplants. . . .

He said that he worked in a busy trauma hospital a decade ago and kept
brain dead patients on life support for organ transplants. Now, after reflecting on the ethics, he thinks he was wrong.

"The problem started when I began to think about the life of the donor.
I assumed that the donor was dead. Once dead, no one will object to any
way we dispose of the body, so long as it is respectful. But now I believe
those patients I looked after in ICU were alive."

Yun said he realizes the whole concept of brain death was created with
one aim in mind—organ harvesting.

"We must not jump to the conclusion that a dubious definition of death—
the medical hypothesis of brain death—is, in fact death."

(Kennedy 1999)

Reflections

Jean Baudrillard argues that the "punctual" or "natural" biological death (the "good" death) of modernity has been made into a quantifiable norm. We practice "risk management" to remain healthy into old age, and we are obsessed with security, a theme that Baudrillard satirizes:

> Car safety: mummified in his helmet, his seatbelt, all the paraphernalia of security, wrapped up in the security myth, the driver is nothing but a corpse. . . . Riveted to his machine, glued to the spot in it, he no longer runs the risk of dying, since he is *already* dead. This is the secret of security, like a steak under cellophane: *to surround you with a sarcophagus in order to prevent you from dying.*
>
> (1993:177)

We fear the loss of control and work to keep chance at bay; we battle against disease and other threats to life, but even so we are doomed. Death is indeed a scandal to reason, as Zygmunt Bauman argues. But we defer it more successful than previously. Highway deaths are down. Motorcycles—"death machines" in the idiom of the transplant world— are not as abundant a source of organ donors as they used to be, and neither are the newly constructed motor vehicles, made safer yet through seat belts and legislation against drunken driving. "There just aren't enough accidents," as one newspaper reporter put it recently, highlighting the "grim irony" of the long lists of patients waiting for organs (Mickleburgh 1993).

Despite all this prudence, "daily life becomes a perpetual rehearsal of death" (Bauman 1992:187). Flirting with death is the spice of life; we push the envelope of chance, with the result that "extreme" sports—the new fad described by some as an addiction—may make up a little for the shortfall of donated organs from motor vehicle accidents (Toynbee 1999). The absurdity of human existence is tested in such circumstances, as it is repeatedly in war and disasters of one kind and another. Michael Herr's *Dispatches* from the Vietnam war show how in extremity death can border on the meaningless:

> In the months after I got back the hundreds of helicopters I'd flown in began to draw together until they'd formed a collective meta-chopper, and in my mind it was the sexiest thing going; saver-destroyer, provider-waster, right hand-left hand, nimble, fluent, canny and human; hot steel, grease, jungle-saturated canvas webbing, sweat cooling and warming up again, cassette rock and roll in one ear and door-gun fire in the other, fuel, heat, vitality and death, death itself, hardly an intruder.
>
> (1977:8–9)

Movies, television programs, books, memoirs, and daily news reporting all encourage us to reduce death to a moment of obliteration. As Octavio Paz puts it, "Catastrophe has become banal and laughable because in the final analysis the Accident is only an accident" (1969: 113). But we know that many survivors and witnesses never forget violent or accidental deaths. Organ donors suffer untimely, traumatic deaths that inevitably incite not only grief but also anxiety; survivors are forced to face human fragility and to recognize that, even with our puny efforts at control, death lurks among us.

The medical world, as many critics have observed, has reinforced a vision of death as scandal, as failure. This is equally true for the profession in the United States, Canada, Japan, and elsewhere. Death is cast as the archenemy (Farmer and Kleinman 1989:148), a condition to be perpetually postponed. Transplant technology, with the assistance of the ventilator, opens the door to a technological transcendence of death—a chance to make meaning out of a "bad" death.

Not everyone is willing to participate in this endeavor. The resistors disagree that death is encapsulated in the moment when the brain becomes irreversibly damaged. For this belief to be palatable, people must first be reassured that clinical judgments and technological recordings accurately reveal the condition of the brain and that errors virtually never happen. They must also agree, tacitly at least, that a permanent loss of consciousness and of the ability to breathe spontaneously signifies death, and acquiesce in the commodification of the body.

Although many doctors assert that brain death represents no radical departure from cardiopulmonary death, not everyone agrees. A living cadaver, exhibiting many signs of life, is redolent with ambiguity. The very facts that the brain-dead machine hybrid is warm, appears animated, and can be kept in this condition for increasing periods raise entirely new issues. So too does the significance given for the first time to the condition of the person's cognitive status in determining death.

The Pervasiveness of Culture

No straightforward answer exists as to why the United States, Canada, and most of Europe accepted the concept of brain death with little difficulty, thus enabling the procurement of organs from brain-dead bodies. No doubt the lengthy history of medical dissection in Europe facilitated the visualization of dead bodies as a resource from which good could come. Medical professionals and many members of the public clearly support this view, even to the extent of bequeathing their bodies to medicine; for them, dead bodies, including their own, have no inherent value apart from their possible worth to science. Even so, many of these people believe that respect is due, as a matter of convention, to dead bodies. This is culture at work, culture as shared values, and it cuts across ethnic groups, religious beliefs, education, birthplace, and place of residence.

Obviously, the general absence of objections from legal and religious bodies in Europe and North America secured the confidence of those physicians who pushed for international recognition of brain death. In Japan, however, the legal profession remains opposed.

Equally important, trust in the medical profession in North America, although tarnished, runs much deeper than it does in Japan. Of course some people, notably those who are economically and socially marginalized, mistrust doctors, but they are in a minority, particularly when it comes to intensive care. A trust in doctors is an extension of a trust in medical science, and it includes a readiness to accept death as a fundamentally measurable, biological event. Understanding death as a moment in time is not counterintuitive in North America, it seems, nor is the idea that death, manifested as an irreversible loss of consciousness, can be located in the brain. This, too, is culture at work.

The responses of medical professionals, philosophers, and the people I have polled informally on the matter suggest that not many would want to be kept on life support once it was clear that they had become permanently unconsciousness. Indeed, most claim that they would rather die than be left severely impaired, possibly even if they were conscious. If these findings hold true for large segments of the population, then the public does not massively oppose the idea of "medical futility." Perhaps Americans and Canadians feel reasonably comfortable with withdrawal of life support from permanently unconscious patients, especially if these patients have indicated in advance that this is what they want. Withdrawal of support can be thought of as a humane move, as can the donation of organs from such individuals, once declared dead, with their prior consent. Culture is also at work here.

The real test of how people react to brain death is in the clinical setting. In North America the majority of involved families are willing to recognize medical judgments as final, despite the ambiguous appearance of brain-dead entities. They apparently think of the body exhibiting signs of life in front of them as a technical artifact and recognize that the machine is doing the necessary work. Perhaps some families rather quickly come to think of continued treatment as futile. Culture is at work here, too. But many families may refuse to donate organs because this entails an active decision on their part, rather than passive acceptance of a medical diagnosis. Relatives in shock are often unwilling to face up to instant commodification of the body after a traumatic death.

Because of the "shortage" of organs, all possible ways of increasing procurement have been considered, and some have been put into practice. One effect has been to force a reconsideration of what exactly we are about. This has led to considerable anxiety in some segments of the medical and bioethical worlds, about which the public knows almost nothing, that brain death, although definitively irreversible, may not be as secure a signifier of the end of *biological* life as was once thought. Some scientists are having second thoughts about the death they helped to make factual among the public not long ago.

Japan, in contrast, has only a relatively brief acquaintance with the donation of bodies to medical science. The history of abuse by doctors in Manchuria, and on a less horrific scale closer to home, causes many people to equivocate about cooperating even with what some see as a good cause. The Wada case, although at first hailed as a medical breakthrough by the media, was quickly retold as a story of unethical medical experimentation and must have triggered memories of the war for many people. (Similarly, hesitation among African Americans to cooperate with organ donation may well be traced in part to fears that stem from reporting of the Tuskegee experiments; see Brandt 1981.)

The media in Japan have fomented anxiety about brain death. Although much of their coverage has been responsible and insightful, hyperbole and bias are also evident. Japanese groups outspokenly opposing brain death have no equivalent at all in North America. Without a legal recognition of brain death, of course, it could not be routinized. Moreover, because of the murder charges brought against doctors, cases that remained undecided until very recently, the entire effort to promote organ transplants was tainted. Trust in emergency medicine doctors and transplant surgeons was severely compromised, and physicians were in no position to try to push through any legislative changes.

Because of the cultural values ascribed to dead bodies in Japan, medical use of cadavers is abhorrent to many, and communal memorialization of deceased relatives remains very important throughout the population. These activities involve less ritual than formerly, but there are distinct signs today of a revival of belief in animism (Natsuishi 1994). Although clearly a minority view, this revival may well influence some individuals as they reflect on the brain-death problem.

The fact that recognition of brain death and transplant technology are thought of by many as foreign imports provides fuel for criticism, especially from conservative commentators. The issue is consciously used, usually by supporters of "tradition," to question Japan's modernization, its loss of values, and blind following of the decadent West.

In the clinical situation, even though styles of medical reasoning and the moral economy of medical science are essentially the same as in North America, death in Japan remains above all a social event; the family is in control, and death with dignity requires family participation (Nakagawa 1995). Because dying is a social process, people feel much more comfortable thinking of death as a process rather than a moment. The concept of brain death is seen by many as a clumsy creation of technological medicine, devised to hasten the end of life. Because the concept of "person" is not usually lodged exclusively in the brain, locating death in the brain causes discomfort. Moreover, as the story of Yasutoshi shows so clearly, it is difficult to entertain the idea that treatment is futile, let alone act on such a concept. Physicians are often unwilling to make a clear declaration of death once brain death is confirmed; nor do many of them feel strongly obliged to try to procure organs. It is not at all surprising, then, that the brain-death problem has persisted so long in Japan or that the transplant enterprise has not prospered.

Japanese attitudes to insensate things may offer some insights into the debate on brain death. The way in which machines in Japan are frequently "animated" comes as a surprise to most outsiders. Cars, subway trains, bank machines, escalators, and so on "talk" to their users in a friendly fashion, offering advice and information in polite language. Moreover, Japanese are sensitive toward their tools and the materials with which they work. Even in large factories, people work *with* their machines; the machine is understood not as an instrument of alienation but on the contrary as an integral part of the human worker (Kondo 1990:245). This attitude appears to be a direct legacy from the everyday lives of skilled workers of all kinds, whose activities have long been explicitly linked with Shinto ritual and with qualities of animism. Spirits reside not only in nature but also in tools and other inanimate objects. Mathews Hamabata notes that workers often understand the machinery they work with as a spiritual extension of themselves (cited in Kondo 1990:245). Human beings and machines inhabit the same world, and working with machines reaffirms the social identity of the human. In a different mode, in science fiction and in *manga*, machines often permit not only an escape from this world but also transcendence.

Whereas in North America the thought of being attached in an unconscious state to a machine is humiliating and demeaning, quite different reactions are common in Japan. Rather than visualize the machine as doing the work for the human, as taking over the empty shell, in Japan some people may conceptualize machine and human as working in partnership, creating an animated hybrid that can overcome all odds.

We still know very little about why people choose not to donate organs in either setting. Both countries are teetering on the edge of major changes. In Japan, the first procurements from brain-dead bodies have now taken place, finally breaking the thirty-year impasse. In North America, possible revisions in the meaning of brain death are emerging, so that in the end brain death may be understood among both the public and medical professionals not as biological death, but as *imminent* death.

Support for keeping patients on ventilators when there is no hope of recovery may not be nearly as widespread in Japan as many assume. A poll conducted by the Mainichi newspaper in the 1980s found that only 27 percent favored prolonging treatment for patients in a persistent vegetative state and that 69 percent would support stopping treatment; the remainder were undecided (*Mainichi Daily News* 1982). Passive euthanasia is not necessarily abhorrent to the majority; perhaps the biggest obstacle is the unwillingness of medical professionals to assert themselves in making such decisions

A "peaceful" death is the desired outcome in Japan, one free of medical intrusions. Unless physicians make clear statements when, in their opinion, the situation is hopeless, families do not feel able to raise the matter themselves. To do so would be a form of disloyalty. As Kimura Reiko put it, describing the experience of standing with her family around the bedside of her brain-dead father, "None of us wanted to be thought of as selfish by being the first to say we should resign ourselves to his death."

Making decisions about persistent vegetative state and other unusual diseases, such as Werdnig-Hoffmann's disease, is extraordinarily difficult, but with brain death the situation is quite different. Physicians could relieve families of the burden of deciding whether the situation is hopeless by making it clear that no one recovers, even temporarily, from brain death. But, until recently, physicians who might do so have been vulnerable to media attacks and possible lawsuits, and many also firmly believe that they should not impose their authority on families coming to terms with death.

Families in North America are comforted by the presence of nurse-clinicians who, unlike attending physicians, can take time, hours if necessary, to discuss the situation with the family. Donation rates have increased threefold in centers where these specially trained nurses work and where the family is given privacy with their dead relative and as much time as they need to come to terms with the situation (Picard 2000). If trained nurse-clinicians took on this responsibility in Japan, the situation might change radically.

Making Death Visible

In North America, we proclaim a shortage of organs, even as we wring our hands at increasing suicide rates and drug overdose deaths among youth. But we do not make associations between these disparate "facts." A lack of public memory about organ donors and their families is part of a deliberate forgetting, a sanitizing of what we are about, contributing perhaps to the feelings of the "uncanny" that so many individuals associate with the transplant enterprise, and to the anthropomorphization

commonly exhibited by organ recipients.[1] This deliberate forgetting also
contributes, no doubt, to the aggressive language so often associated
with drives to procure more organs: a language of entitlement, as though
there *should* be enough to go around.

By encouraging the idea, even inadvertently, that donors "live on" in
the bodies of recipients, donation is individualized. The act of giving
assists personal transcendence. Use of language and metaphors such as
the "gift of life" encourage anthropomorphization and fantasies about
personality changes. No doubt some families create such imagery with
no assistance from the medical profession. I believe, however, that if
anthropomorphism were damped down rather than discreetly encouraged, this could circumvent some of the resistance to donation, permitting donor families to come to terms with the finality of death and grieve
more appropriately. Reconstructing donation as a communal good,
rather than as an individual gift, could transform the way in which organ
donation is thought about. Such a reconstruction is closer to the kind
of communal fecundity generated out of death rituals in premodern societies.

In Japan, a similar difficulty exists, although for different reasons.
With Japan's propensity for collective memorialization of the dead by
families and local communities, reluctance to give to unknown others is
apparent. Potential donors want to know exactly to whom their donated
organs would go, but such a system could easily inject inequalities into
organ distribution, and might lead later to donor families' efforts to
monitor recipients.

Japanese families do not fantasize about individual transcendence of
death but rather worry whether recipients will treat their relatives' organs with due respect. If organ donation is to succeed in Japan, it will
have to be dissociated from tenacious ideas about personalized reciprocity. The metaphor of "life's relay," increasingly used by the Japan
Organ Transplant Society, is a powerful idiom for encouraging people
to think of donation as a social good, one that transcends formalized
exchange at the familial or community level.

Preserving donor anonymity is important. Families of donors should
not have their photographs splashed across the pages of newspapers and
magazines, as was the case in South Africa thirty years ago. Nor should
they be expected to give interviews or have to fend off the media, as

1. Linda Hogle has shown convincingly how transplant coordinators are schooled in
a rhetoric of utility in which emotions and curiosity are repressed (1995, 1996).

happened in Japan in 1999. However, as a group they should receive more public recognition for their generosity to society. At present many receive no thanks beyond a form letter from the transplant procurement agency. However, since 1985, the United States Congress has officially commemorated National Organ and Tissue Donor Awareness Week in April each year. Donor families come together with transplant administrators, doctors, coordinators, and recipients to "celebrate . . . the valuable sacrifice made by those who enabled life" (United Network for Organ Sharing 2000b). Many of the activities are designed to promote donation, including the LifeLink Golf Classic tournament in Florida. In New Jersey, donor family quilts have been made as a tribute to donors, and in one of the biggest transplant centers in the United States, Loyola University Medical Center, candles were lit in the year 2000 to honor donors. Present at this ceremony was Loyola's five-hundredth heart transplant recipient (United Network for Organ Sharing 2000b). It may well be appropriate to further increase recognition of donors and perhaps to bring donor families and recipients together more frequently, not to establish personal ties but to celebrate the social good that emanates from organ donation. But the public at large needs to be better informed about these activities.

In North America, we encourage the idea that donation is a selfless act, but it can also be thought of as the giving away of something no longer of any use. It has been suggested to me that donation is akin to sending used clothes or money to a disaster zone. This may be the case for donors themselves: it takes virtually no effort to sign a donor card. But donor families make a much greater emotional sacrifice. They must usually come to terms with the fact that someone dear to them has been transformed, in the space of a few hours, and often through a violent encounter, from a healthy individual into an irrevocably damaged entity, suspended between life and death. To give selflessly under these circumstances requires courage, as well as faith in the ICU staff and in the truth of their assessments. No wonder some people resort to themes of transcendence to assist them with their decisions.

Second Thoughts about the New Death

Polly Toynbee, in a 1999 article in the *Guardian Weekly,* argues that "superstition and squeamishness have dogged the history of medical progress—nowhere more than in transplantation." She reminds us that the first transplant surgeons were seen as body snatchers and argues that negative public sentiment should not be allowed to outweigh the suffering of those waiting for transplants. An article in the British *Sunday Times,* reacting to proposed institutionalization of presumed consent in the United Kingdom, presents a starkly different view. Melanie Phillips argues that because consciousness remains a mystery and cannot be "tested," there is no scientific or philosophical basis for saying that brain death is death (1999). She adds that the medical establishment appears to think that because a motorcyclist will die anyway, he is virtually dead. "But being virtually dead is not being dead," Phillips argues, "It is being alive. To behave as if this is not so is to treat the dying as disposable."

Can some kind of middle ground be found between these extreme positions? In so many arguments, people start out from the assumption that death is an event that can be medically confirmed. But, as I have argued throughout this book, this is a reductionist position that assumes that death is merely a physical fact and that this is its totality. Even those who argue for biological death as a process usually assume a factual endpoint of death. It is quite possible to conceive of social death as of primary significance and biological demise as secondary to it, as has been the case until relatively recently in most societies. A decaying body will never return to a living condition, and many of us readily agree that a brain-dead body will never revert to consciousness or breathe again, but death and dying are nevertheless social constructs.

The physician and ethicist Steven Miles claims that institutionalizing whole-brain death as the end of individual existence "was an act of reductionistic scientific hegemony" (1999:313). He celebrates the reopening of the discussion, arguing that a precise moment or technological criterion for determining death may be needed or feasible only in certain special circumstances, such as forensic medicine or organ donation. In most cases we do not need to know exactly when death takes place. I agree with this position and with that of Norman Fost (1999) when he states that not only do we not need to know, but we *cannot* know exactly when death takes place. If organs are going to be procured, then this activity must be justified on the basis of something other than complete biological death.

The invention of brain death (the French *coma dépassé,* literally "state beyond coma," is much more descriptive) was indeed a political act. With widespread use of the ventilator, many physicians in North America and Europe considered it imperative that decisions be made expediently as to when to take patients off ventilators and, with appropriate permission, procure organs without repercussions. A death located in the brain would accomplish these ends. However, the ambiguity created by the living cadaver set off a train of events that in some places created ripples of discontent and in other places, such as Japan, storms of protest. The process of biological demise was being interrupted much too abruptly for these dissenters, and the social importance of a gradual recognition of the inexorable workings of fate was being curtailed.

The recognition of biological death has always, as far as we can tell, been based on signs of irreversibility, whether they be putrefaction, holding a feather in front of the nose to see if it moves, the absence of a pulse, or formal tests to establish brain death. It has also been known for centuries that signs of "life" can be found for days after the heart and circulation of the blood have stopped. This residual activity is inevitable, and where rapid burial is customary must surely persist after burial. Hearts taken out of animals continue to beat for hours, as Alexis Carrel showed at the beginning of the twentieth century, and irreversibly damaged brains often exhibit residual electrical and neuroendocrine activity. This is life of a sort, but cannot be described as organized or purposeful, and it is inevitably doomed.

We can no longer sustain the fiction of a radical dichotomy between culture and nature. The presence of living cadavers and other ambiguous entities has forced our hand. Commentators are increasingly critical of the position set out in the Uniform Determination of Death Act, which was emphatic that irreversible cessation of all functions of the *entire* brain, including the brain stem, must be established. Today it is often suggested that the act should never have equated death with whole-brain death because signs of insignificant purposeless activity often remain in the brains of patients who are irreversibly unconscious and will never again breathe spontaneously.[2] Moreover, the body is clearly alive. Obfuscation was created from the outset. Although not a *radical* departure from previous biological definitions of death, irreversible loss of consciousness accompanied by an inability to breathe spontaneously— without the aid of a ventilator—is a "new" death, established earlier than ever before on a continuum of biological breakdown. And, for the first time, we can minutely control the progress of these changes, enabling doctors to procure organs, carry out experiments, or bring fetuses to term.

2. The United Kingdom avoided this problem by making a diagnosis of brain-stem death equivalent to death. Activity may persist in the upper brain, but it is recognized that if the brain stem is irreversibly damaged, then death of the whole brain will inevitably follow in short order.

Many of those interested in reopening the brain death debate argue that an irreversible loss of consciousness alone is the most important signifier—this should be the definitive factor in recognizing death, even though biological death may not be imminent. For such commentators not only brain-dead patients but those who are permanently vegetative count as dead. Others argue that, because the condition of brain-dead and PVS patients as alive or dead is ambiguous, we cannot count them as dead. But, because the prognosis is hopeless, decisions about forgoing treatment and about organ procurement can be based on the application of a concept of futility, and a loss of interest on the part of the patient. Yet others who want further public discussion about brain death remain opposed entirely to the procurement of organs from the brain-dead because they insist that these patients are alive.

Making criteria of irreversibility starkly visible, instead of hiding them behind the euphemism of brain death, is advisable, but my position is different from those set out above. The term *brain death*, with its ambiguity, should be dropped, in my opinion, or used only circumspectly. A diagnosis of an irreversible loss of consciousness together with a permanent loss of spontaneous breathing should be medically and legally recognized as the death of a person. Even though what constitutes the concept of "person" is by no means universal, it seems likely that there would be widespread agreement that individual persons (as opposed to recognition of them as social beings) cease to exist bodily once it is recognized by all concerned that biological death is inevitable. An equation of death with the demise of persons is already made reasonably explicit in intensive care units in North America. In Japan, even though the hopelessness and irreversibility of the condition are discussed, death of the person remains largely tacit and unspoken until such time as the family is prepared to grant that this has happened.

A move to official recognition of death of persons would not include PVS patients. These patients cannot be counted as dead in my opinion. Until such time as this condition is better understood and medically managed so that individuals are not in danger of being taken for good-as-dead, cases such as these should be handled individually and with great caution; although some may in the end be deemed hopeless, and death may then be hastened with appropriate consent.

Nor does an agreement about death of persons in any way affect decisions about organ donation as they stand at present. However, such an agreement might mean that involved health care professionals and certain bereaved families would feel more at ease with the situation, despite the ambiguity associated with brain-dead bodies.

If brain death is no longer recognized as death, but this same medically diagnosable condition is understood to be the death of a *person*, will the public still be willing to donate organs? Will images of body snatching loom large once again, or might they diminish? On the other hand, can we permit the current muddle to continue? All along we have imagined that by clearly demarcating life and death, we would retain objectivity and integrity, ensuring that no one not yet dead could be counted as good-as-dead. The game is up, it seems, leaving us to face another unsavory discovery—that death is not amenable to our efforts at its mastery; it will not be pinned down once and for all.

Bibliography

Ad Hoc Committee of the American Electroencephalographic Society. 1969. Cerebral Death and the Electroencephalogram. *JAMA* 209 (10): 1505–1510.

Ad Hoc Committee of the Harvard Medical School to Examine the Definition of Death. 1968. A Definition of Irreversible Coma. *Journal of the American Medical Association* 205 (6): 85–88.

Agamben, Giorgio. 1998. *Homo Sacer: Sovereign Power and Bare Life.* Stanford: Stanford University Press.

Agger, Ben. 1976. Marcuse and Habermas on New Science. *Polity* 9 (Winter): 158–181.

Akabayashi, Akira, and Masahiro Morioka. 1991. Ethical Issues Raised by Medical Use of Brain-Dead Bodies in the 1990s. *BioLaw* 2 (48): 531–538.

Alexander, Marc. 1980. The Rigid Embrace of the Narrow House: Premature Burial and the Signs of Death. *Hastings Center Report* 10:25–31.

Alexandre, G. P. J. 1966. Discussion, Organ Transplantation: The Practical Possibilities. In *Ethics in Medical Progress: With Special Reference to Transplantation,* edited by G. E. W. Wolstenholme and M. O'Connor, 68–69. Boston: Little, Brown and Company.

Allstetter, Billy. 1991. Cheating Brain Death. *Discover,* August, 24.

Amano Kenichi. 1987. Nōshi o Kangaeru, Zōki Ishoku to no Kanren no naka de (Thoughts on brain death in connection with organ transplants). *Gekkan Naashingu* 15, 13:1949–1953.

American Academy of Pediatrics, Committee on Bioethics. 1992. Infants with Anencephaly as Organ Sources: Ethical Considerations. *Pediatrics* 89 (6): 1116–1119.

Amersi, Farin, Douglas G. Farmer, and Ronald W. Busuttil. 1998. Fifteen-Year Experience with Adult and Pediatric Liver Transplantation at the University of California, Los Angeles. In *Clinical Transplants,* edited by Michael Cecka and Paul Terasaki, 255–257. Los Angeles: UCLA Tissue Typing Laboratory.

Andrews, Keith. 1993a. Should PVS Patients be Treated? *Neuropsychological Rehabilitation* 3:109–119.

———. 1993b. Recovery of Patients after Four Months or More in the Persistent Vegetative State. *British Medical Journal* 306:1597–1600.

———. 1993c. Patients in the Persistent Vegetative State: Problems in their Long Term Management. *British Medical Journal* 306:1600–1602.

Andrews, Keith, Lesley Murphy, Ros Munday, and Clare Littlewood. 1996. Misdiagnosis of the Vegetative State: Retrospective Study in a Rehabilitation Unit. *British Medical Journal* 313:13–16.

Annals of Internal Medicine. 1964. Moral Problems in the Use of Borrowed Organs, Artificial and Transplanted. 60 (2): 309–313.

———. 1968. When Do We Let the Patient Die? 68 (3): 695–700.

Annas, George J. 1988. Brain Death and Organ Donation: You Can Have One without the Other. *Hastings Center Report* 18:28–30.

Annual Registry Report of Japanese Dialysis Therapy. 2000. Dialysis Therapy Conditions in Japan as of December 1998. Tokyo: Japan Society for Dialysis Therapy, 57.

Appadurai, Arjun. 1986. Introduction: Commodities and the Politics of Value. In *The Social Life of Things: Commodities in Cultural Perspective,* edited by Arjun Appadurai, 3–63. Cambridge: Cambridge University Press.

———. 1990. Disjuncture and Difference in the Global Cultural Economy. *Public Culture* 2:1–24.

Appel, James Z. 1968. Ethical and Legal Questions Posed by Recent Advances in Medicine. *JAMA* 205 (7): 101–104.

Ariès, Philippe. 1974. *Western Attitudes toward Death from the Middle Ages to the Present.* Baltimore: Johns Hopkins University Press.

Arnold, John D., Thomas F. Zimmermann, and Daniel C. Martin. 1968. Public Attitudes and the Diagnosis of Death. *JAMA* 206 (9): 1949–1954.

Arnold, Ken. 1997. The Medical Context: Definitions of Death. In *Doctor Death: Medicine at the End of Life,* 19–23. Catalogue of an exhibition at the Wellcome Institute for the History of Medicine, January. London: Wellcome Institute.

Arnold, Robert M., and Stuart J. Youngner. 1995. The Dead Donor Rule: Should We Stretch it, Bend it, or Abandon it? In *Procuring Organs for Transplant,* edited by Robert M. Arnold, Stuart J. Youngner, Renie Shapiro, and Carol Mason Spicer, 219–234. Baltimore: Johns Hopkins University Press.

Arnold, Robert M., Stuart J. Youngner, Renie Shapiro, and Carol Mason Spicer, eds. 1995. Introduction. In *Procuring Organs for Transplant: The Debate over Non-Heart-Beating Cadaver Protocols,* edited by Robert M. Arnold, Stuart J. Youngner, Renie Shapiro, and Carol Mason Spicer, 1–13. Baltimore: Johns Hopkins University Press.

———, eds. 1995. *Procuring Organs for Transplant: The Debate over Non-Heart-Beating Cadaver Protocols.* Baltimore: Johns Hopkins University Press.

Asahi Shinbun. 1968a. Nihon hatsu no shinzō ishoku: Sapporo Idai 18sai no shōnen ni (Japan's first heart transplant to 18-year-old boy at Sapporo Medical University). August 8.

———. 1968b. Shinzō ishoku, teikyōsha wa musuko desu (Heart transplant: The donor is our son). August 11.

———. 1968c. Shinzō ishoku soko ga kikitai, Wada kyōju to ichimon ittō (Heart transplant: Questions and answers with Dr. Wada), August 15.

———. 1968d. Shinzō ishoku no Miyazaki-kun shinu (Mr. Miyazaki, the heart recipient, dies). October 29.

———. 1969. Shinzō ishoku ni kensatsu no mesu (Prosecutors cut into the heart transplant case). October 14.

———. 1987a. Bisoku zenshin, kokunai no zoki ishoku: Ukeire no okure ni iradachi (Light wind, some progress, domestic organ transplant: Doctors irritated by the delay in acceptance). September 23.

———. 1987b. Nōshi to ishoku to ishi e no shinrai (Trust in brain death, transplant, and doctors). March 27.

———. 1988. Nichibenren Nōshi yōnin ni hantai (Japan Federation of Bar Associations opposes accepting brain death). April 17.

———. 1989a. Seimei Rinri wa tsumamigui de wa naku (Taking bioethics seriously). January 16.

———. 1989b. "Jin ishoku o chūkai" to sagi (Fraud: "I'll provide kidney transplant"). April 23.

———. 1991a. Wada shinzō ishoku, Daidōmyakuben "surikae" giwaku, kantei shita Ohta-shi hiteisezu (Suspicion that the main artery valve had been replaced was not denied by the examiner, Dr. Ohta). March 30.

———. 1991b. Hatsu no nōshi kan ishoku (First brain-death liver transplant). July 12.

———. 1991c. Rongi fujūbun to hihan no kenkai (Inadequate discussion, critical view expressed). October 17.

———. 1991d. Teikyō ishi dō kakunin (How to confirm the will to donate). December 27.

———. 1992a. Tōmen wa shisei kaezu (The present stance will be maintained). January 23.

———. 1992b. Nichibenren Nōshi rincho tōshin ni hanron (Japan Federation of Bar Associations objects to the committee report). March 14.

———. 1993a. Yokohama Sōgō Byōin no nōshi ishoku, mukokyū tesuto sezu (Brain death transplant at Yokohama General Hospital did not include apnea test). July 13.

———. 1993b. Shinteishigo ni kanzō tekishutsu (Liver removed after heart stops). October 22.

———. 1993c. Kan ishoku kanja no "dōi" Kyūdai rokuon o kōkai (Kyūshū University makes public the tape-recording of the "consent" of the liver recipient). October 25.

———. 1993d. Nōshi to shinteishi no hazama de: Kyūdai kanzō ishoku o kenshō (Between brain death and heart death: Examining the Kyūshū University liver transplant case). November 26.

———. 1993e. Nōshi ishoku ni hantai, shimin dantai ga shūkai (Opposing brain death transplant, citizens' groups hold a meeting). December 6.

———. 1994a. Nōshi ishoku Kankoku wa ippo saki ni (Brain death transplant: Korea has moved ahead). March 17.

———. 1994b. 'Teishutsu yamete' shiminraga yōsei ("Do not submit," demanded by citizens: Internal organ transplant bill). April 2.

———. 1994c. Zōki ishoku hōan matamo sakiokuri (Organ transplant legislation postponed again). May 25.

———. 1994d. Yokohama Sōgō Byōin no nōshi mukokyō testo sezu (Brain death, organ transplant without apnea test at Yokohama General Hospital). July 13.

———. 1994e. "Nōshi" kanja no jinken o obiyakashi, hito no zōki o mono to shite atsukau Zōki ishoku hō no seitei ni watashitachi wa tsuyoku hantai shimasu (We strongly oppose the enactment of the Organ Transplant Law, which threatens the human rights of "brain-dead" patients and treats human organs as objects). June 23 and 24, July 24.

———. 1994f. Tokyo shitamachi denchū ni bira: "Jinzō urimasu" (Flyer on an electronic pole in downtown Tokyo: "Kidney for sale"). October 10.

———. 1994g. Inochi motomete—101 nin no ishoku tokō: Nihonjin mura "Atarashii kanzō o" ikoku no chi de matsu hibi (101 persons seeking life by going abroad: Days waiting in a foreign land for a "new liver" in a Japanese village). November 7.

———. 1994h. Ishi no setsumei fujūbun (Insufficient explanation by doctor). December 11.

———. 1996a. "Nōshi wa hito no shi" to mitomemasuka? (Do you recognize brain death as human death?). October 1.

———. 1996b. "Nōshi wa hito no shi" 53% (Brain death is human death, 53 percent). October 1.

———. 1996c. Nōshi ishoku kyōryoku de Masui Gakkai ga kenkai (Anesthesiology Association expresses a view for cooperation with brain death transplant). November 16.

———. 1997a. Nōteitaion ryōhō hodokoshita kanja, nōkino no sokushin yaku de shokubutsu jōtai kara kaifuku (A patient treated by hypothermia recovers from a vegetative state). April 6.

———. 1997b. "Nōshi wa shi ka" shinchōron aitsugu ("Is brain death death?" Many cautious arguments made). April 9.

———. 1997c. Zōki ishoku hōan, Chikazuku Shūin Saiketsu (Organ transplantation bill: The coming voting in the Lower House). April 20.

———. 1997d. Sei ka nōshi, shi ka (Is brain death life or death?). April 25.

———. 1997e. Shūkyōkai ni "nōshi" hamon (Brain death ripples spread in the religious world). May 9.

———. 1997f. Nōshi o hito no shi de aru to omouka? (Do you think that brain death is human death?). May 27.

———. 1997g. Zōki Ishoku hōan "Nōshi wa Hito no Shi" kitei, sansei 40%, hantai 42% de nibun (Organ transplant law, "Brain death is human death" divided, 40 percent agree and 42 percent are opposed). May 27.

———. 1998a. "Zōki teikyō" ishi ikizu (Will to "donate organs" went unheeded). January 6.

———. 1998b. Izoku to ishi tsutawaranu kokoro (The deceased's family and doctor failed to communicate). March 24.

———. 1998c. Shinteishimae ni jinzō hozon sochi: Byōin gawa ni baishō meirei

(Preservation measure taken before heart stopped: Hospital to pay compensation). May 21.

———. 1998d. Zōki Ishokuhō shikō 1nen: Ishokutaisei mada nakaba (A year after the Organ Transplant Law: Conditions for transplant still only half ready). November 13.

———. 1999a. Jibun ga nōshi, zōki teikyō wa nozomanu 37%, nozomu 31%, Sōrifu yoron chōsa ("If I were to become brain dead, I would": 37 percent would donate, 31 would not, a national survey by the Prime Minister's Office shows). February 28.

———. 1999b. "Jōhō kaiji wa dōji shinkō de", shimin dantai ("Information should be disclosed simultaneously," citizens groups say). March 4.

Asai, Atsushi, Munetaka Maekawa, Ichirō Akiguchi, Tsuguya Fukui, Yasuhiko Miura, Noboru Tanabe, and Shunichi Fukuhara. 1999. Survey of Japanese Physicians' Attitudes towards the Care of Adult Patients in Persistent Vegetative State. *Journal of Medical Ethics* 25:302–308.

Asquith, Pamela. 1986. Anthropomorphism and the Japanese and Western Traditions in Primatology. In *Primate Ontogeny, Cognition, and Behavior: Developments in Field and Laboratory Research*, edited by J. Elfe and P. Lee, 61–71. New York: Academic Press.

———. 1990. The Japanese Idea of Soul in Animals and Objects as Evidenced by "Kuyō" Services. In *Discovering Japan*, ed. D. V. Daly and T. T. Sekine, 181–88. Toronto: Captus Press.

Asquith, Pamela, and Arne Kalland, eds. 1997. *Japanese Images of Nature: Cultural Perspectives*. Surrey: Curzon.

Bai, Kōichi. 1970. Contemporary Problems of Medical Law in Japan, Parts I and II. *Annals of the Institute of Social Science* 11:17–54.

———. 1990. The Definition of Death: The Japanese Attitude and Experience. *Transplant Proceedings* 22:991–992.

Bai, Kōichi, and K. Hirabayashi. 1984. The Legal Situation in Japan and Whose Consent Shall Make Organ Removal Lawful. *Comparative Law Journal* 46:291–294.

Baird, Patricia A., and Adele D. Sadovnick. 1987. Survival in Liveborn Infants with Anencephaly. *American Journal of Genetics* 28:1019–1020.

Bal, Mieke. 1991. *Reading "Rembrandt": Beyond the Word-Image Opposition*. Cambridge: Cambridge University Press.

Barkan, Leonard. 1996. Cosmas and Damian: Of Medicine, Miracles and the Economics of the Body. In *Organ Transplantation: Meanings and Realities*, edited by Stuart J. Youngner, Renée C. Fox, and Laurence J. O'Connell, 221–251. Madison: University of Wisconsin Press.

Barker, Francis. 1984. *The Tremulous Private Body: Essays on Subjection*. London: Methuen.

Barnard, Christiaan N. 1968. Human Cardiac Transplantation: An Evaluation of the First Two Operations Performed at the Groote Schuur Hospital, Cape Town. *American Journal of Cardiology* 22:584–596.

Barsotti, Anna Maria Bertoli, and Alessandro Ruggeri. 1997. The Skinned Model: A Model for Science Born between Truth and Beauty. *Italian Journal of Anatomy and Embryology* 102:63–69.

Bart, K. J., E. J. Macon and A. L. Humphries. 1979. A Response to the Shortage of Cadavric Kidneys for Transplantation. *Transplantation Proceedings* 11: 455–458.

Bartlett, Edward T., and Stuart J. Youngner. 1988. Human Death and the Destruction of the Neocortex. In *Death: Beyond Whole-Brain Criteria*, edited by Richard M. Zaner. Dordrecht: Kluwer Academic Publishers, 199–216.

Basalla, G. 1988. *The Evolution of Technology*. Cambridge: Cambridge University Press.

Bastien, J. 1985. Qollahuaya-Andean Body Concepts: A Typographical Hydraulic Model of Physiology. *American Anthropology* 87:595–611.

Bataille, George. 1988. *Inner Experience*. Albany: State University of New York Press.

Bauby, Jean-Dominique. 1998. *The Diving-Bell and the Butterfly*. London: Fourth Estate.

Baudrillard, Jean. 1993. *Symbolic Exchange and Death*. London: Sage Publications.

Bauman, Zygmunt. 1992. *Mortality, Immortality, and Other Life Strategies*. Stanford: Stanford University Press.

Becker, Carl B. 1993. *Breaking the Circle: Death and the Afterlife in Buddhism*. Carbondale: Southern Illinois University Press.

———. 1999. Money Talks, Money Kills: The Economics of Transplantation in Japan and China. *Bioethics* 13 (3/4): 236–243.

Becker, Ernest. 1973. *The Denial of Death*. New York: Free Press.

Becker, Lawrence C. 1975. Human Being: The Boundaries of the Concept. *Philosophy and Public Affairs* 4:335–359.

Beecher, Henry K. 1969. After the "Definition of Irreversible Coma." *New England Journal of Medicine* 281 (19): 1070–1071.

Beidel, Deborah C. 1987. Psychological Factors in Organ Transplantation. *Clinical Psychology Review* 7:677–694.

Benjamin, Walter. 1969. *Illuminations*. New York: Schocken.

Bernat, James L. 1992. The Boundaries of the Persistent Vegetative State. *Journal of Clinical Ethics* 3 (3): 176–180.

Bernat, James L., Charles M. Culver, and Bernard Gert. 1981. On the Definition and Criteria of Death. *Annals of Internal Medicine* 94:389–391.

Bessert, I., W. Buschart, K. Horatz, et al. 1970. On the Numerical Relation between Reanimation Patients, Patients with Dissociated Brain Death, and Potential Organ Donors in a Reanimation Center. *Electroencephalography and Clinical Neurophysiology* 29:210–211.

Beyene, Yewoubdar. 1989. *From Menarche to Menopause: Reproductive Lives of Peasant Women in Two Cultures*. Albany: State University of New York Press.

Binski, Paul. 1996. *Medieval Death: Ritual and Representation*. Ithaca: Cornell University Press.

Bion, J. 1995. Rationing Intensive Care. *British Medical Journal* 310: 682–683.

Black, Peter. 1978. Brain Death (2 parts). *New England Journal of Medicine* 229 (7): 338–344 and 229 (8): 393–401.

————. 1980. Editorial: From Heart to Brain: The New Definitions of Death. *American Heart Journal* 99:279–281.

————. 1986. Comment. *Neurosurgery* 18:567.

Black, Peter McL., and Nicholas T. Zervas. 1984. Declaration of Brain Death in Neurosurgical and Neurological Practice. *Neurosurgery* 15 (2): 170–174.

Bloch, Maurice. 1982. Death, Women and Power. In *Death and the Regeneration of Life,* edited by Maurice Bloch and Jonathan Parry. Cambridge: Cambridge University Press, 211–230.

Bloch, Maurice, and Jonathan Parry, eds. 1982. *Death and the Regeneration of Life,* Cambridge: Cambridge University Press.

Boltanski, Luc. 1993. *La souffrance à distance.* Paris: Metailie.

Borges, Jorge Luis. 1964. The Immortal. In *Labyrinths: Selected Stories and Other Writings.* New York: New Directions.

Bourdieu, Pierre. 1990a. *In Other Words: Essays towards a Reflective Sociology.* Stanford: Stanford University Press.

————. 1990b. *The Logic of Practice,* trans. R. Nice. Cambridge: Polity; Stanford: Stanford University Press.

————. 1997. *Outline of a Theory of Practice.* Cambridge: Cambridge University Press.

Bradley, David J., and David C. Warhurst. 1995. Malaria Prophylaxis: Guidelines for Travellers from Britain. *British Medical Journal* 310: 709–714.

Brandt, Allan. 1981. Racism and Research: The Case of the Tuskegee Syphilis Study. In *The Social World,* edited by Ian Robertson. New York: Worth, 186–195.

Brante, Thomas, and Margareta Hallberg. 1991. Brain or Heart? The Controversy over the Concept of Death. *Social Studies of Science* 21:389–413.

British Medical Association. 1992. *Medicine Betrayed: The Participation of Doctors in Human Rights Abuse — Report of a Working Party.* London: Zed Books.

Bronfen, Elisabeth, and Sarah Webster Goodwin. 1993. Introduction. In *Death and Representation,* edited by Sarah Webster Goodwin and Elisabeth Bronfen. Baltimore: Johns Hopkins University Press, 3–25.

Brouardel, Pierre. 1897. *Death and Sudden Death,* translated by B. Y. F. Lucas Benham. New York: Wood.

Brown, Elizabeth A. R. 1981. Death and the Human Body in the Later Middle Ages: The Legislation of Boniface VIII on the Division of the Corpse. *Viator* 12:221–270.

Brown, James A. C. 1961. *Freud and the Post-Freudians.* Harmondsworth: Penguin Books Ltd.

Brown, Keith. Ms. The Importance of Culture: A Lesson Learned from Robert J. Smith. University of Pittsburgh.

Bukkyō Dendō Kyōkai. 1975. *The Teaching of Buddha.* Tokyo: Bukkyō Dendō Kyōkai.

Bulletin of Medical Ethics. 1996. Editorial. No. 115. February.

Bynum, Caroline Walker. 1991. *Fragmentation and Redemption: Essays on Gender and the Human Body in Medieval Religion.* New York: Zone Books.

Byrne, Paul, and Richard Nilges. 1993. The Brain Stem in Brain Death: A Critical Review. *Issues in Law and Medicine* 9:3–21.

Byrne, Paul A., Sean O'Reilly, and Paul M. Quay. 1979. Brain Death—An Opposing Viewpoint. *JAMA* 242:1985–1990.

Callon, Michel. 1986. Some Elements of a Sociology of Translation: Domestication of the Scallops and the Fishermen of St. Brieux Bay. In *Power, Action and Belief: A New Sociology of Knowledge?* edited by John Law. London: Routledge and Kegan Paul, 196–229.

Calne, Roy. 1966. Discussion, Organ Transplantation: The Practical Possibilities. In *Ethics in Medical Progress: With Special Reference to Transplantation*, edited by G. E. W. Wolstenholme and M. O'Connor, 73. Boston: Little, Brown and Company.

Campbell, John Creighton, and Naoki Ikegami. 1998. *The Art of Balance in Health Policy: Maintaining Japan's Low-Cost, Egalitarian System*. Cambridge: Cambridge University Press.

Camporesi, Piero. 1988. Decay and Rebirth. Chapter 5 in *The Incorruptible Flesh: Bodily Mutation and Mortification in Religion and Folklore*. Cambridge: Cambridge University Press, 67–89.

Canadian Medical Association Journal. 1987. Guidelines for the Diagnosis of Brain Death: A CMA Position. *Canadian Medical Association Journal* 136 (January 15): 200a–b.

Canadian Organ Replacement Register. 1996. *Annual Report, Vol. 2: 1996. Organ Donation and Transplantation*. Ottawa: Canadian Institute for Health Information.

———. 2000. Number of Liver Transplants by Pediatric Age Groups (0–5 Years): Canada and Provinces. Toronto: Canadian Organ Replacement Register/Canadian Institute for Health Information.

Canadian Pediatric Society. 1990. Transplantation of Organs from Newborns with Anencephaly. *Canadian Medical Association Journal* 142 (7): 715–717.

Canetti, Elias. 1973. *Crowds and Power*. London: Penguin Books.

Caplan, Arthur L. 1987. Measuring Brain Function Difficult Because There's No Brain to Measure. *Medical Ethics Advisor* 3 (12): 164.

———. 1988. Professional Arrogance and Public Misunderstanding. *Hastings Center Report* April/May 18:34–37.

Capps, Lisa L. 1994. Change and Continuity in the Medical Culture of the Hmong in Kansas City. *Medical Anthropology Quarterly* 8 (2): 161–177.

Capron, A. M., and L. R. Kass. 1972. A Statutory Definition of the Standards for Determining Human Death. *University Pennsylvania Law Review* 121: 87–118.

Carnevale, Franco A. 1998. The Utility of Futility: The Construction of Bioethical Problems. *Nursing Ethics* 5 (6): 509–517.

Casper, Monica J. 1994. At the Margins of Humanity: Fetal Positions in Science and Medicine. *Science, Technology & Human Values* 19 (3): 307–323.

Choron, Jacques. 1964. *Death and Modern Man*. New York: Collier Books.

Christison, Robert. 1885–1886. *The Life of Sir Robert Christison*. Edinburgh: Blackwood.

Cohen, Kathleen. 1973. *Metamorphosis of a Death Symbol: The Transi Tomb in the Late Middle Ages and the Renaissance*. Berkeley: University of California Press.

Cohen, Lawrence. Ms. Organ Sales.

Comaroff, Jean. 1984. Medicine, Time, and the Perception of Death: Listening. *Journal of Religion and Culture* 19:155–169.

Conference of Medical Royal Colleges and Their Faculties in the United Kingdom. 1976. Diagnosis of Death. *British Medical Journal* 2: 1187–1188.

Conrad, Peter. 1994. Wellness as Virtue: Morality and the Pursuit of Health. *Culture, Medicine and Psychiatry* 18:385–401.

Cooper, Theodore, and Sheila C. Mitchell. 1969. Cardiac Transplantation: Current Status. *Transplantation Proceedings* 1:755–757.

Cornell, Laurel. 1996. Infanticide in Early Modern Japan? Demography, Culture and Population Growth. *Journal of Asian Studies* 55:22–50.

Council on Ethical and Judicial Affairs, American Medical Association. 1995. The Use of Anencephalic Neonates as Organ Donors. *JAMA* 273:1614–1618.

Crane, Diana. 1976. Physicians' Attitude toward the Treatment of Critically Ill Patients. *Radcliffe Quarterly* 62:18–21.

Cranford, Ronald. 1996. Misdiagnosing the Persistent Vegetative State. *British Medical Journal* 313: 5–6.

———. 1998. Even the Dead Are Not Terminally Ill Anymore. *Neurology* 51 (6): 1530–1531.

Cronon, William, ed. 1996. *Uncommon Ground: Rethinking the Human Place in Nature*. New York: W. W. Norton.

Crowley, Megan. Ms. The Brain Dead Body: Carnivalesque, Transgressive and Eminently Productive.

Culver, C. M., and B. Gert. 1982. *Philosophy in Medicine: Conceptual and Ethical Issues in Medicine and Psychiatry*. Oxford: Oxford University Press.

Cummings, Bruce. 1993. Japan's Position in the World System. In *Postwar Japan as History*, edited by Andrew Gordon, 34–95. Berkeley: University of California Press.

Cunningham, Clark. 1973. Order in the Atoni House. In *Right and Left: On Dual Symbolic Classification*, edited by Rodney Needham, 204–238. Chicago: University of Chicago Press.

Dallas, H. A. 1927. What Is Death? *The Living Age* 332:354–359.

Daniel, Valentine. 1991. Is There a Counterpoint to Culture? Wertheim Lecture, 1991. Amsterdam: Centre for Asian Studies.

Daston, Lorraine. 1992. Objectivity and the Escape from Perspective. *Social Studies of Science* 22:597–618.

———. 1995. The Moral Economy of Science. *Osiris* 10:3–26.

Davidson, Arnold. 1996. Styles of Reasoning, Conceptual History, and the Emergence of Psychiatry. In *The Disunity of Science: Boundaries, Contexts and Power*, edited by P. Galison and D. Stump, 75–100. Stanford: Stanford University Press.

Davidson, Henry. 1968. Transplantation in the Brave New World. *Mental Hygiene* 5:46–78.

De Coppet, Daniel. 1981. The Life-Giving Death. In *Mortality and Immortality: The Anthropology and Archeology of Death*, edited by S. C. Humphreys and Helen King, 175–204. London: Academic Press.

Delmonico, Francis L., and Judson G. Randolph. 1973. Death: A Concept in Transition. *Pediatrics* 51 (2): 234–239.

Descartes, René. 1968 [1637]. *Discourse on Method and the Meditations*. London: Penguin Books.

Dickson, David. 1988. Human Experimentation Roils French Medicine. *Science* 239:1370.

Dominguez, Virginia R. 1992. Invoking Culture: The Messy Side of "Cultural Politics." *South Atlantic Quarterly* 91:19–42.

Doniger, Wendy. 1996. Transplanting Myths of Organ Transplants. In *Organ Transplantation: Meanings and Realities*, edited by S. J. Youngner, R. C. Fox, and L. J. O'Connell, 194–220. Madison: University of Wisconsin Press.

Dorff, Elliot. 1996. Choosing Life: Aspects of Judaism Affecting Organ Transplantation. In *Organ Transplantation: Meanings and Realities*, edited by Stuart J. Youngner, Renée C. Fox, and Laurence J. O'Connell, 168–193. Madison: University of Wisconsin Press.

Dougherty, John Jr., F. Rawlinson, David E. Levy, and Fred Plum. 1981. Hypoxic-Ischemic Brain Injury and the Vegetative State: Clinical and Neuropathologic Correlation. *Neurology* 31:991–997.

Douglas, Mary. 1990. Foreword: No Free Gifts. In Marcel Mauss, *The Gift*, 7–18. New York: W. W. Norton.

Douglass, W. A. 1969. *Death in Murelaga: Funerary Rituals in a Spanish Basque Village*. Seattle: University of Washington Press.

Dyer, Clare. 1997. Hillsborough Victim "Awakes": PVS Man Aware after Eight Years. *The Guardian*. March 17.

Ebony. 1968. The Telltale Heart. March, 118–119.

Elias, Norbert. 1985. *The Loneliness of Dying*, translated by Edmond Jephcott. Oxford: Blackwell.

Ellul, Jacques. 1964. *The Technological Society*, translated by John Wilkinson. New York: Alfred A. Knopf.

Emanuel, Linda L. 1995. Reexamining Death: The Asymptotic Model and a Bounded Zone Definition. *Hastings Center Report* 25 (4): 27–35.

Engelhardt, Karlheinz. 1998. Correspondence. Organ Donation and Permanent Vegetative State. *Lancet* 351:211.

Epstein, Steven. 1997. Activism, Drug Regulation, and the Politics of Therapeutic Evaluation in the AIDS Era: A Case Study of ddC and the "Surrogate Markers" Debate. *Social Studies of Science* 27:691–726.

Evans-Pritchard, E. E. 1937. *Witchcraft, Oracles, and Magic Among the Azande*. Oxford: Clarendon.

Evans-Wenz, W. Y., comp. and ed. 1981. *The Tibetan Book of the Dead*. Oxford: Oxford University Press.

Fabian, Johannes. 1972. How Others Die: Reflections on the Anthropology of Death. In *Death in American Experience*, edited by Arien Mack, 177–201. New York: Schocken Books.

Fagot-Largeault, Anne. 1989. *Les causes de la mort: Histoire naturelle et facteurs de risque.* Paris: Librairie Philosophique J. Vrin.

Falk, R. H. 1999. Physical and Intellectual Recovery Following Prolonged Hypoxia Coma. *Postgraduate Medical Journal* 66:384–386.

Farmer, Paul, and Arthur Kleinman. 1989. AIDS as Human Suffering. *Daedalus* 118 (Spring): 135–160.

Feldman, Eric. 1994. Over My Dead Body: The Enigma and Economics of Death in Japan. In *Containing Health Care Costs in Japan,* edited by Naoki Ikegami and John C. Campbell, 234–247. Ann Arbor: University of Michigan Press.

Fetters, Michael D. 1998. The Family in Medical Decision Making: Japanese Perspectives. *Journal of Clinical Ethics* 9:143–157.

Field, David R., Elena A. Gates, Robert K. Creasy, Albert R. Jonsen, and Russell K. Laros Jr. 1988. Maternal Brain Death During Pregnancy: Medical and Ethical Issues. *JAMA* 260 (6): 816–822.

Field, Norma. 1991. *In the Realm of a Dying Emperor: A Portrait of Japan at Century's End.* New York: Pantheon Books.

Figal, Gerald. 1996. How to *jibunshi:* Making and Marketing Self-Histories of Shōwa among the Masses in Postwar Japan. *Journal of Asian Studies* 55 (4): 902–933.

Finucane, R. C. 1981. Sacred Corpses, Profane Carrion: Social Ideals and Death Rituals in the Later Middle Ages. In *Mirrors of Mortality: Studies in the Social History of Death,* edited by Joachim Whaley, 40–60. London: Europa Publications.

Fost, Norman. 1986. Ethical Problems in Pediatrics. *Current Problems in Pediatrics* 6:12 (October), 1–31.

———. 1988. Organs from Encephalic Infants: An Idea Whose Time Has Not Yet Come. *Hastings Center Report* 18:5–10.

———. 1999. The Unimportance of Death. In *The Definition of Death: Contemporary Controversies,* edited by Stuart J. Youngner, Robert M. Arnold, and Renie Shapiro, 161–178. Baltimore: Johns Hopkins University Press.

Foucault, Michel. 1970. *The Order of Things: An Archeology of the Human Sciences.* New York: Random House.

———. 1980. *The History of Sexuality, Volume 1: An Introduction.* Trans. Robert Hurley. New York: Vintage Books.

Fox, E., and C. Stocking. 1993. Ethics Consultants' Recommendation for Life-Prolonging Treatments of Patients in Persistent Vegetative State. *JAMA* 270: 2578–2582.

Fox, Renée. 1978. Organ Transplantation: Sociocultural Aspects. In *Encyclopedia of Bioethics,* vol. 3, edited by W. T. Reich. New York: Free Press, 1166–1169.

Fox, Renée, and Judith P. Swazey. 1978. *The Courage to Fail: A Social View of Organ Transplants and Dialysis.* Chicago: University of Chicago Press.

———. 1992. *Spare Parts: Organ Replacement in American Society.* Oxford: Oxford University Press.

Francis, Robert. 1995. A Legal Comment. *British Medical Journal* 310: 718.

Freedman, Maurice. 1958. *Lineage Organization in Southeastern China.* London: Athlone Press.

Freud, Sigmund. 1939. *Civilization, War, and Death: Selections from Three Works by Sigmund Freud,* edited by J. Richman. London: Hogarth Press and the Institute of Psychoanalysis.

———. 1959. The "Uncanny." In *Collected Papers, Volume IV, Papers on Metapsychology, Papers on Applied Psycho-Analysis,* 368–407. London: Basic Books.

Fukaura, Asato, Hiroki Tazawa, Hiroaki Nakajima, and Mitsuru Adachi. 1995. Occasional Notes—Do-Not-Resuscitate Orders at a Teaching Hospital in Japan. *New England Journal of Medicine* 333 (12): 805–808.

Fukuda, Masaaki. 1975. A Survey Research of Doctors' Attitudes toward Euthanasia in Boston and in Tokyo. *Osaka University Law Review* 22:19–77.

Fukumoto, Eiko. 1989. *Seibutsugaku jidai sei to shi* (Life and death in the era of the biological sciences). Tokyo: Gijitsu no Ningen sha.

Fulton, Robert. 1965. *Death and Identity.* New York: John Wiley and Sons.

Garcia-Ballester, Luis. 1995. Artifex factivus sanitatis: Health and Medical Care in Medieval Latin Galenism. In *Knowledge and the Scholarly Medical Traditions,* edited by Don Bates, 127–150. Cambridge: Cambridge University Press.

Gaylin, Willard. 1974. Harvesting the Dead. *Harpers* 52:23–30.

Geary, Patrick J. 1994. *Living with the Dead in the Middle Ages.* Ithaca: Cornell University Press.

Geertz, Clifford. 1973. *The Interpretation of Cultures.* New York: Basic Books, 360–411.

———. 2000. *Available Light: Anthropological Reflections on Philosophical Topics.* Princeton: Princeton University Press.

Gervais, Karen Grandstand. 1986. *Redefining Death.* New Haven: Yale University Press.

Giacomini, Mita. 1997. A Change of Heart and a Change of Mind? Technology and the Redefinition of Death in 1968. *Social Science of Medicine* 44 (10): 1465–1482.

Gianakos, Dean. 1995. Terminal Weaning. *Chest* 108:1405–1406.

Gianelli, Diane M. 1987. Anencephalic Heart Donor Creates New Ethics Debate. *American Medical News* 3 (November 6): 47–49.

Gibbs, Nancy. 1993. Angels among Us. *Time,* December 27.

Gilligan, Timothy, and Thomas A. Raffin. 1995. Rapid Withdrawal of Support. *Chest* 108:1407–1408.

——— ———. 1996. Withdrawing Life Support: Extubation and Prolonged Terminal Weaning are Inappropriate. *Critical Care Medicine* 24 (2): 352–353.

Ginsburg, Faye, and Rayna Rapp, eds. 1995. *Conceiving the New World Order: The Global Politics of Reproduction.* Berkeley: University of California Press.

Globe and Mail. 1999a. Intensive Scare. January 30.

———. 1999b. Low Organ Donation Rate Blamed on Reluctance to Ask. April 20.

Gluck, Carol. 1990. "The Meaning of Ideology in Modern Japan." In *Rethink-*

ing Japan, edited by A. Boscaro, F. Gatti, and M. Raveri, 283–297. Folkestone: Japan Library.

———. 1993. The Past in the Present. In *Postwar Japan as History,* edited by Andrew Gordon, 64–95. Berkeley: University of California Press.

Good, Mary-Jo Delvecchio, Paul E. Brodwin, Byron J. Good, and Arthur Kleinman, eds. 1992. *Pain as Human Experience: An Anthropological Perspective.* Berkeley: University of California Press.

Goodwin, W. E. 1966. Final Discussion. In *Ethics in Medical Progress: With Special Reference to Transplantation,* edited by G. E. W. Wolstenholme and M. O'Connor. Boston: Little, Brown and Company, 211.

Gorer, Geoffrey. 1956. The Pornography of Death. *Berkeley Book of Modern Writing* 3:56–62.

———1965. *Death, Grief, and Mourning in Contemporary Britain.* London: Cresset Press.

Granet, Marcel. 1930. *Chinese Civilization.* London: K. Paul, Trench, Trubner, and Co.

Green, Michael B., and Daniel Wikler. 1980. Brain Death and Personal Identity. *Philosophy & Public Affairs* 9 (2): 105–133.

Grenvik, Ake, David J. Powner, James V. Snyder, Michael S. Jastremski, Ralph A. Babcock, and Michael G. Loughhead. 1978. Cessation of Therapy in Terminal Illness and Brain Death. *Critical Care Medicine* 6:284–291.

Griaule, M. 1965. *Conversations with Ogotemmeli.* Oxford: Oxford University Press.

Grubb, Andrew, Pat Walsh, Neil Lambe, Trevor Murrells, and Sarah Robinson. 1997. *Doctors' Views on the Management of Patients in Persistent Vegetative State (PVS): A UK Study.* Occasional Papers, series 1. London: Centre of Medical Law & Ethics, King's College London.

Grundel, J. 1968. Ethics of Organ Transplantation. In *Organ Transplantation Today: Symposium Held on the Occasion of the Official Opening of the Sint Lucas Ziekenhuis by H.R.H. The Prince of the Netherlands* (Amsterdam 6–8, 1968), 333–354. Amsterdam: Excerpta Medica Foundation.

Guardian Weekly. 1996a. Japanese are Dying for a Transplant. August 4.

———. 1996b. Thwarting the Grim Reaper. January 14.

———. 1996c. Untitled letter. January 21.

Habermas, Jürgen. 1970. *Toward a Rational Society.* Boston: Beacon Press.

Hacking, Ian. 1990. *The Taming of Chance.* Cambridge: Cambridge University Press.

———. 1996. The Disunities of Science. In *The Disunity of Science: Boundaries, Contexts and Power,* edited by P. Galison and D. Stump, 37–74. Stanford: Stanford University Press.

Halevy, A., and B. Brody. 1993. Brain Death: Reconciling Definitions, Criteria and Tests. *Annals of Internal Medicine* 119:519–525.

Haller, Jordan, and Marcial Cerruti. 1969. Heart Transplantation in Man: Compilation of Cases, II, January 23, 1964, to June 22, 1969. *American Journal of Cardiology* 24:554–563.

Hamano, Kenzo. 1997. A Report from Japan: Human Rights and Japanese Bioethics. *Bioethics* 11 (3–4): 328–335.

Hamburger, J., and J. Crosnier. 1968. Moral and Ethical Problems in Transplantation. In *Human Transplantation,* edited by F. T. Rapaport and J. Dausset, 37–44. New York: Grune and Stratton.

Haraway, Donna. 1990. A Manifesto for Cyborgs: Science, Technology, and Socialist Feminism in the 1980's. In *Feminism/Postmodernism,* edited by L. J. Nicholson, 190–233. London: Routledge.

————. 1991. A Cyborg Manifesto: Science, Technology, and Socialist-Feminism in the Late Twentieth Century. Chapter 8 in *Simians, Cyborgs, and Women: The Reinvention of Nature.* New York: Routledge, 149–181.

Harcourt, Glenn. 1987. Andreas Vesalius and the Anatomy of Antique Sculpture. *Representations* 17 (Winter): 28–61.

Hardacre, Helen. 1994. The Response of Buddhism and Shintō to the Issue of Brain Death and Organ Transplants. *Cambridge Quarterly of Healthcare Ethics* 3:585–601.

————. 1997. *Marketing the Menacing Fetus in Japan.* Berkeley: University of California Press.

Hardy, James D., and Carlos M. Chavez. 1968. The First Heart Transplant in Man: Developmental Animal Investigations with Analysis of the 1964 Case in the Light of Current Clinical Experience. *American Journal of Cardiology* 22:772–781.

Harootunian, H. D. 1988. *Things Seen and Unseen: Discourse and Ideology in Tokugawa Nativism.* Chicago: University of Chicago Press.

————. 1989. Visible Discourses/Invisible Ideologies. In *Postmodernism and Japan,* edited by M. Miyoshi and H. D. Harootunian, 63–92. Durham, N.C.: Duke University Press.

Harris, Olivia. 1982. The Dead and the Devils among the Bolivian Laymi. In *Death and the Regeneration of Life,* edited by Maurice Bloch and Jonathan Parry. Cambridge: Cambridge University Press, 45–73.

Harris, Sheldon H. 1994. *Factories of Death: Japanese Biological Warfare, 1932–45, and the American Cover-Up.* London: Routledge.

Harvey, David. 1996. *Justice, Nature, and the Geography of Difference.* Oxford: Blackwell.

Healy, David. 1998. *The Antidepressant Era.* Cambridge: Harvard University Press.

Heelas, Paul, and Andrew Lock. 1981. *Indigenous Psychologies: The Anthropology of Self.* London: Academic Press.

Heidegger, Martin. 1962. *Being and Time.* New York: Harper & Row.

Heilbroner, Robert L. 1967. Do Machines Make History? *Technology and Culture* 8:335–345.

Hendrick, Burton J. 1913. On the Trail of Immortality. *McClure's* 40:304–317.

Herr, Michael. 1977. *Dispatches.* New York: Alfred A. Knopf.

Hertz, Robert. 1960. *Death and the Right Hand,* translated and with an introduction by E. E. Evans-Pritchard. New York: Free Press.

Hirano, Ryūichi. 1997. Sanpō ichiryōzon teki kaiketsu: Sofuto randingu no tame no zanteiteki sochi (Tentative measures for a soft landing). *Jurist* 1121: 30–38.

Hirosawa, Kōshichirō. 1992. Junkanki senmoni no tachiba kara mita nōshi to shinzō ishoku (Brain death and heart transplants from the point of view of a circulatory system specialist). In *Nōshi to zōki-ishoku* (Brain death and organ transplants), edited by Takeshi Umehara. Tokyo: Asahi Shinbunsha.

Hobsbawm, Eric, and Terence Ranger. 1983. *The Invention of Tradition.* Cambridge: Cambridge University Press.

Hoffenberg, Raymond, Margaret Lock, Nick Tilney, C. Casabona, Abdullah S. Daar, Ronald D. Guttmann, I. Kennedy, S. Nundy, Janet Radcliffe-Richards, and Robert A. Sells, for the International Forum for Transplant Ethics. 1997. Should Organs from Patients in Permanent Vegetative State Be Used for Transplantation? *Lancet* 350:1320–1321.

Hogle, Linda. 1995. Standardization across Non-Standard Domains: The Case of Organ Procurement. *Science, Technology & Human Values* 20:482–500.

———. 1996. Transforming "Body Parts" into Therapeutic Tools: A Report from Germany. *Medical Anthropology Quarterly* 10 (4): 675–682.

———. 1999. *Recovering the Nation's Body: Cultural Memory, Medicine and the Politics of Redemption.* New Brunswick, N.J.: Rutgers University Press.

Hosaka, Masayasu. 1992. *Zōki ishoku to nihonjin* (Japanese and organ transplants). Tokyo: Asahi Sonorama.

Hōsō bunka kenkyūjo Yoron chōsabu (NHK Public Poll Section). 1996. *Zenkoku kenmin ishiki chōsa kekka no gaiyō* (Overview of the results from an NHK nationwide survey on the awareness of residents in each prefecture). Tokyo: NHK.

Hughes, J. R. 1978. Limitations of the EEG in Coma and Brain Death. *Annals of the New York Academy of Sciences* 315:121–136.

Hughes, R., and G. McGuire. 1997. Neurologic Disease and the Determination of Brain Death: The Importance of a Diagnosis. *Critical Care Medicine* 25: 1923–1924.

Hughes, Thomas. 1983. *Networks of Power: Electrification of Western Society, 1880–1930.* Baltimore: Johns Hopkins University Press.

Humphreys, S. C. 1981. Introduction: Comparative Perspectives on Death. In *Mortality and Immortality: The Anthropology and Archaeology of Death,* edited by S. C. Humphreys and Helen King. London: Academic Press, 1–13.

Huntington, R., and P. Metcalf. 1979. *Celebrations of Death: The Anthropology of Mortuary Ritual.* Cambridge: Cambridge University Press.

Hyde, Alan. 1997. *Bodies of Law.* Princeton: Princeton University Press.

Iga, Mamoru. 1975. Tradition and Modernity in Japanese Suicide: The Case of Yasunari Kawabata. In *Modernization and Stress in Japan,* edited by Toyomasa Fusé, 62–73. Leiden: E. J. Brill.

Ikeda Mitsuho. 1993. Kindai Byōin no naka no Dentōteki "Shi": Makki Kanja to kōzō ka sareta Patanarizumu (Traditional "death" in modern hospitals: Terminal patients and structured paternalism). In *Jirei o chūshin to shita taminaru kea* (Case-centered terminal care), edited by Kazuyo Yotsumoto and Reiko Kawaguchi, 11–26. Tokyo: Hirokawa Shuppan.

Ikegami, Naoki. 1988. Health Technology Development in Japan. *International Journal of Technology Assessment in Health Care* 4:239–254.

Illich, Ivan. 1992. *In the Mirror of the Past: Lectures and Addresses, 1978–1990.* New York: Marion Boyars Publishers.

Itō, Kimio. 1998. The Invention of *Wa* and the Transformation of the Image of Prince Shōtoku in Modern Japan. In *Mirror of Modernity: Invented Traditions of Modern Japan,* edited by Stephen Vlastos, 37–47. Berkeley: University of California Press.

Ivy, Marilyn. 1995. *Discourses of the Vanishing: Modernity, Phantasm, Japan.* Chicago: University of Chicago Press.

Iwasaki, Y., K. Fukao, and H. Iwasaki. 1990. Moral Principles of Kidney Donation in Japan. *Transplantation Proceedings* 22:963.

Japan Echo. 1991. Attitudes toward Death. 18 (1): 67.

Japan Times. 1997. Brain-Dead May Feel Pain: Expert Wary of New Transplant Law. October 17.

———. 1999a. Brain Death Tests Taken in Wrong Order—Doctor. April 12.

———. 1999b. Overseas Best Option for Organ Transplants. March 2.

Jennett, B. 1992. Severe Head Injuries: Ethical Aspects of Management. *British Journal of Hospital Medicine* 47 (5): 354–357.

Jennett, B., and F. Plum. 1972. Persistent Vegetative State after Brain Damage. *Lancet* 1:734–737.

Jonas, Hans. 1974. *Philosophical Essays: From Ancient Creed to Technological Man.* Englewood Cliffs, N.J.: Prentice-Hall, Inc.

Jones, Michael A. 1995. The Legal Background. *British Medical Journal* 310: 717–718.

Joralemon, Donald. 1995. Organ Wars: The Battle for Body Parts. *Medical Anthropology Quarterly* 9 (3): 335–356.

Jordon, Mary. 1996. Japanese Are Dying for a Transplant. *Washington Post,* August 4.

Journal of the American Medical Association. 1968a. What and When Is Death? 204:219–220.

———. 1968b. When Is a Patient Dead? 204:142.

Jouvet, M. 1959. Diagnostic électro-sous-corticographique de la mort du système nerveux central au cours de certains comas. *Electroencephalography and Clinical Neurophysiology* 11:805.

Kaga Otohiko. 1991. *Ikiteiru shinzō* (A living heart). Tokyo: Kōdansha.

Kaji Nobuyuki. 1990. *Jukyō to wa nanika* (What is Confucianism?). Chukō Shinsho.

Kalland, Arne, and Brian Moeran. 1992. *Japanese Whaling: End of an Era?* London: Curzon.

Kaneko, Satoru. 1990. Dimensions of Religiosity among Believers in Japanese Folk Religion. *Journal for the Scientific Study of Religion* 29:1–18.

Kantō Chiku Kōchōkai. 1992. Rinji Nōshi oyobi Zōkiishoku Chōsa Kai (Special investigation into Brain Death and Organ Transplant Committee).

Karatani, Kōjin. 1993. *Origins of Modern Japanese Literature.* Translated by Brett de Bary. Durham, N.C.: Duke University Press.

Kass, Leon. 1992. Organs for Sale? Propriety, Property, and the Price of Progress. *Public Interest,* April, 65–84.

Kaufman, Howard H. 1990. The Acute Care of Patients with Gunshot Wounds to the Head. *Neurotrauma Medical Reports* Spring, 1.

Kaufman, Sharon. 2000. In the Shadow of Death with Dignity: Medicine and Cultural Quandaries of the Vegetative State. *American Anthropologist* 102: 69–83.

Kawakita, Yoshio, and Chikara Sasaki. 1992. *Dialogue between History of Medicine and History of Mathematics.* Tokyo: Chūōkōron.

Kawano, Satsuki. In press. "Finding Common Ground: Family, Gender, and Burial in Contemporary Japan." In *Demographic Change and the Family in Japan's Aging Society,* edited by J. W. Traphagan and John Knight. Albany: State University of New York Press.

Kawashima, T., T. Hasegawa, K. Fuse, Y. Sohara, S. Endo, T. Yamaguchi, and M. Ohta. 1994. Organ Transplantation from Brain-Dead Individuals in Japan: Results of a Questionnaire in Families of Brain-Dead Patients. *Transplantation Proceedings* 26:977–979.

Kennedy, Ian. 1971. The Kansas Statute on Death: An Appraisal. *New England Journal of Medicine* 285:946–950.

———. 1973. The Legal Definition of Death. *Medico-Legal Journal* 41 (1): 36–41.

Kennedy, Mark. 1999. Brain Dead Donors "Alive": MD's Debate Ethics of Transplant. *Ottawa Citizen.* March 3, A3.

Kerner, Karen. 1974. The Malevolent Ancestor: Ancestral Influence in a Japanese Religious Sect. In *Ancestors,* edited by William H. Newell. Paris: Mouton Publishers.

Kikan Medicaru Toritomento Henshūbū, ed. 1992. *Yottsu no shibōjikoku: Handai Byōin "nōshi" ishoku satsujin jiken no shinsō* (Four Deaths: The Truth about the Murder of the Brain-Dead Organ Donor at the Osaka University Hospital). Osaka: Sairosha.

Kilbrandon, Hon. Lord. 1966. Chairman's Opening Remarks. In *Ethics in Medical Progress: With Special Reference to Transplantation,* edited by G. E. W. Wolstenholme and M. O'Connor, 2. Boston: Little, Brown and Company.

Kimbrell, Andrew. 1993. *The Human Body Shop: The Engineering and Marketing of Life.* San Francisco: Harper San Francisco.

Kimura Bin. 1992. *Seimei no katachi/katachi no seimei* (Form of life/life of form). Tokyo: Seido-sha.

Kimura Hiroshi. 1989. *Shi: Bukkyō to minzoku* (Death: Buddhism and ethnic groups). Tokyo: Meichō Shuppan.

King, T. T. 1998. Correspondence: Organ Donation and Permanent Vegetative State. *Lancet* 351:211.

Kleinman, Arthur. 1988. *The Illness Narratives: Suffering, Healing, and the Human Condition.* New York: Basic Books.

Kleinman, Arthur, and Byron Good. 1985. *Culture and Depression: Studies in the Anthropology of Cross-Cultural Affect and Disorder.* Berkeley: University of California Press.

Kolata, Gina. 1984. New Neurons Form in Adulthood. *Science* 224:1325.

Komatsu, Yoshihiko. 1993. Sentaku gijutsu to nōshironsō no shikaku (The blind spot in advanced technology and brain death debates). *Gendai Shisō* (Modern thought) 21:198–212.

———. 1996. *Shi wa kyōmeisuru: Nōshi zōkiishoku no fukami e* (Death reverberations: To the depths of brain death and organ transplants). Tokyo: Keisō Shobō.

Kondo, Dorinne K. 1990. *Crafting Selves: Power, Gender, and Discourses of Identity in a Japanese Workplace.* Chicago: University of Chicago Press.

Kopytoff, Igor. 1986. The Cultural Biography of Things: Commoditization as Process. In *The Social Life of Things: Commodities in Cultural Perspective,* edited by Arjun Appadurai, 64–91. Cambridge: Cambridge University Press.

Korein, Julius. 1978. Terminology, Definitions, and Usage. In *Brain Death: Interrelated Medical and Social Issues,* edited by Julius Korein. Annals of the New York Academy of Science, vol. 315, 9. New York: New York Academy of Science.

Kosaku, Yoshino. 1992. *Cultural Nationalism in Contemporary Japan: A Sociological Inquiry.* London: Routledge.

Kōseishō (Ministry of Health and Welfare). 1985. *Kōseishō kenkyūhan ni yoru nōshi no hantei kijun* (Brain death determination criteria of the Ministry of Health and Welfare). Tokyo.

Kōseishō seikatsu eisei kyoku kikakuka. 1988. *Bochi, Maisō ni kansuru hōritsu kaiseiban* (Law Regarding Cemetery and Burial) (Revised). Tokyo: Daiichi hōki shuppan.

Kōsei tōkei kyōkai. 1998. Kokumin Eisei no Dōkō (Statistics on Hygiene). Special Issue of *Kōsei no Shihyō* (Journal of Health and Welfare Statistics), 321.

Kovacs, Maureen Gallery, trans. 1989. *The Epic of Gilgamesh.* Stanford: Stanford University Press.

Krais, Beate. 1993. Gender and Symbolic Violence: Female Oppression in the Light of Pierre Boudieu's Theory of Social Practice. In *Bourdieu: Critical Perspectives,* edited by Craig Calhoun, Edward LiPuma, and Moishe Postone, 156–177. Chicago: University of Chicago Press.

Kunii, Irene. 1997. Where the Heart Isn't. *Time Asian Edition.* March 12, 20.

Kuriyama, Shigehisa. 1992. Between Mind and Eye: Japanese Anatomy in the Eighteenth Century. In *Paths to Asian Medical Knowledge,* edited by Charles Leslie and Allan Young, 21–43. Berkeley: University of California Press.

———. 1999. *The Expressiveness of the Body and the Divergence of Greek and Chinese Medicine.* New York: Zone Books.

Kuss, R., and P. Bourget. 1992. *Illustrated History of Organ Transplantation.* Rueil Mal Maison: Laboratoire Sandoz.

Lamb, David. 1985. *Death, Brain Death, and Ethics.* London: Croom Helm.

———. 1990. *Organ Transplants and Ethics.* London: Routledge.

Lancet. 1974. Editorial: Brain Damage and Brain Death. Vol. 1:341–342.

La Puma, John. 1988. Discovery and Disquiet: Research on the Brain-Dead. *Annals of Internal Medicine* 109:606–608.

Latour, Bruno. 1993. *We Have Never Been Modern*. Cambridge: Harvard University Press.

Law, J. 1991. Introduction: Monsters, Machines and Sociotechnical Relations. In *A Sociology of Monsters: Essays on Power, Technology and Domination*, edited by J. Law. New York: Routledge, 1–23.

Lawrence, Susan C. 1998. Beyond the Grave—The Use and Meaning of Human Body Parts: A Historical Introduction. In Robert F. Weir, ed. *Stored Tissue Samples: Ethical, Legal, and Public Policy Implications*. Iowa City: University of Iowa Press, 111–142.

Leach, E. R. 1961. Two Essays Concerning the Symbolic Representation of Time. In *Rethinking Anthropology*. London: Athlone Press.

Leflar, Robert B. 1996. Informed Consent and Patients' Rights in Japan. *Houston Law Review* 33 (1): 1–112.

Le Goff, Jacques. 1989. Head or Heart? The Political Use of Body Metaphors in the Middle Ages. In *Fragments for a History of the Human Body*, edited by M. Feder. New York: Urzone Inc., 13–26.

Lewis, Thomas. 1988. On the Science and Technology of Medicine. Reprinted in *Deadalus* 117 (3) (Summer): 299–316.

Lienhardt, G. 1961. *Divinity and Experience: The Religion of the Dinka*. Oxford: Oxford University Press.

Life. 1967. Gift of a Heart 63:24a–24c.

———. 1969. People with other People's Hearts 66:82–85.

Lifton, Robert Jay, Shūichi Katō, and Michael R. Reich. 1979. *Six Lives, Six Deaths: Portraits from Modern Japan*. New Haven: Yale University Press.

Lindenbaum, Shirley, and Margaret Lock, eds. 1993. *Knowledge, Power and Practice: The Anthropology of Medicine and Everyday Life*. Berkeley: University of California Press.

Linebaugh, Peter. 1975. The Tyburn Riot: Against the Surgeons. In *Albion's Fatal Tree: Crime and Society in Eighteenth-Century England*, edited by Douglas Hay, Peter Linebaugh, John Rule, E. P. T. Thompson, and Cal Winslow. London: Allen Lane, 65–117.

Lipovenko, Dorothy. 1988. Malformed Infants Upset MD's Theories. *Toronto Globe and Mail*, May 2nd, A8.

Liptak, Gregory. 1986. In Reply. *Journal of the American Medical Association* 255 (April 18): 2028.

Literary Digest. 1931. Heart-Beats after Death. August 15, 110 (7): 28.

Lock, Margaret. 1980. *East Asian Medicine in Urban Japan: Varieties of Medical Experience*. Berkeley: University of California Press.

———. 1993. *Encounters with Aging: Mythologies of Menopause in Japan and North America*. Berkeley: University of California Press.

———. 1994. Menopause in Cultural Context. *Experimental Gerontology* 29 (3/4): 307–317.

———. 1995. Contesting the Natural in Japan: Moral Dilemmas and Technologies of Dying. *Culture, Medicine, and Psychiatry* 19:1–38.

———. 1997. Displacing Suffering: The Reconstruction of Death in North America and Japan. In *Social Suffering*, edited by Arthur Kleinman, Veena Das, and Margaret Lock, 271–295. Berkeley: University of California Press.

———. 1998a. Perfecting Society: Reproductive Technologies, Genetic Testing, and the Planned Family in Japan. In *Pragmatic Women and Body Politics,* edited by Margaret Lock and Patricia Kaufert. Cambridge: Cambridge University Press, 206–239.

———. 1998b. Anomalous Women and Political Strategies for Aging Societies. In *The Politics of Women's Health: Exploring Agency and Autonomy,* edited by Susan Sherwin, 178–204. Philadelphia: Temple University Press.

———. 1998c. Breast Cancer: Reading the Omens. *Anthropology Today* 14:7–16.

———. 1998d. Situating Women in the Politics of Health. In *The Politics of Women's Health: Exploring Agency and Autonomy,* edited by Susan Sherwin, 48–63. Philadelphia: Temple University Press.

———. 1999. Genetic Diversity and the Politics of Difference. *Chicago Kent Law Review* 75 (1): 83–111.

———. 2000. Deadly Disputes: The Calculation of Meaningful Life. In *Intersections: Living and Working with the New Medical Technologies,* edited by Margaret Lock, Allan Young, and Alberto Cambrosio, 233–262. Cambridge: Cambridge University Press.

———. In press. On Being as-Good-as Dead in a World Short of Organs. Santa Fe: School of American Research.

Lock, Margaret, and Christina Honde. 1990. Reaching Consensus about Death: Heart Transplants and Cultural Identity in Japan. In *Social Sciences Perspectives on Medical Ethics,* edited by George Weisz, 99–119. Dordrecht: Kluwer Academic Publishers.

Lock, Margaret, and Patricia Kaufert, eds. 1998. *Pragmatic Women and Body Politics.* Cambridge: Cambridge University Press.

Lock, Margaret, and Edward Norbeck, eds. 1987. *Health, Illness, and Medical Care in Japan: Cultural and Social Dimensions.* Honolulu: University of Hawaii Press.

Lock, Margaret, Allan Young, and Alberto Cambrosio. 2000. *Living and Working with the New Medical Technologies: Intersections of Inquiry.* Cambridge: Cambridge University Press.

Long, Susan O. 1997. Reflections on Becoming a Cucumber: Images of the Good Death in Japan and the United States. Paper presented at the Center for Japanese Studies, University of Michigan, Ann Arbor, September 11.

———. 2000. Living Poorly or Dying Well: Decisions about Life. Support and Treatment Termination for American and Japanese Patients. *Journal of Clinical Ethics* 11:27–41.

Long, Susan O., and B. Long. 1982. Curable Cancers and Fetal Ulcers. *Social Science and Medicine* 16:2102–2108.

Louis, M. Antoine. 1752. *Lettres sur la certitude des signes de la mort.* Paris: M. Lambert.

Louw, J. H. 1967. Ex Unitate Vires. *South African Medical Journal* 41:1257.

Low, Morris F. 1996. Medical Representations of the Body in Japan: Gender, Class, and Discourse in the Eighteenth Century. *Annals of Science* 53:345–359.

Machado, Nora. 1996. The Swedish Transplant Acts: Sociological Considerations on Bodies and Giving. *Social Science & Medicine* 42 (2): 159–168.

———. 1998. *Using the Bodies of the Dead: Legal, Ethical, and Organizational Dimensions of Organ Transplantation.* Brookfield, Vt.: Ashgate Publishing.

Machino, Saku. 1996. *Hanzai Kakuron no Genzai* (Current theories of crime). Tokyo: Yuhikaku.

Machino, Saku, and Etsuko Akiba, eds. 1993. *Nōshi to zōki ishoku dai nihan* (Brain death and organ transplant, second edition). Tokyo: Shinanosha.

Mainichi Daily News. 1982. 80% of the People Expect "Peaceful" Death Rather than the Life-Prolonging Treatment of Terminal Cancer. November 10.

———. 1985a. Basic Guidelines of Brain Death. September 7.

———. 1985b. Definition of Brain Death Needs Review. September 6.

———. 1991a. Kidney Transplant from Brain-Dead Man Revealed. May 30.

———. 1991b. Family Not Told of Donor's Brain Death. May 30.

Mainichi Shinbun. 1985. Nōshi nintei o dō kangaeru ka (How to think about the recognition of brain death). February 8.

———. 1988. Tsukuba Dai no Zōki Ishoku, Kensatsu ga shobun "tōketsu" (Organ transplant at Tsukuba University: Public Prosecutor's Office decides to "freeze" the case). January 11.

———. 1991. Nōshi Ishoku 55% sansei (55 percent approve transplants from brain-dead). October 16.

———. 1994. Zōki Ishoku Hōan wa aimai "Ishi 159 nin ga seimei" ("The organ transplant bill is too vague," a statement by 159 doctors), June 1.

———. 1999. Nōshi ishoku "yokatta" 66% (Brain death is "good." 66 percent). March 4.

Malinowski, Bronislaw. 1922. *Argonauts of the Western Pacific.* London: Routledge and Kegan Paul.

Manninen, D., and R. Evans. 1985. Public Attitudes and Behavior Regarding Organ Donation. *Journal of the American Medical Association* 253:21.

Mantel, Hilary. 1998. *The Giant, O'Brien.* Toronto: Doubleday Canada Limited.

Mappes, Thomas, and Jane Zembaty. 1981. *Biomedical Ethics.* New York: McGraw-Hill Book Company.

Martin, Lester W., Luis L. Gonzalez, and Clark D. West. 1969. Homotransplantation of Both Kidneys from an Anencephalic Monster to a 17-Pound Boy with Eagle-Barrett Syndrome. *Surgery* 66(3): 603–607.

Martyn, Susan R. 1986. Using the Brain Dead for Medical Research. *Utah Law Review* 1: 1–28.

Maruyama, Kumiko, F. Hayashi, and H. Kamisasa. 1981. A Multivariate Analysis of Japanese Attitudes toward Life and Death. *Behaviormetrika* 10:37–48.

Maslin, Janet. 1999. Buoyed by the Strangeness of Kinship. *New York Times.* September 24.

Matsumoto, Akira. 1993. *Nihon no miira botoke* (Mummy-Buddhas in Japan). Kyoto: Rinkawa Shoten.

Mauss, Marcel. 1990 [1950]. *The Gift*. New York: W. W. Norton.

May, William. 1973. Attitudes towards the Newly Dead. *Hastings Center Report* 1:3–13.

McIlroy, Anne. 1999. "From One Who's Been There: Don't Alter Organ-Donation Law." *Globe and Mail*. March 3.

McMenamin, Brigid. 1996. Why People Die Waiting for Transplants. *Forbes*. March 11, 140–148.

Meckler, Laura. 1999. Nurses Better at Procuring Organ Donation. http://lw7fd.law7.hotmail.msn.com. Retrieved November 6.

Meinke, Sue A. 1989. Anencephalic Infants as Potential Organ Sources: Ethical and Legal Issues. *Scope Note 12*, 1–11. Washington, D.C.: National Reference Center for Bioethics Literature.

Mejia, Rodrigo E., and Murray M. Pollack. 1995. Variability in Brain Death Determination Practices in Children. *Journal of the American Medical Association* 274 (7): 550–553.

Metchnikoff, Elie, and Henry Smith Williams. 1912. Why Not Live Forever? *Cosmopolitan* 53:436–446.

Mickleburgh, Rod. 1993. Safer Roads Give Death 2nd Chance. *Globe and Mail*. April 1.

Middleton, John. 1982. Lugbara Death. In *Death and the Regeneration of Life*, edited by Maurice Bloch and Jonathan Parry, 134–154. Cambridge: Cambridge University Press.

Miles, Steven. 1999. Death in a Technological and Pluralistic Culture. In *The Definition of Death: Contemporary Controversies*, edited by Stuart J. Youngner, Robert M. Arnold, and Renie Shapiro, 311–318. Baltimore: Johns Hopkins University Press.

Miller, Jonathan. 1971. *McLuhan*. London: Fontana.

Mitchell, Alanna. 1995. Down's Transplant Bid Poses Dilemma. *Globe and Mail*. April 29.

Miura, Shumon. 1991. Attitudes towards Death. *Japan Echo* 18:67.

Miyaji, Naoko T. 1994. Informed Consent, Cancer, and Truth in Prognosis. *New England Journal of Medicine* 331:810.

Miyazaki Tetsuya and Yamaori Tetsuo. 1999. Noshi giron no ookina keturaku (Significant shortcomings in the brain death debates). *Ronza*. May.

Miyoshi, M., and H. D. Harootunian, eds. 1989. *Postmodernism and Japan*. Durham, N.C.: Duke University Press.

Moeran, Brian. 1984. Individual, Group and Seishin: Japan's Internal Cultural Debate. *Man* 19:252–266.

Mohandas, A., and Shelley N. Chou. 1971. Brain Death: A Clinical and Pathological Study. *Journal of Neurosurgery* 35:211–218.

Mollaret, P., and M. Goulon. 1959. Coma dépassé et nécroses nerveuses centrales massives. *Revue Neurologique* 101:116–139.

Montreal Gazette. 1989. Two-Year-Old's Voice Woke Grandfather from Coma. January 22.

Moore, Francis D. 1964. *Give and Take: The Development of Tissue Transplantation*. Philadelphia: W. B. Saunders.

Mörch, E. Trier. 1985. History of Mechanical Ventilation. In *Mechanical Ven-*

tilation, edited by Robert R. Kirby, Robert A. Smith, and David A. Desautels, 1–58. New York: Churchill Livingstone.

Morin, Edgar. 1970. *L'homme et la mort.* Paris: Seuil.

Morioka Masahiro. 1989. *Nōshi no hito* (The brain-dead person). Tokyo: Tokyo Shoseki.

———. 1995. Bioethics and Japanese Culture: Brain Death, Patient Rights, and Cultural Factors. *Eubios* 5:87–91.

Morison, R. S. 1971. Death: Process or Event? *Science* 173:694–698.

Morris-Suzuki, Tessa. 1995. The Invention and Reinvention of "Japanese Culture." *Journal of Asian Studies* 54:759–780.

Moseley, John I., Gaetano F. Molinari, and A. Earl Walker. 1976. Respirator Brain: Report of a Survey and Review of Current Concepts. *Archives of Pathology and Laboratory Medicine* 100:61–64.

Mulkay, Michael, and John Ernst. 1991. The Changing Profile of Social Death. *Archives of European Sociology* 32:172–196.

Multi-Society Task Force on PVS. 1994a. Medical Aspects of the Persistent Vegetative State, part 1. *New England Journal of Medicine* 330 (21): 1499–1508.

———. 1994b. Medical Aspects of the Persistent Vegetative State, part 2. *New England Journal of Medicine* 330 (22): 1572–1579.

Mumford, Lewis. 1934. *Technics and Civilization.* New York: Harcourt Brace.

Nagamine, Takahiko. 1988. Attitutes toward Death in Rural Areas of Japan. *Death Studies* 12:61–68.

Naikaku Sōri Daijin kanbō kōhōshitsu, ed. 1998. Zenkoku yoron chōsa no genjō (Results of national public polls). Tokyo.

Najita, Tetsuo. 1978. Perspectives in Tokugawa Intellectual History. In *Japanese Thought in the Tokugawa Period,* edited by Tetsuo Najita and Irving Scheiner, 4–38. Chicago: University of Chicago Press.

———. 1989. On Culture and Technology in Postmodern Japan. In *Postmodernism and Japan,* edited by M. Miyoshi and H. D. Harootunian, 3–20. Durham, N.C.: Duke University Press.

Naka Yoshitomo. 1996. *Jinishoku tōseki kōchō funtōki* (Kidney transplant: A record of the struggles of a school principal on dialysis). Tokyo: Sanseidō.

Nakagawa, Yonezo. 1995. Death with Dignity in the Japanese Culture. *Psychiatry and Clinical Neurosciences* 49: S161–163.

Nakajima Michi. 1985. *Mienai shi: Nōshi to zōki ishoku* (Invisible death: Brain death and organ transplants). Tokyo: Bungei Shunju.

———. 1994. "Nōshi rippō o isogaseta Kyūshūdai igakubu no kan ishoku hōdō" (Media reporting of liver transplant at Kyūshū University Medical School, which has called for legislation of brain death). *Shokun* 26 (2).

Namihira Emiko. 1988. *Nōshi, zōki ishoku, Gan kokuchi* (Brain death, organ transplants, revealing a diagnosis of cancer). Tokyo: Fukutake Shoten.

Natsuishi Banya. 1994. Fukkatsu suru animizum Nihon bungaku no baai (Revival of animism in Japanese literature). In *Animizum o yomu: Nihon bungaku ni okeru shizen, seimei, jiko* (Reading animism: Nature, life, self in Japanese literature), edited by Hirakawa Sukehiro and Tsuruta Kinya, 125–148. Tokyo: Shinyakusha.

Neuberger, Julia. 1995. The Lay View. *British Medical Journal* 310:715–716.

Newman, B. M. 1940. What is Death? *Scientific American* 162:336–337.

Newsweek. 1967. When are you Really Dead? December 18.

————. 1968a. Surgery and Show Biz. January 15.

————. 1968b. Time of the Transplants. May 13.

————. 1968c. Redefining Death. May 20.

Newsweek Nihon Han. 1993. Zōki ishoku no saizensen (The frontline in transplants). February 25.

New York Times. 1967a. Heart Transplant Keeps Man Alive in South Africa. December 4.

————. 1967b. Patient Progresses after Heart Transplant. December 5.

————. 1967c. Growing Shortage of Organs Worrying Doctors. December 5.

————. 1967d. Editorial: Historic Heart Experiment. December 5.

————. 1967e. Editorial: Living Transplants—1984. December 24.

————. 1996. Hope Offered for "Permanent" Unconsciousness. January 4.

————. 1998. Japan's Blossoms Soothe a P.O.W. Lost in Siberia. April 12.

Nihon Ishikai Seimei Rinri Kondankai (Japan Medical Association Life Ethics Round Table Conference). 1990. Unpublished report. Tokyo.

Nihon Ishoku Gakkai. 2000. Jinzo Ishoku Rinsho Tōroku shūkei Hōkoku. *Ishoku* 35:43–48.

Nihon Ishoku Gakkai Shakai Mondai Kentō Tokubetsu Iinkai, ed. 1991. *Zōki Ishōku e no apurōchi IV: Zōki ishoku to hōdō; Zōki ishoku to rinri i inkai* (Approches to organ transplant, IV: Organ transplant and media report, organ transplant and ethics committees). Osaka: Medika Shuppan.

Nihon Keizai Shinbun. 1985a. "Nōshi" to "shinzōshi" no hazama no kadai (Issues regarding the border between "brain death" and "heart death"). May 20.

————. 1985b. Seimei kagaku to shakai rinri to no konpon kadai (Fundamental issues in life science and social ethics). September 3.

————. 1990a. Shinteishi mae ni migiashi sekkai: Nōshi "shibō" shindan no dansei (Right leg incised before heart death: The time of brain death entered as the death time for the man). September 7.

————. 1990b. Nōshi rinchō no ōshu shisatsu, nōshi zōki ishoku yōnin shisei ni katamuku (The Brain Death Special Committee's overseas inspection tour: Toward approving brain death and organ transplant). January 23.

————. 1990c. Nōshi rinchō no shingi honkakuka (The Special Committee's discussion deepens). November 8.

————. 1992. Nōshi rinchō saishu tōshin: "Nōshi ishoku" michisuji nao futōmei (Final committee report: The path toward brain-death transplant still unclear). January 23.

————. 1993. Tekishutsu, jijitsujō no nōshi dankai: Shinteishimae ni hozoneki, kanzo kinō iji nerai tōnyū e (Removal done virtually at the brain death stage: Preservative liquid injected before cardiac arrest in order to maintain liver function). October 23.

————. 1994a. Nichibenren, zōki ishoku hōan ni taisaku "Honnin no ishi" zettai jōken (Japan Bar Association proposes counterproposal bill: Prior will is the absolute condition). May 7.

———. 1994b. Seikyū na zōki ishoku rippōka ni hantai (Opposing hasty leg-islation of organ transplant). May 25.

———. 1994c. Seitai jin ishoku no kibōsha, chirashi de hiroku boshū (Recruit-ing for live-donor kidney transplant through ads). June 4.

———. 1997. Supido saiketsu "musekinin" no koe (Speedy vote criticized as "irresponsible"). June 17.

Nishioka Hideki. 1989. Nōshi, zōki ishoku mondai to jinken (The brain death and organ transplant problem and human rights). In Nōshi to zōki ishoku o kangaeru: Arata na sei to shi no kōsatsu (Thinking about brain death and organ transplants: Approaches to the new life and death), edited by Kōbe Seimei, Rinri Kenkyūkai 114:103–131. Osaka: Medica Shuppan.

Norgren, Tiana. 1998. Abortion before Birth Control: The Interest Group Pol-itics behind Postwar Japanese Reproduction Policy. Journal of Japanese Studies 24 (1): 59–94.

Nudeshima Jirō. 1991a. Nōshi, zōki ishoku to nihon shakai (Brain death, organ transplants, and Japanese society). Tokyo: Kōbundō.

———. 1991b. Obstacles to Brain Death and Organ Transplantation in Japan. Lancet 338:1063–1064.

Nuland, Sherwin. 1990. Transplanting a Heart. New Yorker, February, 82–94.

Oe Kenzaburo. 1995. A Healing Family. Tokyo: Kodansha International.

Ohara, Shin. 1997. The Brain-Death Controversy: The Japanese View of Life, Death, and Bioethics. Japan Foundation Newsletter 15 (2): 1–5.

Ohi, Gen, Tomonori Hasegawa, Hiroyuki Kumano, Ichiro Kai, Nobuyuki Tak-enaga, Yoshio Taguchi, Hiroshi Saito, and Tsuinamasa Ino. 1986. Why are Cadaveric Renal Transplants So Hard to Find in Japan? An Analysis of Eco-nomic and Attitudinal Aspects. Health Policy 6:269–278.

Ohkubo, Michikata. 1995. The Quality of Life after Kidney Transplantation in Japan: Results from a Nationwide Questionnaire. Transplantation Proceed-ings 27:1452–1457.

O'Malley, C. D. 1964. Andreas Vesalius of Brussels, 1514–1564. Berkeley: Uni-versity of California Press.

Ōmine, Akira. 1991. Right and Wrong in the Brain-Death Debate. Japan Echo 18 (1): 68–71.

O'Neill, John. 1985. Five Bodies: The Human Shape of Modern Society. Ithaca: Cornell University Press.

Ooms, Herman. 1967. The Religion of the Household: A Case Study of Ancestor Worship in Japan. Contemporary Religions in Japan 8:201–333.

Ota, Kazuo, Satoshi Teraoka, and Tatsuo Kawai. 1995. Donor Difficulties in Japan and Asian Countries. Transplantation Proceedings 27:83–86.

Palgi, Phyllis, and Henry Abramovitch. 1984. Death: A Cross-Cultural Per-spective. Annual Review of Anthropology 13:385–417.

Pallis, Christopher. 1987. Brain Stem Death: The Evolution of a Concept. Med-ico Legal Journal 2:84–104.

———. 1990. Brainstem Death. In Handbook of Clinical Neurology, vol. 57, edited by P. J. Vinken and G. W. Bruyn, 441–496. Amsterdam: Elsevier.

Park, Katherine. 1994. The Criminal and the Saintly Body. *Renaissance Quarterly* 47:1–33.

———. 1995. The Life of the Corpse: Division and Dissection in Late Medieval Europe. *Journal of the History of Medicine and Allied Sciences* 50:114.

Pasternak, Joseph F., and Joseph J. Volpe. 1979. Full Recovery from Prolonged Brainstem Failure Following Intraventricular Hemorrhage. *Journal of Pediatrics* 95 (6): 1046–1049.

Paton, Alec. 1971. Life and Death: Moral and Ethical Aspects of Transplantation. *Seminars in Psychiatry* 3 (1): 161–168.

Patterson, Orlando. 1982. *Slavery and Social Death: A Comparative Study.* Cambridge: Harvard University Press.

Paulette, Lesley. 1993. A Choice for K'aila. *Humane Medicine* 9 (1): 13–17.

Paulme, D. 1940. *Organisation sociale des Dogons.* Paris: Institut de Droit Comparé: Études de sociologie et d'ethnologie juridique, 32.

Payne, K., R. M. Taylor, C. Stocking, and G. A. Sachs. 1996. Physicians' Attitudes about the Care of Patients in Persistent Vegetative State: A National Survey. *Annals of Internal Medicine* 125:104–110.

Paz, Octavio. 1969. *Conjunctions and Disjunctions: A Study of the Human Condition.* New York: Viking.

Perkins, Henry S., and Susan W. Tolle. 1992. Letter to the Editor. *New England Journal of Medicine* 326:1025.

Pernick, Martin S. 1988. Back from the Grave: Recurring Controversies over Defining and Diagnosing Death in History. In *Death: Beyond Whole-Brain Criteria,* edited by Richard M. Zaner, 17–74. Dordrecht: Kluwer Academic Publishers.

———. 1999. Brain Death in the Cultural Context: The Reconstruction of Death 1967–1981. In *The Definition of Death: Contemporary Controversies,* edited by Stuart J. Youngner, Robert M. Arnold, and Renie Schapiro, 3–33. Baltimore: Johns Hopkins University Press.

Peters, T. G. 1991. Life or Death: The Issue of Payment in Cadaveric Organ Donation. *Journal of the American Medical Association* 265:1302.

Pfaffenberger, Bryan. 1988. Fetishised Objects and Humanized Nature: Towards an Anthropology of Technology. *Man* (n.s.) 23:236–252.

———. 1992. Social Anthropology of Technology. *Annual Review of Anthropology* 21:491–516.

Phillips, Melanie. 1999. Making the Dying a Disposable Asset. *Times.* February 21.

Picard, André. 2000. Easing the Choice over the Ultimate Gift. *Globe and Mail.* January 3.

Pickering, Andrew. 1992. From Science as Knowledge to Science as Practice. In *Science as Practice and Culture,* edited by Andrew Pickering. Chicago: University of Chicago Press, 1–26.

Pinkus, Rosa Lynn. 1984. Families, Brain Death, and Traditional Medical Excellence. *Journal of Neurosurgery* 60:1192–1194.

Plum, Fred. 1999. Clinical Standards and Technological Confirmatory Tests in Diagnosing Brain Death. In *The Definition of Death: Contemporary Con-*

troversies, edited by Stuart J. Youngner, Robert M. Arnold, and Renie Shapiro, 34–66. Baltimore: Johns Hopkins University Press.

Poe, Edgar Allan. 1991. The Premature Burial. In *Tales of Edgar Allan Poe.* New York: William Morrow and Company, 61–80.

Pollack, David. 1992. *Reading against Culture: Ideology and Narrative in the Japanese Novel.* Ithaca: Cornell University Press.

Pollock, William. 1978. "Cognitive" and "Sapient": Which Death is the Real Death? *American Journal of Surgery* 136:3–7.

The Pope Speaks. 1958. The Prolongation of Life: An Address of Pope Pius XII to an International Congress on Anesthesiologists, 24 November 1957. *The Pope Speaks* 4: 393–398.

Poses, R. M., C. Bekes, F. J. Copare, and W. E. Scott. 1989. The Answer to "What are my chances, doctor?" Depends on Who Is Asked: Prognostic Disagreement and Inaccuracy for Critically Ill Patients. *Critical Care Medicine* 17 (8): 827–833.

Post, Stephen G. 1995. Alzheimer Disease and the "Then" Self. *Kennedy Institute of Ethics Journal* 5 (4): 307–321.

Potter, Paul. 1976. Herophilus of Chalcedon: An Assessment of his Place in the History of Anatomy. *Bulletin of the History of Medicine* 50:45–60.

Poulton, Thomas J. 1986. Spontaneous Movements in Brain-Dead Patients. *Journal of the American Medical Association* 255 (April 18): 2028.

Powner, David J., Bruce M. Ackerman, and Ake Grenvik. 1996. Medical Diagnosis of Death in Adults: Historical Contributions to Current Controversies. *Lancet* 348:1219–1223.

President's Commission on the Uniform Determination of Death. 1981. *Defining Death: Medical, Legal, and Ethical Issues in the Determination of Death.* Washington, D.C.: U.S. Government Printing Office.

Prottas, Jeffrey. 1994. *The Most Useful Gift: Altruism and the Public Policy of Organ Transplants.* San Francisco: Jossey-Bass Publishers.

Provisional Commission for the Study on Brain Death and Organ Transplants. 1992. Translation of Report by Nōshi oyobi Ishoku Chōsa Kai. Osaka: Osaka Kidney Foundation.

Puccetti, R. 1976. The Conquest of Death. *Monist* 59 (2): 249–263.

Pyle, Kenneth. 1987. In Pursuit of a Grand Design: Nakasone betwixt the Past and Future. *Journal of Japanese Studies* 13:243–270.

Rabinow, Paul. 1996. *Essays on the Anthropology of Reason.* Princeton: Princeton University Press.

Rachels, James. 1986. *The End of Life.* Oxford: Oxford University Press.

Ragosta, K. 1993. Miller Fisher Syndrome, a Brainstem Encephalitis, Mimics Brain Death. *Clinical Pediatrics* 32 (11): 685–687.

Ramsay, Sarah. 1996. News: British Group Presents Vegetative-State Criteria. *Lancet* 347:817.

Randall, T. 1991. Too Few Human Organs for Transplantation, Too Many in Need . . . and the Gap Widens. *Journal of the American Medical Association* 265:1223–1227.

Reading, Ian. 1991. *Religion in Contemporary Japan.* London: Macmillan.

Reeves, Robert B. 1969. The Ethics of Cardiac Transplantation in Man. *Bulletin of the New York Academy of Medicine* 45 (5): 404–411.

Reichel-Dolmatoff, G. 1971. *Amazonian Cosmos: The Sexual and Religious Symbolism of the Tukano Indians.* Chicago: University of Chicago Press.

Revillard, J. P. 1966. Discussion, Organ Transplantation: The Practical Possibilities. In *Ethics in Medical Progress: With Special Reference to Transplantation,* edited by G. E. W. Wolstenholme and M. O'Connor, 70. Boston: Little, Brown and Company.

Reynolds, D. K. 1976. *Morita Psychotherapy.* Berkeley: University of California Press.

Riad, Hany, and Anthony Nicholls. 1995. Elective Ventilation of Potential Organ Donors. *British Medical Journal* 310:714–715.

Richardson, Ruth. 1988. *Death, Dissection, and the Destitute.* London: Routledge.

———. 1996. Fearful Symmetry: Corpses for Anatomy, Organs for Transplantation. In *Organ Transplantation: Meaning and Realities,* edited by Stuart J. Youngner, Renée C. Fox, and Laurence J. O'Connell, 66–100. Madison: University of Wisconsin Press.

Richardson, Ruth, and Brian Hurwitz. 1987. Jeremy Bentham's Self-Image: An Exemplary Bequest for Dissection. *British Medical Journal* 295:195–198.

———. 1995. Donors' Attitudes towards Body Donation for Dissection. *Lancet* 346:277–279.

———. 1997. Death and the Doctors. In *Doctor Death: Medicine at the End of Life.* Catalogue of an Exhibition at the Wellcome Institute for the History of Medicine, 6–13. London: Wellcome Institute.

Rivers, W. H. R. 1926. The Primitive Conception of Death. In *Psychology and Ethnology,* edited by W. H. R. Rivers, 36–50. London: Kegan Paul.

Rix, Bo Andreassen. 1999. Brain Death, Ethics, and Politics in Denmark. In *The Definition of Death: Contemporary Controversies,* edited by Stuart J. Youngner, Robert M. Arnold, and Renie Shapiro, 227–238. Baltimore: Johns Hopkins University Press.

Robertson, Jennifer. 1991. *Native and Newcomer: Making and Remaking a Japanese City.* Berkeley: University of California Press.

———. 1998. It Takes a Village: Internationalization and Nostalgia in Postwar Japan. In *Mirror of Modernity: Invented Traditions of Modern Japan,* edited by Stephen Vlastos, 110–132. Berkeley: University of California Press.

Robertson, John A. 1988. Relaxing the Death Standard for Organ Donation in Pediatric Situations. In *Organ Substitution Technology: Ethical, Legal, and Public Policy Issues,* edited by D. Mathieu, 69–76. Boulder, Colo.: Westview Press.

Roelofs, Richard. 1978. Some Preliminary Remarks on Brain Death. In *Brain Death: Interrelated Medical and Social Issues,* edited by Julius Korein. Annals of the New York Academy of Science, vol. 315. New York: New York Academy of Science.

Rohlen, Thomas. 1974. *For Harmony and Strength: Japanese White-Collar Organization in Anthropological Perspective.* Berkeley: University of California Press.

————. 1978. The Promise of Adulthood in Japanese Spiritualism. In *Adult-hood*, edited by E. Erikson, 125–143. New York: Norton.

Rorty, Richard. 1988. Is Science a Natural Kind? In *Construction and Con-straint: The Shaping of Scientific Rationality*, edited by E. McMullin, 49–74. Notre Dame: University of Notre Dame Press.

Rosenberg, G. A., S. F. Johnson, and R. P. Brenner. 1977. Recovery of Cogni-tion after Prolonged Vegetative State. *Annals of Neurology* 2:167–168.

Rosenfeld, Albert. 1968. Search for an Ethic. *Life* 64:75–81.

Ross, Catrien. 1995. Towards Acceptance of Organ Transplantation? *Lancet* 346: 41–42.

Rothman, David. 1991. *Strangers at the Bedside: A History of How Law and Bioethics Transformed Medicinal Decision Making*. New York: Basic Books.

Ruggeri, Alessandro, and Anna Maria Bertoli Barsotti. 1997. The Birth of Wax-work Modelling in Bologna. *Italian Journal of Anatomy and Embryology* 102 (2): 99–107.

Sabata Toyoyuki. 1990. *Kasō no bunka* (The culture of cremation). Tokyo: Shinchōsha.

Sahlins, Marshall. 1972. *Stone Age Economics*. Chicago: Aldine Press.

————. 1976. *Culture and Practical Reason*. Chicago: University of Chicago Press.

Sakai, Naoki. 1991. *Voices of the Past: The Status of Language in Eighteenth-Century Japanese Discourse*. Ithaca: Cornell University Press.

Sakai Shizu. 1982. *Nihon no iryōshi* (Japanese medical history). Tokyo: Tokyo Shoseki.

Sakakihara, Yoichi, Tatsuhiro Yamanaka, Motofumi Kajii, and Shigehiko Ka-moshita. 1996. Long-Term Ventilator-Assisted Children in Japan: A Na-tional Survey. *Acta Paediatrica Japonica* 38:137–142.

Sanderson, Christine, and D. M. B. Hall. 1995. The Outcomes of Neonatal In-tensive Care. *British Medical Journal* 310:681–682.

Sanger, David E. 1991. A Noh Drama Poses New Questions in Old Forms. *New York Times*. March 31.

Sanner, Margareta. 1994. A Comparison of Public Attitudes toward Autopsy, Organ Donation, and Anatomic Dissection. *Journal of the American Medical Association* 271:284–288.

Saturday Review of Literature. 1968. Transplanting the Heart. January 6, 98–101.

Savage, Douglas. 1980. After Quinlan and Saikewicz: Death, Life, and God Committees. *Critical Care Medicine* 8 (2): 87–93.

Schaniel, W. 1988. New Technology and Cultural Change in Traditional Soci-eties. *Journal of Economics Issues* 22:493–498.

Scheper-Hughes, Nancy. 1998. Truth and Rumor on the Organ Trail. *Natural History* 107 (8): 48–56.

————. 2000. The Global Traffic in Organs. *Current Anthropology* 41:191–224.

Schleifer, Ronald. 1993. Afterword. Walter Benjamin and the Crisis of Repre-sentation: Multiplicity, Meaning, and Athematic Death. In *Death and Rep-

resentation, edited by S. W. Goodwin and E. Bronfen, 312–333. Baltimore: Johns Hopkins University Press.

Schmeck, Harold M. 1969. Transplantation of Organs and Attitudes: The Public's Attitude Toward Clinical Transplantation. *Transplantation Proceedings* 1 (1): 670–674.

Schöne-Seifert, Bettina. 1999. Defining Death in Germany: Brain Death and its Discontents. In *The Definition of Death: Contemporary Controversies,* edited by Stuart J. Youngner, Robert M. Arnold, and Renie Shapiro, 257–271. Baltimore: Johns Hopkins University Press.

Schumaker, John F., William G. Warren, and Gary Groth-Marnat. 1991. Death Anxiety in Japan and Australia. *Journal of Social Psychology* 131 (4): 511–518.

Schwab, R. S., F. Potts, and A. Bonazzi. 1963. EEG as an Aid in Determining Death in the Presence of Cardiac Activity (Ethical, Legal, and Medical Aspects). *Electroencephalography and Clinical Neurophysiology* 15: 147.

Schwager, Robert L. 1978. Life, Death, and the Irreversibly Comatose. In *Ethical Issues in Death and Dying,* edited by T. L. Beauchamp and S. Perlin, 38–51. Englewood Cliffs, N.J.: Prentice-Hall.

Seiden, Howard. 1987. Schoutens are Inspiration to All. *Montreal Gazette.* December 19.

Sells, Robert A. 1995. Practical Implications. *British Medical Journal* 310: 717.

Selzer, Richard. 1993. *Raising the Dead: A Doctor's Encounter with His Own Mortality.* New York: Viking.

Seremetakis, C. Nadia. 1991. *The Last Word: Women, Death, and Divination in Inner Mani.* Chicago: University of Chicago Press.

Shapiro, Hillel A., ed. 1969a. *Experience with Human Heart Transplantation.* Proceedings of the Cape Town Symposium, 13–16 July 1968. Durban: Butterworths.

———. 1969b. New Hearts for Old? *Journal of Forensic Medicine* 16 (4): 117–119.

Sharp, Lesley A. 1995. Organ Transplantation as a Transformative Experience: Anthropological Insights into the Restructuring of the Self. *Medical Anthropology Quarterly* 9 (3): 357–389.

Shewmon, D. Alan. 1988. Commentary on Guidelines for the Determination of Brain Death in Children. *Annals of Neurology* 24 (6): 789–791.

———. 1998. Chronic "Brain Death": Meta-Analysis and Conceptual Consequences. *Neurology* 51 (6): 1538–1545.

Shewmon, D. Alan, Alexander M. Capron, Warwick J. Peacock, and Barbara L. Schulman. 1989. The Use of Anencephalic Infants as Organ Sources: A Critique. *Journal of the American Medical Association* 261:1773–1781.

Shōwa 54 Nenban yoron chōsa nenkan (Yearbook of opinion polls). 1979. Zenkoku kenmin ishiki chōsa (Research on the consciousness of the Japanese prefectural populations), edited by Naikaku Sōri Daijin Kanbō Kōhōshitsu, 585–591. Tokyo: NHK hōsō yoron chōsacho.

Shōwa 55 Nenban yoron chōsa nenkan (Yearbook of opinion polls). 1986.

Yomiuri zenkoku yoron chōsa (59 nen 7 gatsu) (Opinion poll of the Yomiuri publishing house for all of Japan—July 1984), edited by Naikaku Sōri Daijin Kanbō Kōhōshitsu, 507–512. Tokyo: Yomiuri Shinbunsha.

Shōwa 61 Nenban yoron chōsa nenkan (Yearbook of opinion polls). 1987. Kokoro no jidai. Zenkoku yoron chōsa (The era of the heart. Opinion poll by the Mainichi publishing house for all of Japan), edited by Naikaku Sōri Daijin Kanbō Kōhōshitsu, 508–510. Tokyo: Mainichi Shinbunsha.

Shrader, Douglas. 1986. On Dying More Than One Death. *Hastings Center Report* 16 (1): 12–17.

Simmons, Roberta G., Susan K. Marine, and Richard L. Simmons. 1987. *Gift of Life: The Effect of Organ Transplantation on Individual, Family, and Societal Dynamics.* New Brunswick, N.J.: Transaction Books.

Simpson, Keith. 1967. The Moment of Death: A New Medico-Legal Problem. *South African Medical Journal* 41:1188–1191.

Sivin, Nathan. 1988. Science and Medicine in Imperial China: The State of the Field. *Journal of Asian Studies* 47:41–90.

Smith, David Randolph. 1988. Legal Issues Leading to the Notion of Neocortical Death. In *Death: Beyond Whole-Brain Criteria,* edited by Richard M. Zaner, 111–144. Dordrecht: Kluwer Academic Publishers.

Smith, Desmond. 1968. The Heart Market: Someone Playing God. *Nation,* December 30, 719–721.

Smith, Robert J. 1974. *Ancestor Worship in Contemporary Japan.* Stanford: Stanford University Press.

———. 1999. The Living and the Dead in Japanese Popular Religion. In *Lives in Motion: Composing Circles of Self and Community in Japan,* edited by S. O. Long. Ithaca, N.Y.: East Asia Program, Cornell University.

Starr, Douglas. 1998. *Blood: An Epic History of Medicine and Commerce.* New York: Alfred A. Knopf.

Starzl, Thomas E. 1966. General Discussion. In *Ethics in Medical Progress: With Special Reference to Transplantation,* edited by G. E. W. Wolstenholme and M. O'Connor, 155. Boston: Little, Brown and Company.

Stephenson, Peter H. 1983. "He Died Too Quick!" The Process of Dying in a Hutterian Colony. *Omega* 14 (2): 127–134.

Strathern, Marilyn. 1992. *Reproducing the Future: Anthropology, Kinship, and the New Reproductive Technologies.* New York: Routledge.

———. 1996. Cutting the Network. *Journal of the Royal Anthropological Institute* 2 (n.s.): 517–535.

Suzuki, Hikaru. 1998. Japanese Death Rituals in Transit: From Household Ancestors to Beloved Antecedents. *Journal of Contemporary Religion* 13 (2): 171–188.

Sweeting, Helen, and Mary Gilhooly. 1997. Dementia and the Phenomenon of Social Death. *Sociology of Health & Illness* 19 (1): 93–117.

Tachibana Takashi. 1986. *Nōshi* (Brain death). Tokyo: Chūo Bunko.

———. 1988. *Nōshi sairon* (Rethinking brain death). Tokyo: Chūo Kōronsha.

———. 1992. *Nōshi rinchō hihan* (Criticism of the brain death Special Committee). Tokyo: Chūo Kōronsha.

———. 1994. *Shi no rehaasaru: Rinshi taiken kenkyu de yawaraida watashi jishin no shi e no kyofu* (Death rehearsal: My own fear of death has become mitigated after the study of near-death experiences). *Bungei Shunjū* (Literature spring and autumn) 72: 280–295.

Tachikawa, Shōji. 1979. *Kinsei yamai zōshi: Edo jidai no byōki to iryō* (The modern book of illness: Illness and medicine in the Edo Period). Tokyo: Heibonsha.

Tada, Tomio. 1994. Asking the Dead if They're Dead: A Modern Noh Drama. *Japan Society Newsletter*, March, 2–3.

Takeshi, Yōrō. 1992. Book review of Takeshi Umehara's "Nōshi to Zōki ishoku" (Brain death and organ transplants). *Japan Foundation Newsletter* 20 (3): 13–14.

Takeuchi, Kazuo. 1990. Evolution of Criteria for Determination of Brain Death in Japan. *Acta Neurochirurgia* 105:82–84.

Takeuchi, K., H. Takeshita, K. Takakura, Y. Shimazono, H. Handa, F. Gotoh, Sh. Manaka, and T. Shiogai (Brain Death Study Group, Ministry of Health and Welfare, Tokyo). 1987. Evolution of Criteria for Determination of Brain Death in Japan. *Acta Neurochirurgica* 87:93–98.

Tamanoi, Mariko Asano. 1998. *Under the Shadow of Nationalism: Politics and Poetics of Rural Japanese Women.* Honolulu: University of Hawaii Press.

Tambiah, Stanley J. 1990. *Magic, Science, Religion, and the Scope of Rationality.* Cambridge: Cambridge University Press.

Taussig, Michael. 1987. *Shamanism, Colonialism, and the Wild Man: A Study in Terror and Healing.* Chicago: University of Chicago Press.

Taylor, Charles. 1989. *Sources of the Self: The Making of Modern Identity.* Cambridge: Harvard University Press.

Taylor, Robert. 1997. Re-examining the Definition and Criteria of Death. *Seminars in Neurology* 17 (3): 265–270.

Tebb, William Edward, and Perry Vollum. 1905. *Premature Burial and How It May Be Prevented.* London: Swan Sonnenschein & Co.

Tetsuo, Yamaori. 1986. The Metamorphosis of Ancestors. *Japan Quarterly* 33 (1): 50.

Thomas, L.-V. 1975. *Anthropologie de la mort.* Paris: Payot.

Thomas, Nicholas. 1991. *Entangled Objects: Exchange, Material Culture, and Colonialism in the Pacific.* Cambridge: Harvard University Press.

Thomson, Elizabeth H. 1963. The Role of Physicians in the Humane Societies of the Eighteenth Century. *Bulletin of the History of Medicine* 37:43–51.

Tierney, Thomas F. 1997. Death, Medicine, and the Right to Die: An Engagement with Heidegger, Bauman, and Baudrillard. *Body & Society* 3 (4): 51–77.

Time. 1941. What is Death? June 2.

———. 1966. Thanatology. May 27.

———. 1967. Surgery: The Ultimate Operation. December 15.

———. 1968a. Public Affairs. January 5.

———. 1968b. Surgery. January 12.

Timmermans, Stefan. 1999. *Sudden Death and the Myth of CPR.* Philadelphia: Temple University Press.

Timmermans, Stefan, and Marc Berg. 1997. Standardization in Action: Achieving Local Universality through Medical Protocols. *Social Studies of Science* 27:273–305.

Titmuss, Richard. 1971. *The Gift Relationship*. London: Allen and Unwin.

Todeschini, Maya. 1999. Bittersweet Crossroads: Women of Hiroshima and Nagasaki. Ph.D. thesis, Department of Anthropology, Harvard University.

Tokyo Shinbun. 1985. Nōshi hantei wa seimitsu, meikaku ni (For a precise and clear brain death diagnosis), May 15.

———. 1986. Nōshi no atsukai shinchō (Cautious treatment of brain death). October 4.

———. 1988a. Fushinkan nuguenu zoki ishoku yōnin (Distrust hard to shake off concerning the recognition of organ transplant). January 12.

———. 1988b. Shinzō ishoku Wada-shi no shujutsu, nōha sokutei uso datta (Heart transplant by Dr. Wada: It was a lie that the brain wave was measured). January 7.

———. 1994. Zōki ishoku no seikyū na rippōka hantai renrakukai ga hossoku (Opposition group formed against the hasty legislation of organ transplant). May 27.

Tolstoy, Leo. 1960. *The Death of Ivan Ilyich and Other Stories*. London: Penguin Books.

Toynbee, Polly. 1999. You Can't Take it With You. *Guardian Weekly*. July 15–21, 12.

Transplant News. 1994. OIG Report on Tissue Banking. June 30.

Traweek, Sharon. 1988. *Beamtimes and Lifetimes: The World of High Energy Physics*. Cambridge: Harvard University Press.

Treat, John Whittier. 1995. *Writing Ground Zero: Japanese Literature and the Atomic Bomb*. Chicago: University of Chicago Press.

Trémolières, F. 1991. Description of a Ventilator. In *Mechanical Ventilation*, edited by François Lemaire, 1–18. New York: Springer-Verlag.

Truog, Robert. 1997. Is it Time to Abandon Brain Death? *Hastings Center Report* 27 (1): 29–37.

———. 1999. Letter. *Hastings Center Report* 29:4.

Turner, Victor W. 1969. *The Ritual Process: Structure and Anti-structure*. Chicago: Aldine Publishing Company.

Ueno, Chizuko. 1997. Reproductive Rights/Health and Japanese Feminism. *Review of Japanese Culture and Society* 9:79–92.

Umeda, Toshirō. 1989. Transplants Forbidden. *Japan Quarterly* 36:146–154.

Umehara Takeshi. 1991. Tasūiken wa ronriteki ni hatan shite iru (The majority opinion is theoretically a failure). *Asahi Journal* 33:21–22.

———. 1997. Seiji ga shi o kettei shitemo yoika (Should politics determine death?) *Asahi Shinbun*. June 2.

Umehara Takeshi, ed. 1992. Hajime ni (Introduction). In *Nōshi to zōki-ishoku* (Brain Death and Organ Transplants), 1–7. Tokyo: Asahi Shinbunsha.

Umehara Takeshi and Nakajima Michi. 1992. Soredemo nōshi wa shi de wa nai (Yet brain death is not death). *Bungei Shunjū*. March, 302–312.

United Network for Organ Sharing. 1995. Critical Data. http://www.unos.org/newsroom/critdata. Retrieved October 26.

———. 1999. Critical Data. http://www.unos.org/newsroom/critdata. Retrieved October 26.

———. 2000a. Critical Data. http://www.unos.org/patients/tpd. Retrieved January 14.

———. 2000b. Organ Donors Remembered Nationwide During NOTDAW.

Uozumi, Tōru. 1992. Nōshi mondai ni kansuru shikan to teian (My opinion and proposals on the brain death issue). In Nōshi to zōki-ishoku (Brain death and organ transplants), edited by Takeshi Umehara, 80–99. Tokyo: Asahi Shinbunsha.

Van Gennep, A. 1960. The Rites of Passage, translated by by M. B. Vizedom and G. L. Caffee. Chicago: University of Chicago Press.

Veatch, Robert M. 1975. The Whole-Brain-Oriented Concept of Death: An Outmoded Philosophical Formulation. Journal of Thanatology 3:13–30.

———. 1978. The Definition of Death: Ethical, Philosophical, and Policy Confusion. In Brain Death: Interrelated Medical and Social Issues, edited by Julius Korein. Annals of the New York Academy of Science, vol. 315. New York: New York Academy of Science.

———. 1993. The Impending Collapse of the Whole-Brain Definition of Death. Hastings Center Report 23 (4): 18–24.

Vesalius, Andreas. 1543. De humani corporis fabrica.

Vidal, John. 1999. Call of the Wild. Guardian Weekly. August 5, 21.

Vlastos, Stephen, ed. 1998. Mirror of Modernity: Invented Traditions of Modern Japan. Berkeley: University of California Press.

Von Staden, Heinrich. 1989. Herophilus: The Art of Medicine in Early Alexandria. Cambridge: Cambridge University Press.

Walters, James W. 1987. Should the Law be Changed? Loma Linda University Ethics Center Update 3 (November): 3–6.

Walters, James W., and Stephen Ashwal. 1988. Organ Prolongation in Anencephalic Infants: Ethical and Medical Issues. Hastings Center Report 18:19–27.

Watanabe Junichi. 1976. Shiroi Utage (White banquet). Tokyo: Kadokawa Shuppan.

Watanabe Toyō. 1988. Ima, naze "shi" ka (Why "death" now?). Tokyo: Futago Shuppan.

Watanabe, Yoshio. 1994. Why Do I Stand Against the Movement for Cardiac Transplantation in Japan? Japanese Heart Journal 35:701–714.

Watts, Jonathan. 1998a. One Year On, Japan Has Yet to Accept Organ Transplantation. Lancet 352:1837.

———. 1998b. Concept of Brain Death to be Accepted in South Korea. Lancet 352:1996.

———. 1998c. Japanese Clinic Employees Arrested. Lancet 325:1368.

———. 1999. Media Coverage of First Transplantations Fuels Public Distrust in Japan. Lancet 354 (July 17): 229.

Weijer, Charles, and Carl Elliott. 1995. Pulling the Plug on Futility. British Medical Journal 310: 683–684.

Weiner, Annette B. 1992. Inalienable Possessions: The Paradox of Keeping While Giving. Berkeley: University of California Press.

Weisbard, Alan. 1995. A Polemic on Principles: Reflections on the Pittsburgh Protocol. In *Procuring Organs for Transplant: The Debate over Non-Heart-Beating Cadaver Protocols,* edited by Robert M. Arnold, Stuart J. Youngner, Renie Shapiro, and Carol Mason Spicer, 141–154. Baltimore: Johns Hopkins University Press.

Weiss, Brad. 1996. *The Making and Unmaking of the Maya Lived World: Consumption, Commoditization, and Everyday Practice.* Durham, N.C.: Duke University Press.

Werbner, Pnina, and Tariq Modood, eds. 1997. *Debating Cultural Hybridity.* London: Zed Books.

Wetzel, Randall C. 1985. Hemodynamic Responses in Brain Dead Organ Donor Patients. *Anesthesia & Analgesia* 64:125–127.

Whaley, Joachim, ed. 1981. *Mirrors of Mortality: Studies in the Social History of Death.* London: Europa Publications.

Wikler, Daniel, and Alan J. Weisbard. 1989. Editorial: Appropriate Confusion over "Brain Death." *Journal of the American Medical Association* 261 (15): 2246.

Willats, Sheila M. 1995. Transplantation and Interventional Ventilation on the Intensive Therapy Unit. *British Medical Journal* 310: 716–717.

Willems, Dick. Ms. Medical Practices around Death and the Dying Body.

Williams, Raymond. 1976. *Keywords: A Vocabulary of Culture and Society.* London: Fontana.

Willke J. C., and Dave Andrusko. 1988. Personhood Redux. *Hastings Center Report* 18:30–33.

Winner, Langdon. 1977. *Autonomous Technology: Technics-out-of-Control as a Theme in Political Thought.* Cambridge: MIT Press.

———. 1986. *The Whale and the Reactor: A Search for Limits in an Age of High Technology.* Chicago: University of Chicago Press.

Wolf, Zane Robinson. 1991. Nurses' Experiences Giving Post-Mortem Care to Patients Who Have Donated Organs: A Phenomenological Study. *Scholarly Inquiry for Nursing Practice* 5:73–87.

Wolstenholme, G. E. W., and M. O'Connor. 1966. *Ethics in Medical Progress: With Special Reference to Transplantation.* Boston: Little, Brown and Company.

Woodburn, James. 1982. Social Dimensions of Death in Four African Hunting and Gathering Societies. In *Death and the Regeneration of Life,* edited by Maurice Bloch and Jonathan Parry. Cambridge: Cambridge University Press.

Wöss, Fleur. 1992. When Blossoms Fall: Japanese Attitudes towards Death and the Other World: Opinion Polls, 1953–1967. In *Ideology and Practice in Modern Japan,* edited by R. Goodman and K. Refsing, 72–100. London: Routledge.

Yamaguchi, Kenichirō. 1995. *Seimei o moteasobu gendai no iryō* (Contemporary medicine that plays with life). Tokyo: Shakai Hyōronsha.

Yamaori, Tetsuo. 1986. The Metamorphosis of Ancestors. *Japan Quarterly* 33: 50–53.

Yamauchi, Masaya. 1990. Transplantation in Japan. *British Medical Journal* 301:507.

Yanagida Kunio. 1994. Sakurifaisu: waga musuko nōshi no 11 nichi (Sacrifice: our son and eleven days with brain death). *Bungei Shunjū* 72:144–162.

———. 1995. Nōshi: watashi no teigen (Brain death: My proposal). *Bungei Shunjū* 73:164–174.

———. 1999. Nōshi ishoku no kūhakuiki (A void in the brain death/organ transplant debate). *Mainichi Shinbun*. March 30.

———. 2000. *Nōchiro kakumei no Asa* (The dawning revolution of treatment of the brain). Tokyo: Bungei Shunjū.

Yeats, W. B. 1966. The Tower. In *The Variorum Edition of the Poems of W. B. Yeats,* edited by Peter Allt and Russell K. Alspach, 415. New York: Macmillan.

Yokota, Gerry. 1991. If Only a Voice Would Emerge. *Japan Quarterly* 38:436–444.

Yomiuri Shinbun. 1983. Noshi hantei wa shōsō (Too early for brain death diagnosis), January 7.

———. 1984. Lawyers with conflicting opinions. August 15.

———. 1986. Daisansha kikan mōkeyo (Third-party inspection should be instituted). March 4.

———. 1987. Kyōiku to shite no "I no rinri o" ("Medical ethics" as education). July 4.

———. 1988a. Nōshi juyō niwa shinrai ga fukaketsu (Trust indispensable for recognition of brain death). January 13.

———. 1988b. Okaruto būmu: Nezuyoi higōri shikō (The occult boom: The firmly rooted intention to be irrational). November 6.

———. 1990a. Nōshi jōtai kara shinteishi no chokugo jin o tekishutsu, ishoku shujutsu (Kidney removed immediately after the heart stopped from the brain-dead and transplanted). September 6.

———. 1990b. Shihō kaibō chū ni jinzō tekishutsu (Kidney removed during autopsy). September 8.

———. 1992. Songenshi kara jin ishoku, 53 sai josei "Sengensho" ikasu (Kidney transplant from a death with dignity: Fifty-three-year-old woman's "living will" respected). October 18.

———. 1996a. Nōshi jōtai ni nattara shi to hanteishitemo yoi to omoimasuka? (Do you think it is all right to recognize brain death as death?). January 10.

———. 1996b. Nōshi yōnin 50 percent wari masu (More than 50 percent approve of brain death). January 10.

———. 1999a. Nōshi hatsu hantei shikisha zadankai: hataraita chekku kino (First brain-death diagnosis—specialists' discussion: Check system worked). February 26.

———. 1999b. "31nen, nagai jikan datta" (Thirty-one years has been a long time). March 1.

———. 1999c. Zōki ishoku hō puraibash—hogo kyōka (Privacy issues to be emphasized in the revision of the law). March 2.

———. 1999d. "Nōshi ishoku" kadai to hyōka: Shikisha zadankai ("Brain death transplant" issues and evaluations: Specialists' discussions). March 2.

Yomiuri Shinbun Henshūbu. 1984. *Inochi Saisentan: Nōshi to zōki ishoku* (The leading edge of life: Brain death and organ transplants). Tokyo: Yomiuri.

Yonemoto Shōhei. 1985. *Baioesshikusu* (Bioethics). Tokyo: Kodansha, Gendai Shinsho.

Yōrō Takeshi. 1992a. *Kami to hito no kaibōgaku* (Anatomy of the gods and humans). Kyoto: Hōzōkan.

———. 1992b. Review of *Nōshi to Zōki Ishoku* (Brain death and organ transplants), edited by T. Umehara. *Japan Foundation Newsletter* 20:13–14.

Yoshida, Teigo. 1984. Spirit Possession and Village Conflict. In *Conflict in Japan,* edited by E. S. Krauss, T. P. Rohlen, and P. G. Steinhoff, 85–104. Honolulu: University of Hawaii Press.

Yoshioka, T., H. Sugimoto, M. Uenishi, T. Sakamoto, D. Sadamitsu, T. Sakano, and T. Sugimoto. 1986. Prolonged Hemodynamic Maintenance by the Combined Administration of Vasopressin and Epinephrine in Brain Death: A Clinical Study. *Neurosurgery* 18:565–567.

Young, Allan. 1995. *The Harmony of Illusions: Inventing Posttraumatic Stress Disorder.* Princeton: Princeton University Press.

Young, P. V., and B. F. Matta. 2000. Anaesthesia for Organ Donation in the Brain Stem Dead—Why Bother? *Anaesthesia* 55:105–106.

Youngner, Stuart. 1992. Brain Death: A Superficial and Fragile Consensus. *Archives of Neurology* 49:570–572.

———. 1996. Some Must Die. In *Organ Transplantation: Meanings and Realities,* edited by Stuart J. Youngner, Renée C. Fox, and Laurence J. O'Connell, 32–55. Madison: University of Wisconsin Press.

Youngner, Stuart, Martha Allan, Edward Bartlett, Helmut Cascorbi, Toni Han, David Jackson, Mary Mahowald, and Barbara Martin. 1985. Psychological and Ethical Implications of Organ Retrieval. *New England Journal of Medicine* 313:321–324.

Youngner, S. J., S. Landfeld, C. J. Coulton, et al. 1989. Brain Death and Organ Retrieval: A Cross Sectional Survey of Knowledge and Concept among Health Professionals. *Journal of the Medical American Association* 261: 2205–2210.

Zaner, Richard M. 1988. Introduction. In *Death: Beyond Whole-Brain Criteria,* edited by Richard M. Zaner, 1–14. Dordrecht: Kluwer Academic Publishers.

Zepeda, Rodrigo Salvador. 1998. A Comparative Analysis of Brain Death and Organ Transplantation in the UK and Japan. LL.B. dissertation, University of Wales, Cardiff.

Legal Cases

Gray v. Sawyer, 247 SW2d 496 (1952).
In the matter of Karen Quinlan, 355 A.2d 647 (1976).
Saskatchewan v. Paulette, 69 DLR 4th, 134 Saskatchewan Minister of Social Services (1990).
Schmidt v. Pierce, 344 SW2d 120 (1961).
Smith v. Smith, 317 SW2d 275 (1958).
Vaegemast v. Hess, 280 NW 641 (1938).

Index

Text: 10/13 Sabon
Display: Sabon
Compositor: Binghamton Valley Composition
Printer/binder: Thomson-Shore
Index: Carol Roberts